Musculoskeletal Disorders: The Basis of Diagnosis and Treatment

Musculoskeletal Disorders: The Basis of Diagnosis and Treatment

Editor: Benjamin West

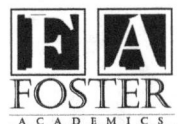

FOSTER
ACADEMICS

www.fosteracademics.com

www.fosteracademics.com

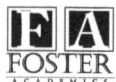

Cataloging-in-Publication Data

Musculoskeletal disorders : the basis of diagnosis and treatment / edited by Benjamin West.
    p. cm.
Includes bibliographical references and index.
ISBN 978-1-63242-583-6
1. Musculoskeletal system--Diseases. 2. Musculoskeletal system--Diseases--Diagnosis.
3. Musculoskeletal system--Diseases--Treatment. 4. Musculoskeletal system--Wounds and injuries.
I. West, Benjamin.
RC925 .M87 2019
616.7--dc23

© Foster Academics, 2019

Foster Academics,
118-35 Queens Blvd., Suite 400,
Forest Hills, NY 11375, USA

ISBN 978-1-63242-583-6 (Hardback)

Contents

Preface

In my initial years as a student, I used to run to the library at every possible instance to grab a book and learn something new. Books were my primary source of knowledge and I would not have come such a long way without all that I learnt from them. Thus, when I was approached to edit this book; I became understandably nostalgic. It was an absolute honor to be considered worthy of guiding the current generation as well as those to come. I put all my knowledge and hard work into making this book most beneficial for its readers.

Musculoskeletal disorders refer to injuries or pain in the human musculoskeletal system that includes joints, tendons, nerves, ligaments and muscles. Carpal tunnel syndrome, tension neck syndrome, tendinitis, back pain and epicondylitis are some common musculoskeletal disorders. These injuries can be sudden or generated due to repeated strain or exposure to force and vibration. These disorders can arise due to psychological, ergonomic, social and occupational factors. The diagnosis of these conditions is based on a comprehensive understanding of the patient's history, recreational and occupational hazards and various medical examinations. X-rays and MRI are used for the diagnosis of musculoskeletal conditions. This book contains some path-breaking studies in the area of musculoskeletal disorders. It also discusses the fundamentals as well as modern approaches of diagnosis and treatment of musculoskeletal disorders. It is a complete source of knowledge on the present status of this important field.

I wish to thank my publisher for supporting me at every step. I would also like to thank all the authors who have contributed their researches in this book. I hope this book will be a valuable contribution to the progress of the field.

Editor

Paradoxical tunnel enlargement after ACL reconstruction with hamstring autografts when using β-TCP containing interference screws for tibial aperture fixation-prospectively comparative study

Joon Ho Wang[1,2,3], Eun Su Lee[4] and Byung Hoon Lee[5*]

Abstract

Background: Tibial aperture fixation with a bioabsorbable interference screw is a popular fixation method in anterior cruciate ligament reconstruction (ACLR). An interference screw containing β-tricalcium phosphate (β-TCP) to improve bony integration and biocompatibility was recently introduced. This study aims to compare the clinical outcomes and radiological results of tunnel enlargement effect between the 2 bioabsorbable fixative devices of pure poly-L-lactic acid (PLLA) interference screws and β-TCP-containing screws, for tibial interference fixation in ACLR using hamstring autografts.

Methods: Eighty consecutive patients who had undergone double-bundle ACLR between 2011 to 2012 were prospectively reviewed and randomly divided into two groups based on the type of tibial interference screw: 28 were assigned to the pure PLLA screw group (Group A), while the other 29 were assigned to the β-TCP-containing screw fixation group (Group B). Clinical evaluations and radiological analyses were conducted in both groups with a minimum 2- year follow-up.

Results: There was no significant difference in subjective or objective clinical outcome between the 2 groups. In radiological analyses, the use of a β-TCP-containing screw reduced tunnel widening in the portion of the tunnel with screw engagement compared to the pure PLLA screw, while the use of a β-TCP-containing screw resulted in greater tunnel enlargement in the proximal portion of the tunnel without screw engagement than use of a pure PLLA screw.

Conclusion: Use of a β-TCP-containing interference screw in tibial aperture fixation reduced tunnel enlargement in the vicinity of the screw, whereas greater enlargement occurred proximal to the screw end relative to use of a pure PLLA interference screw. These paradoxical enlargements in use of β-TCP containing screws suggest that for reducing tunnel enlargement, the length of the interference screw should be as fit as possible with tunnel length in terms of using soft grafts.

Level of Evidence: II, Prospectively comparative study.

Trial registration: Retrospectively registered with ClinicalTrials.gov. (NCT02754674), Date of trial registration: February 10, 2016.

Keywords: ACL, Tunnel enlargement, Interference screw, Plla, β-TCP, Hamstring autograft

---

* Correspondence: oselite@naver.com
[5]Department of Orthopaedic Surgery, Kang-Dong Sacred Heart Hospital, Hallym University Medical Center, Gil-dong, Seoul 134-701, South Korea
Full list of author information is available at the end of the article

Background

Interference screws are commonly used for fixation in orthopedic surgery, especially in tibial aperture fixation for ACL reconstruction. Biodegradable cannulated interference fixation screws made of poly-L-lactic acid (PLLA) were introduced in the early 1990s to improve postoperative imaging, decrease stress shielding, avoid graft laceration, and make revision easier [1, 2]. These screws have a fixation strength equivalent to that of metal screws [3–5]. Bioabsorbable fixation devices offer advantages over metallic devices in that they can be substituted for bone contrary to metal screws; bone tunnel remodeling is not possible when metal interference screws are in place.

However, there are concerns that explanted pure PLLA biodegradable interference screws may not degrade, and that replacement with bone may be incomplete [1, 6–8], and the incidence of tunnel enlargements following the use of resorbable devices has been shown to be higher than metallic devices [9–11]. A variety of biodegradable screws with different material compositions have therefore been introduced. Not all bioabsorbable materials have the same compositions, absorption rates, or tissue reactions. Some of the bioabsorbable materials commonly used for interference screws are polyglycolic acid (PGA), polylactic acid (PLA), polyparadioxanone (PDS), polymers of PGA/PLA, and various stereoisomers of lactic acid (PDLA).

The Matryx® (Linvatec Corp, Largo, FL, USA) screw, made of 96 L/4D poly lactic acid (PLA) and 30% β-tricalcium phosphate (β-TCP), was introduced to enhance osteoconduction and to be more biocompatible with bone than existing screw materials. However, to the best of our knowledge, the effect of this screw against tunnel widening effect by osteoconduction and bony integration around tunnels has not been investigated in a clinical setting. Therefore, we sought to investigate the clinical advantages of β-TCP containing biodegradable screws under their theoretical advantages.

We hypothesized that use of β-TCP-containing interference screws would improve coaptation of the graft to the tunnel with replacement of the degraded screw by new bone formation, and result in better tunnel remodeling by preventing tunnel widening. The purpose of this study was to evaluate whether use of a β-TCP-containing interference screw resulted in superior clinical and radiological outcomes (esp, the preventive effect on tunnel enlargement during in vivo degradation within the tunnel) in ACL reconstruction using autologous hamstring grafts compared to a commercially available pure PLLA biodegradable screw.

Methods

Level of Evidence II, prospectively comparative study

From February 2011 to June 2012, a total of 119 patients with ACL injury were enrolled in this study. Inclusion criteria were patients who underwent a primary anatomical double bundle ACL reconstruction with tibial aperture fixation by Bioscrew® (Linvatec Corp, Largo, FL, USA), which is made of 100% poly-L-lactic acid (PLLA) or Matryx® (Linvatec Corp), which is made of 70% 96 L/4D poly lactic acid (PLA) & 30% β-TCP, and who were at least 20 years of age; patients younger than 20 years of age were treated on the basis of adolescent ACL and single-bundle reconstruction with no interference screw placed in the tibial tunnel if open physis. Of these 119 patients, 39 were excluded for the following reasons: single-bundle reconstruction (4), revisional ACL reconstruction (7), combined surgeries such as meniscal allograft transplantation (2), any previous ligament surgery or bony procedure in the area of graft attachment (10), degenerative arthritic knee (1), pregnancy (1), and other reasons (14) (Fig. 1). After exclusion, 80 patients underwent DB-ACLR according to a trial comparing two different interference screws. Eighty patients were randomly assigned to either the PLLA screw group or the β-TCP screw group on the day of surgery using permuted block randomization [12], and 74 underwent knee computed tomography (CT) immediately and 1-year after the operation (Fig. 1).

To assess differences in tibial tunnel widening according to fixation device, the cross sectional areas at four locations were compared between the two groups on the immediate postoperative and 1- year follow-up CT images. All operations were performed by a single surgeon (J.H.W.) experienced in ACLR using both the transportal and outside-in techniques. All patients underwent CT examination twice on the same CT device using the same protocol within 3 days after the initial surgery and at the postoperative 1-year follow-up. The current study received Institutional Review Board approval from our institution (Samsung Medical Center 2010–08-116) before study onset, and our protocol was also approved. Informed consent was obtained from all participants (ClinicalTrials.gov identifier: NCT02754674).

Surgical technique and rehabilitation

All operations were performed using an arthroscopic-assisted technique. Femoral and tibial tunnels were created in the centers of the respective anatomic insertions. Semitendinosus and gracilis tendons were harvested from the affected limb. The tunnels were prepared to be the same size as the graft, and the femoral tunnel was drilled to this diameter by matching the drill and/or dilator to the graft size while accounting for the size of the native insertion site. The drill diameter for the femoral and tibial tunnels was determined based on the diameter

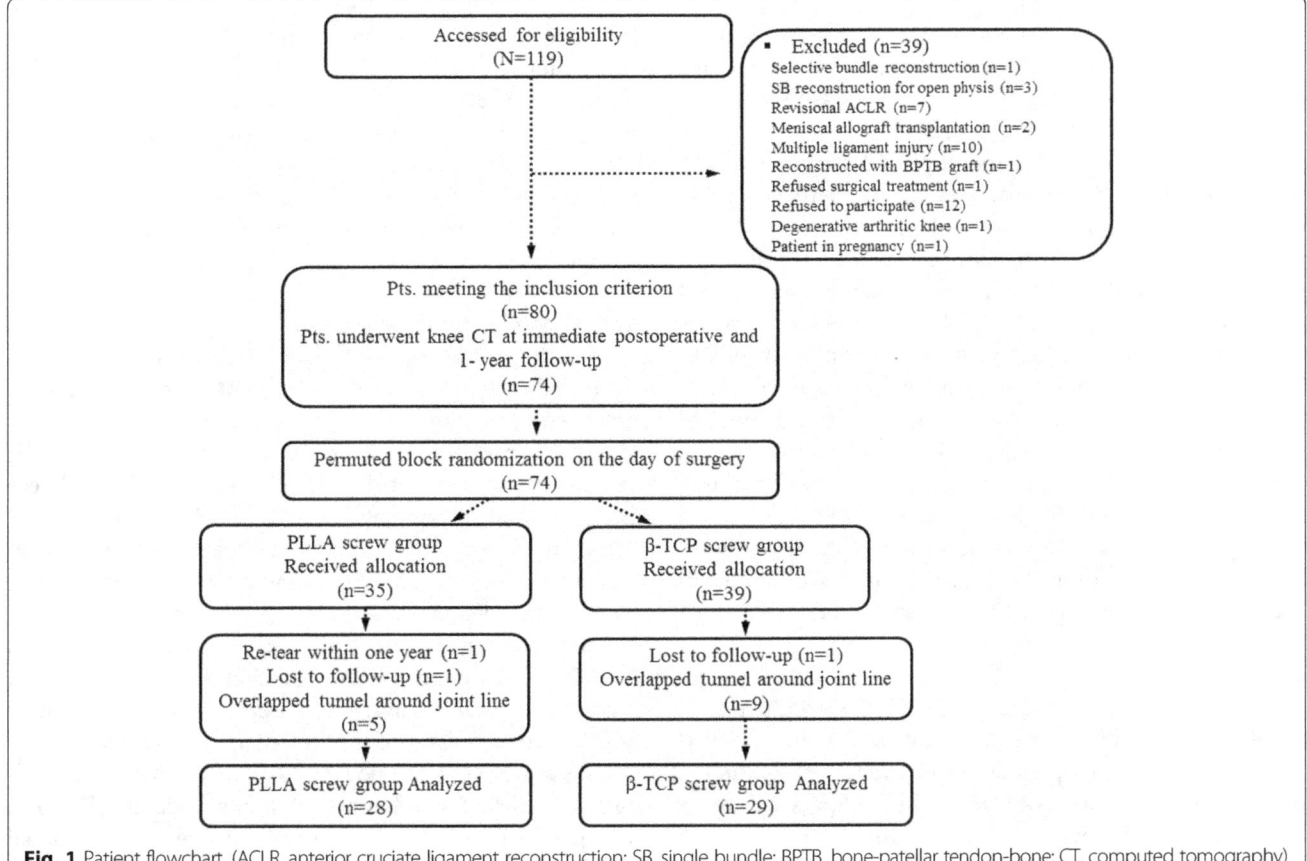

Fig. 1 Patient flowchart. (ACLR, anterior cruciate ligament reconstruction; SB, single bundle; BPTB, bone-patellar tendon-bone; CT, computed tomography)

of the prepared graft. Grafts were inserted retrograde via the tibial tunnel into the femoral tunnel, and fixed with a cortical suspension system using the shortest possible loop (10 to 15 mm) to ensure maximal contact between the graft and the tunnel walls on the femoral side, and with bioabsorbable interference screws with a post tie on the tibial side for all cases.

Graft was normally trimmed to retain its original size with a length of 26 to 30 cm. Then, it was folded and sutured together with the use of no. 1 absorbable sutures to form two triple-strand grafts. A 6-stranded graft, composed of triple semitendinosus (6.5 to 9.5 mm) for the anteromedial (AM) bundle and triple gracilis (4.5 to 7 mm) for the posterolateral (PL) bundle, was created for each group.

Anatomic tibial insertion sites of both bundles were marked with an ArthroCare device (ArthroCare, Sunnyvale, CA, USA), and the tip of the guide was aimed at the centers of the AM and PL bundle remnant tibial insertion sites. A 3.2-mm guide pin was inserted into the bases of the AM and PL tibial insertion sites. The AM and PL tibial tunnels were then drilled with a cannulated drill. Bioscrew® or Matryx® (length 30 mm) with a diameter 1 mm larger than the tunnel diameter was used for tibial aperture fixation at

0° of knee flexion and applying a 30–35 N tension to the graft using the dedicated tie tensioner [13], and an additional extracortical screw with a spike washer was applied. Interference screws eccentrically compress the graft against the wall of the tibial bone tunnel. The type of all screws was blinded at insertion to surgeon for randomized allocation.

All patients began active quadriceps isometric exercise and active range-of-motion exercise immediately after surgery. Four to 5 days after surgery, an ACL limited-motion brace was applied, and joint motion exercise was carried out at 15° increments per week. At 4 and 6 weeks after surgery, 90° and 135° of motion, respectively, were allowed. A pair of crutches was used to allow partial weight bearing from 3 days to 6 weeks after surgery. Patients were educated on performing proprioceptive balancing exercise at 3 months after surgery. Return to competitive sports involving jumping, pivoting, or sidestepping was prohibited until 6 months after the reconstruction [14].

CT evaluation & measurement

A CT scanner Light Speed VCT (GE Medical Systems, Milwaukee, WI, USA) was used for all examinations. All patients were placed in a supine position with knee full extension. The collimation was 16 × 0.625 mm, the tube parameters were 120 kVp and 200 mA, and the acquisition matrix was 512 × 512 pixels. Images were processed for multiplane reconstruction, and cross-sectional area (CSA) was measured using Osirix (version 3.5.1; Pixeo, Geneva, Switzerland). We measured CSAs in the plane perpendicular to the long axis of the tibial tunnel using Osirix at the following four cutting levels (Fig. 2): (1) joint line, which was just below the proximal joint line, (2) center level of the tunnel without screw engagement (mid-tunnel), (3) center level of the tunnel with screw engagement (mid-screw), and (4) tunnel aperture outlet. The difference in CSA at each of the four cutting levels was compared between the two groups on immediate postoperative and postoperative 1-year CT scans (Fig. 3). CSA measurements were performed by two training fellows in sports medicine. If the AM and PL tunnels overlapped around the joint line, the CSA of the joint line was excluded from the statistical analysis because of the inability to measure each value separately.

Clinical evaluation

Clinical follow-up evaluations were then conducted at 12 and 24 months and made by an independent examiner (ARK). The preoperative evaluation was conducted by the Lysholm knee score, Hospital for Special Surgery (HSS) score, Tegner score, the International Knee

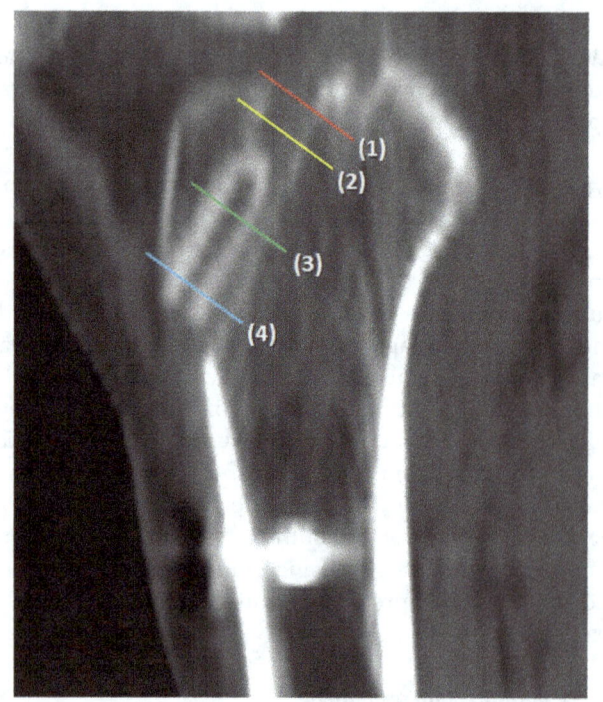

Fig. 2 Cross-sectional area was measured at the four cutting levels of tibial tunnel in the plane perpendicular to the long axis of the tunnel: (1) joint line, (2) mid-tunnel, (3) mid-screw, and (4) outlet

Documentation Committee Score (IKDC) [15–17] and a ligament stability assessment by KT-2000® arthrometer (MEDmetric, San Diego, CA) testing with a side-to-side difference of 30 lb. with the knee at 20° of knee flexion. The differences of ligament stability between both legs were calculated by subtracting the laxity measurement of the uninjured knee from the laxity measurement of the injured knee. Intraoperative and postoperative complications were recorded.

Reliability and statistical analysis

Two orthopedic surgeons (independent observers) developed and agreed to the measurement methods together; however, they were blinded to each other's measurements and their previous measurements. They measured the cross-sectional areas at the four cutting levels for all knees twice with an interval of 2 weeks. Reliability of the measurements was assessed by an independent statistician who examined interobserver reliability using the intraclass correlation coefficient. A priori power analysis was performed to determine the sample size using the two-sided hypothesis test at an α level of 0.05 and a power of 0.8. A post hoc power analysis was performed to determine whether the results of our study of 25 cases indicated adequate power, and the power was 85.21%, which was adequate to detect a difference of 1 mm widening [18, 19]. The paired t-test was applied to compare cross-sectional area at the four cutting levels between both groups on immediate postoperative and 1-year follow-up CT scans. $P < 0.05$ was considered significant (95% confidence intervals). The 2-sample t-test was applied to compare the cross-sectional areas of "mid-tunnel" and "mid-screw". The difference of clinical outcome scales between two groups was evaluated with a 2-sample t test or Mann-Whitney test. Statistical analyses were executed using SAS version 9.3 (SAS Institute, Cary, NC).

Results

Demographics

The mean age was 34.7 years (range, 20 to 60 years) and the mean body mass index (BMI) was 24.6 kg/m² (range, 19.1 to 35.2 kg/m²). The mean duration of postoperative follow-up was 33 months (range, 24 to 60 months). There were no significant differences between groups in age, gender, BMI, femoral tunneling technique, and tunnel diameter, values of which are shown in Table 1. On immediate postoperative CT, CSA at each cutting level was not significantly different between the two groups in either the AM or PL tunnels. AM and PL tunnel overlap around the joint line was found in five cases in group A and nine cases in group B.

No cases of complete absorption and replacement of the interference screw with new bone were observed at the 1-year follow-up CT in either group. No clinical

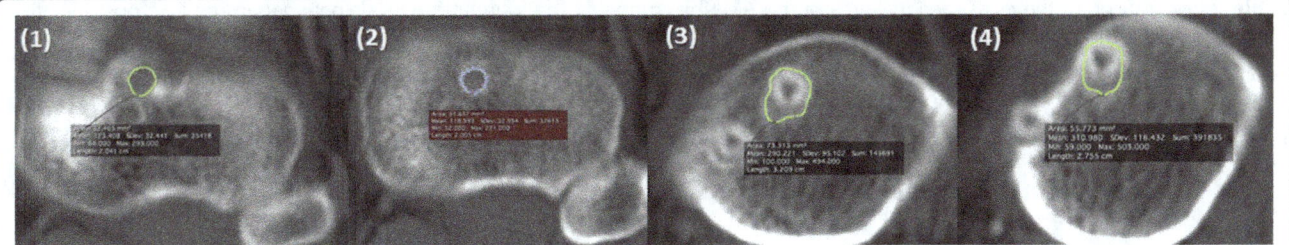

Fig. 3 Cross-sectional view and area (mm²) measurement of (1) the joint line, (2) the mid-tunnel, (3) the mid-screw, and (4) the outlet cutting level

evidence of any adverse events related to these interference fixation screws was observed, and degenerative radiographic changes were not noted.

Radiological results (tunnel enlargement)

In both AM and PL tunnels, the average CSAs at the four cutting levels were significantly greater at postoperative 1 year than immediately post-operatively, and the most increased CSAs were observed at the mid-tunnel level (Tables 2 and 3). There were significant inter-group differences in increments of CSAs of the AM tunnel 1 year after surgery at the mid-tunnel and mid-screw cutting levels. At the mid-screw level, mean increase in CSA after 1 year was significantly smaller in group B (β-TCP screw) than in group A (PLLA screw) (16.8% vs. 27.2%, p = 0.024). At the mid-tunnel level, the mean increase in CSA after 1 year was significantly larger in group 2 (β-TCP screw) than in group 1 (PLLA screw) (66.9% vs. 40.1%, p = 0.028) (Table 2). In PL tunnel analysis, there was no significant difference in average increments of CSAs at the four cutting levels (Table 3). The measurement of CSAs at the four cutting levels showed a good reliability (an appendix is available as a Additional file 1: Table S-1).

Clinical results

Mean Lysholm score, HSS and IKDC values and KT-2000 measurements values are reported in Table 4. At 2 years, the mean side-to-side difference for anterior displacement at 30° flexion was 2.1 mm (SD ± 1.1 mm) in group A and 1.8 mm (SD ± 1.5 mm) in group B. The mean Lysholm score was 94.4 (SD ± 6.8) in group A and 94.1 (SD ± 6.3) in group B. In group A, the mean IKDC subjective score was 85 (SD ± 11.7) in group A and 86.4 (SD ± 9.5). At the last follow-up, both groups reached a satisfactory pain relief and functional improvements, without significant differences. KT-2000 side-to-side differences (p = n.s.) were similar between the two types of screw fixation. In our experience, the difference of tibial tunnel enlargement did not affect clinical results at 2 years.

Discussion

The principal findings of our study were as follows: (1) the use of a β-TCP-containing screw reduced tunnel widening in the portion of the tunnel with screw engagement compared to the pure PLLA screw, while (2) the use of a β-TCP-containing screw resulted in greater tunnel enlargement in the proximal portion of the tunnel

Table 1 Patient demographics[a]

	Group A [PLLA screw] (n = 28)	Group B [β-TCP screw] (n = 29)	p - value
Age, y	36.1 ± 8.9	32.7 ± 12.3	0.225
Sex, male/female, n	21:7	24:5	0.473
BMI, kg/m^2	24.2 ± 2.6	24.7 ± 3.9	0.848
Femoral tunneling technique, n TP: OI	11:17	17:12	0.144
Tunnel diameter (drill size, mm)			
AM	7.5 ± 0.6 (6.5–9.5)	7.4 ± 0.6 (6.0–9.0)	0.387
PL	5.7 ± 0.5 (4.5–7.0)	5.7 ± 0.5 (4.5–7.0)	0.675
Tunnel length (mm)			
AM	39.6 ± 3.9 (34–50)	40.0 ± 2.9 (34–45)	0.661
PL	43.7 ± 3.5 (35–50)	44.8 ± 3.0 (38–50)	0.228

BMI body mass index, *TP* transportal, *OI* outside-in
[a]Value are presented as mean ± standard deviation, with range in parentheses

Table 2 Comparison of the cross-sectional area of the AM tibial tunnel at the four cutting levels between immediate postoperative and postoperative 1 year CT scans

Cutting level	Group	Cross sectional area (mm²)			$^\dagger P$
		Immediate postop.	1YR	Difference	
Joint line	1	41.5 ± 6.6	54.6 ± 11.3	13.2 (31.7%)	< 0.001
	2	42.0 ± 9.1	57.3 ± 12.1	15.4 (36.6%)	< 0.001
$^*P$				0.523	
Mid-tunnel	1	41.8 ± 7.2	58.6 ± 11.6	16.8 (40.1%)	< 0.001
	2	41.9 ± 8.7	70.0 ± 19.5	28.1 (66.9%)	< 0.001
$^*P$				**0.028**	
Mid-screw	1	61.0 ± 10.5	77.6 ± 13.3	16.6 (27.2%)	< 0.001
	2	63.3 ± 9.8	73.9 ± 14.2	10.6 (16.8%)	< 0.001
$^*P$				**0.024**	
Outlet	1	62.0 ± 10.6	69.2 ± 15.1	7.3 (11.7%)	< 0.001
	2	61.6 ± 11.3	68.4 ± 14.4	6.8 (11.0%)	< 0.001
$^*P$				0.833	

1YR; postoperative 1 year
*Comparison of the increments in cross-sectional area 1 year after surgery between the two groups at the each cutting level
†Comparison of the cross-sectional area between immediate postoperative and postoperative 1 year CT scans
*Values of $P < 0.05$ are displayed in bold

without screw engagement than use of a pure PLLA screw. These findings might be explained that in the screw-bone contact area, particles during degradation of β-TCP led to less local reactivity or inflammatory responses under their neutralizing effects, whereas they activated osteoclasts and resulted in osteolysis with mechanical stress or synovial fluid influx in proximal portion without screw engagement.

The use of biodegradable interference screws is widely accepted because of their ease of handling and effective fixation. Ideally, a biodegradable interference screw should degrade with minimal or no host-bone reaction. It is reasonable to assume that the faster a material degrades, the earlier the osseous replacement takes place [20, 21]. However, tissue reaction occurs only during and after degradation of the implant [22]. In fact, use of interference screws made of other, more rapidly degrading polymers has been reported to result in collection of fluid at the top of the femoral bone tunnel and significant tunnel widening [23].

Table 3 Comparison of the cross-sectional area of the PL tibial tunnel at the four cutting levels between immediate postoperative and postoperative 1 year CT scans

Cutting level	Group	Cross-sectional area (mm²)			$^\dagger p$
		Immediate postop.	1YR	Difference	
Joint line	1	21.1 ± 6.3	28.8 ± 10.5	7.7 (36.3%)	0.002
	2	24.5 ± 4.1	34.6 ± 7.5	10.1 (41.5%)	< 0.001
$^*P$				0.411	
Mid-tunnel	1	23.0 ± 6.6	30.7 ± 11.8	7.7 (33.5%)	< 0.001
	2	25.0 ± 3.8	36.0 ± 10.0	11.0 (44.2%)	< 0.001
$^*P$				0.179	
Mid-screw	1	36.6 ± 8.58	42.4 ± 12.8	5.8 (15.8%)	< 0.001
	2	40.0 ± 6.83	46.7 ± 13.3	6.7 (16.8%)	0.003
$^*P$				0.734	
Outlet	1	33.3 ± 9.4	34.1 ± 11.0	0.8 (2.5%)	0.445
	2	36.1 ± 8.0	36.6 ± 10.0	0.5 (1.4%)	0.647
$^*P$				0.845	

1YR; postoperative 1 year
*Comparison of the increments in cross-sectional area 1 year after surgery between two groups at each cutting level
†Comparison of the cross-sectional area between immediate postoperative and postoperative 1 year CT scans

Table 4 Clinical outcomes

	Group A [PLLA screw] (n = 28)	Group B [β-TCP screw] (n = 29)	p - value
KT-2000™ side-to-side difference (mm)			
Baseline	4.5 ± 2.2	4.5 ± 2.2	0.964
24 months	2.1 ± 1.1	1.8 ± 1.5	0.334
Lysholm knee score			
Baseline	71.6 ± 21.7	61.9 ± 22.8	0.102
24 months	94.4 ± 6.8	94.1 ± 6.3	0.848
HSS score (/100)			
Baseline	92.1 ± 11.8	86.6 ± 15.7	0.131
24 months	99.4 ± 1.7	99.6 ± 1.9	0.691
IKDC subjective score			
Baseline	58.2 ± 16.2	51.6 ± 19.0	0.157
24 months	85.0 ± 11.7	86.4 ± 9.5	0.610
Tegner score			
Baseline	3.7 ± 1.4	3.8 ± 1.9	0.706
24 months	6.3 ± 1.5	6.3 ± 1.6	0.977

Values are expressed as median ± standard deviation
ROM range of motion, *IKDC* International Knee Documentation Committee

In terms of bone-patellar tendon-bone (BPTB) grafts, interference screws have the benefit of reducing the potential space created in bone by the compaction method, which forms the walls of the container [24]. Several MRI studies have showed no signs of container phenomenon or pathologic signals at long-term follow-up. In terms of autologous hamstring tendons, the use for ACL reconstruction has increased in popularity over the recent years [25]. However, even the use of an interference screw with a size matching that of the tunnel diameter will not totally prevent synovial fluid from infiltrating into the tunnel during the biologic transition of thin fibrous tissue into dense fibrous tissue. Practically, although we used only interference screws with a diameter 1 mm larger than the tunnel diameter for tibial aperture fixation in our study, significantly increased CSAs were observed at all four cutting levels at postoperative 1 year in both AM and PL tunnels.

However, our finding of a smaller increase in tunnel widening in the portion of the tunnel with β-TCP screw engagement has demonstrated a better behavior in clinical settings. Our hypothesis was that early degradation and the osteoconduction-promoting effect of β-TCP screws would enhance bony integration and reduce tunnel enlargement. As hypothesized, the tunnel was less enlarged in the section with screw engagement in the β-TCP-containing screw group than the PLLA screw group. The addition of β-TCP to a degradable polymer such as PLLA creates an inorganic osteoconductive scaffold and changes the properties of the scaffold. During

degradation, β-TCP breaks down into calcium ions and phosphates, which maintain an elevated pH around the implant [26–28]. This could act as a buffer to acidic degradation products of lactic acid or glycolic acid. These neutralizing effects around screws could result in less local reactivity or inflammatory responses, thereby reducing tunnel enlargement [29]. In the reconstructed oblique axial view on CT, bony integration was observed in the screw-bone contact area in the mid-tunnel area in the β-TCP-containing interference screw group. There was no gap between the adjacent native bone and implanted screw, and the screw tract was corticated as densely as cancellous bone (Fig. 4). Meanwhile, an enlarged tunnel and sclerotic margin without bony integration around the screw was observed in group A. Furthermore, no ingrowth of neo-bone tissue from the adjacent native bone was observed (Fig. 5). We attributed this to the presence of nondegradable poly L-lactide polymer, which could hinder the ingrowth of new bone from the native adjacent cancellous bone tissue.

Meanwhile, abruptly increased tunnel enlargement was observed in the proximal portion to β-TCP containing screw relative to a PLLA screw (Fig. 6). This conflicts with previous findings in patellar tendon autografts; bone tunnels in the tibia began to increase in size from the distal end [24]. Most probable explanation for this paradoxical enlargement is the cellular response to calcium phosphate (β-TCP). Particles proximally degraded from β-TCP by mechanical stress or synovial fluid influx likely activated osteoclasts and resulted in osteolysis, similar to the role of wear debris in aseptic loosening in arthroplasty. Many environmental factors are known to be involved in the osteointegration and degradation of calcium phosphate ceramics after implantation, including physiochemical processes and various cell activating molecules and cytokines [30–32].

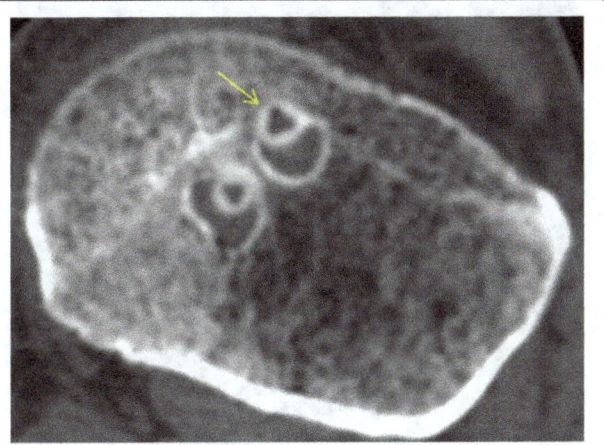
Fig. 4 Bony integration was observed in the screw-bone contact area in group B

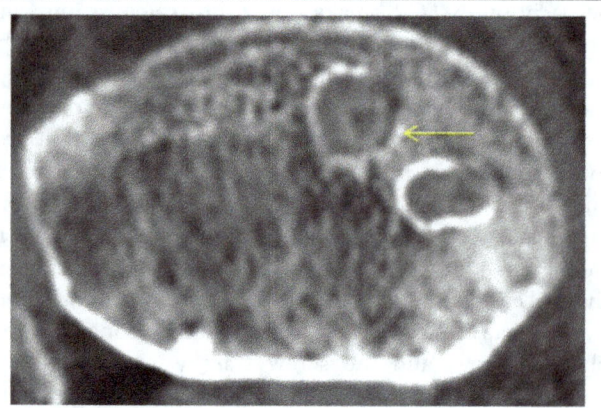

Fig. 5 Sclerotic margin without bony integration in the screw-bone contact area was observed in group A

Almost studies of explanted biodegradable interference screws have been overstated regarding to concerns about whether claims of bio-absorbability because of limited evidences of degradation [21, 33, 34]. It would be resulted from almost studies have been designed using patellar bone graft with little effect of container phenomenon with interference screw. However, when using hamstring grafts, the effects of the biodegradable interference screw on early tunnel widening must be considered. Despite these radiological observations, the clinical evaluation showed no significant difference, with good outcomes in both groups at the postoperative 2-year follow-up in current study. However, this could stem from the use of an additional extra-cortical screw with a spike washer for tibial aperture fixation.

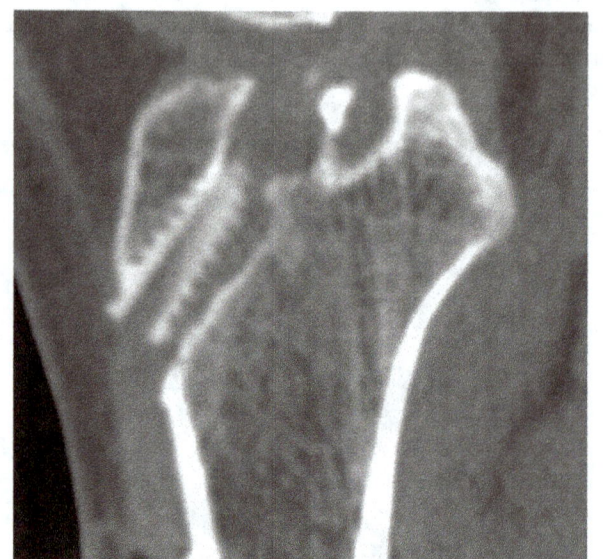

Fig. 6 In group B, the degree of tunnel enlargement increased abruptly proximal to the screw end

Several studies have reported that use of β-TCP-containing screws reduces tunnel enlargement [13]. However, to the best of our knowledge, this is the first study to report the paradoxical tunnel enlargement in the proximal portion of tibial tunnel following fixation with the β-TCP-containing fixation screw. Further studies are needed to clarify the factors aggravating tunnel enlargement in ACL reconstruction.

The strength of this study is that to evaluate bone tunnel widening, immediate and postoperative 1- year CT scans were used instead of digital plan radiograph. Tunnel enlargement is believed to occur both intraoperatively and postoperatively. Intraoperative enlargement may be due to eccentric reaming, graft and reamer diameter mismatch, or use of the press-fit technique, so a difference in CSA between the reamer and actual tunnel is inevitable. In the current study, immediate postoperative CT images were used to obtain baselines values, so postoperative enlargement could be evaluated without intraoperative change bias. Furthermore, the tunnel was segmented into four different sections for more precise analysis; this enabled us to observe paradoxical enlargement in the area of the tunnel without screw engagement.

Nevertheless, the present study had some limitations. First, no histologic data were obtained to confirm complete degradation of the PLLA screws. Second, the follow-up period was relatively short. However, several studies have shown that most tunnel widening occurs during the first 3 months [35–39]. According to these studies, a one-year follow-up period is sufficient to observe enlargement of the tunnel itself, but tunnel remodeling and screw resorption are still occurring. A longer-term follow-up study is required to obtain a thorough understanding of tunnel enlargement and the fate of the implant and tunnel ossification. Third, the current study is limited by its small sample size. However, a post hoc power analysis was performed to determine whether the sample size had sufficient power. Fourth, we did not account for other confounding factors such as bone mineral density, screw and tunnel length ratio, or variations in tunnel location. However, there were no significant differences in age, gender, or BMI between the two groups of subjects. Another limitation is the lack of a comprehensive review of patients who underwent patellar tendon autograft ACL reconstruction. We investigated only the patients underwent DB-ACLR, might not the standard technique in some countries, not single-bundle method.

Conclusion

Use of a β-TCP-containing interference screw in tibial aperture fixation reduced tunnel enlargement in the vicinity of the screw, whereas greater enlargement occurred proximal to the screw end relative to use of a pure PLLP interference screw. These paradoxical enlargements in use of β-TCP containing screws suggest that for reducing tunnel enlargement, the length of the interference screw should be as fit as possible with tunnel length in terms of using soft grafts.

Abbreviations
ACLR: anterior cruciate ligament reconstruction; AM: anteromedial; BMI: body mass index; BPTB: bone-patellar tendon-bone; CSA: cross-sectional area; CT: computed tomography; DB-ACLR: double bundle anterior cruciate ligament reconstruction; HSS: Hospital for Special Surgery; IKDC: International Knee Documentation Committee Score; PDS: polyparadioxanone; PGA: polyglycolic acid; PL: posterolateral; PLA: polylactic acid; PLLA: poly-L-lactic acid; β-TCP: β-tricalcium phosphate

Acknowledgements
The authors thank all members of the Sports Medicine Center, Samsung Medical Center for their great scientific debates.

Funding
This work was supported by the National Research Foundation of Korea(NRF) grant funded by the Korea government(MSIP) (2015R1A2A1A15054779), and this research was supported by a grant of the Korea Health Technology R&D Project through the Korea Health Industry Development Institute (KHIDI), funded by the Ministry of Health & Welfare, Republic of Korea (grant number: HI10C2020).

Authors' contributions
JHW and BHL participated in the study design and helped to draft the manuscript. BHL as a consultant for statistical analysis performed the statistical analysis. ESL conceived of the study, and participated in its design and coordination and helped to draft the manuscript. All authors participated in the development of and approved the final manuscript, and agreed to be accountable for the integrity of the content.

Competing interests
The authors declare that they have no competing interests.

Author details
[1]Department of Orthopaedic Surgery, Samsung Medical Center, Sungkyunkwan University School of Medicine, Seoul 06351, South Korea. [2]Department of Health Sciences and Technology, SAIHST, Sungkyunkwan University, Seoul, South Korea. [3]Department of Medical Device Management and Research, SAIHST, Sungkyunkwan University, Seoul, South Korea. [4]Department of Orthopaedic Surgery, Dongbu Jaeil Hospital, Seoul, Republic of Korea. [5]Department of Orthopaedic Surgery, Kang-Dong Sacred Heart Hospital, Hallym University Medical Center, Gil-dong, Seoul 134-701, South Korea.

References
1. McGuire DA, Barber FA, Elrod BF, Paulos LE. Bioabsorbable interference screws for graft fixation in anterior cruciate ligament reconstruction. Arthroscopy. 1999;15:463–73.
2. Barber FA. Flipped patellar tendon autograft anterior cruciate ligament reconstruction. Arthroscopy. 2000;16:483–90.
3. Drogset JO, Grontvedt T, Tegnander A. Endoscopic reconstruction of the anterior cruciate ligament using bone-patellar tendon-bone grafts fixed with bioabsorbable or metal interference screws: a prospective randomized study of the clinical outcome. Am J Sports Med. 2005;33:1160–5.
4. Kaeding C, Farr J, Kavanaugh T, Pedroza A. A prospective randomized comparison of bioabsorbable and titanium anterior cruciate ligament interference screws. Arthroscopy. 2005;21:147–51.
5. Laxdal G, Kartus J, Eriksson BI, Faxen E, Sernert N, Karlsson J. Biodegradable and metallic interference screws in anterior cruciate ligament reconstruction surgery using hamstring tendon grafts: prospective randomized study of radiographic results and clinical outcome. Am J Sports Med. 2006;34:1574–80.
6. Barber FA, Dockery WD. Long-term absorption of poly-L-lactic acid interference screws. Arthroscopy. 2006;22:820–6.
7. Ma CB, Francis K, Towers J, Irrgang J, Fu FH, Harner CH. Hamstring anterior cruciate ligament reconstruction: a comparison of bioabsorbable interference screw and endobutton-post fixation. Arthroscopy. 2004;20:122–8.
8. Warden WH, Chooljian D, Jackson DW. Ten-year magnetic resonance imaging follow-up of bioabsorbable poly-L-lactic acid interference screws after anterior cruciate ligament reconstruction. Arthroscopy. 2008;24(370): e371–3.
9. Bourke HE, Salmon LJ, Waller A, Winalski CS, Williams HA, Linklater JM, Vasanji A, Roe JP, Pinczewski LA. Randomized controlled trial of osteoconductive fixation screws for anterior cruciate ligament reconstruction: a comparison of the Calaxo and Milagro screws. Arthroscopy. 2013;29:74–82.
10. Foldager C, Jakobsen BW, Lund B, Christiansen SE, Kashi L, Mikkelsen LR, Lind M. Tibial tunnel widening after bioresorbable poly-lactide calcium carbonate interference screw usage in ACL reconstruction. Knee Surg Sports Traumatol Arthrosc. 2010;18:79–84.
11. Moisala AS, Jarvela T, Paakkala A, Paakkala T, Kannus P, Jarvinen M. Comparison of the bioabsorbable and metal screw fixation after ACL reconstruction with a hamstring autograft in MRI and clinical outcome: a prospective randomized study. Knee Surg Sports Traumatol Arthrosc. 2008; 16:1080–6.
12. Doig GS, Simpson F. Randomization and allocation concealment: a practical guide for researchers. J Crit Care. 2005;20:187–91. discussion 191-183
13. Carulli C, Matassi F, Soderi S, Sirleo L, Munz G, Innocenti M. Resorbable screw and sheath versus resorbable interference screw and staples for ACL reconstruction: a comparison of two tibial fixation methods. Knee Surg Sports Traumatol Arthrosc. 2017;25(4):1264–71.
14. Ahn JH, Wang JH, Lee YS, Kim JG, Kang JH, Koh KH. Anterior cruciate ligament reconstruction using remnant preservation and a femoral tensioning technique: clinical and magnetic resonance imaging results. Arthroscopy. 2011;27:1079–89.
15. Hanley ST, Warren RF. Arthroscopic meniscectomy in the anterior cruciate ligament-deficient knee. Arthroscopy. 1987;3:59–65.
16. Buss DD, Warren RF, Wickiewicz TL, Galinat BJ, Panariello R. Arthroscopically assisted reconstruction of the anterior cruciate ligament with use of autogenous patellar-ligament grafts. Results after twenty-four to forty-two months. J Bone Joint Surg Am. 1993;75:1346–55.
17. Iorio R, Vadala A, Argento G, Di Sanzo V, Ferretti A. Bone tunnel enlargement after ACL reconstruction using autologous hamstring tendons: a CT study. Int Orthop. 2007;31:49–55.
18. Aga C, Wilson KJ, Johansen S, Dornan G, La Prade RF, Engebretsen L. Tunnel widening in single- versus double-bundle anterior cruciate ligament reconstructed knees. Knee Surg Sports Traumatol Arthrosc. 2017;25:1316–27.
19. Nebelung W, Becker R, Merkel M, Ropke M. Bone tunnel enlargement after anterior cruciate ligament reconstruction with semitendinosus tendon using Endobutton fixation on the femoral side. Arthroscopy. 1998;14:810–5.
20. Hovis WD, Bucholz RW. Polyglycolide bioabsorbable screws in the treatment of ankle fractures. Foot Ankle Int. 1997;18:128–31.
21. Stahelin AC, Weiler A, Rufenacht H, Hoffmann R, Geissmann A, Feinstein R. Clinical degradation and biocompatibility of different bioabsorbable interference screws: a report of six cases. Arthroscopy. 1997;13:238–44.
22. Bergsma JE, de Bruijn WC, Rozema FR, Bos RR, Boering G. Late degradation tissue response to poly(L-lactide) bone plates and screws. Biomaterials. 1995;16:25–31.
23. Lajtai G, Noszian I, Humer K, Unger F, Aitzetmuller G, Orthner E. Serial magnetic resonance imaging evaluation of operative site after fixation of patellar tendon graft with bioabsorbable interference screws in anterior cruciate ligament reconstruction. Arthroscopy. 1999;15:709–18.
24. Lajtai G, Humer K, Aitzetmuller G, Unger F, Noszian I, Orthner E. Serial magnetic resonance imaging evaluation of a bioabsorbable interference screw and the adjacent bone. Arthroscopy. 1999;15:481–8.
25. Aga C, Rasmussen MT, Smith SD, Jansson KS, LaPrade RF, Engebretsen L, Wijdicks CA. Biomechanical comparison of interference screws and combination screw and sheath devices for soft tissue anterior cruciate

ligament reconstruction on the tibial side. Am J Sports Med. 2013;41:841–8.

26. Kamitakahara M, Ohtsuki C, Miyazaki T. Review paper: behavior of ceramic biomaterials derived from tricalcium phosphate in physiological condition. J Biomater Appl. 2008;23:197–212.

27. Honda Y, Kamakura S, Sasaki K, Suzuki O. Formation of bone-like apatite enhanced by hydrolysis of octacalcium phosphate crystals deposited in collagen matrix. J Biomed Mater Res B Appl Biomater. 2007;80:281–9.

28. Okuda T, Ioku K, Yonezawa I, Minagi H, Kawachi G, Gonda Y, Murayama H, Shibata Y, Minami S, Kamihira S, Kurosawa H, Ikeda T. The effect of the microstructure of beta-tricalcium phosphate on the metabolism of subsequently formed bone tissue. Biomaterials. 2007;28:2612–21.

29. Agrawal CM, Athanasiou KA. Technique to control pH in vicinity of biodegrading PLA-PGA implants. J Biomed Mater Res. 1997;38:105–14.

30. Braux J, Velard F, Guillaume C, Bouthors S, Jallot E, Nedelec JM, Laurent-Maquin D, Laquerriere P. A new insight into the dissociating effect of strontium on bone resorption and formation. Acta Biomater. 2011;7:2593–603.

31. Penolazzi L, Lambertini E, Tavanti E, Torreggiani E, Vesce F, Gambari R, Piva R. Evaluation of chemokine and cytokine profiles in osteoblast progenitors from umbilical cord blood stem cells by BIO-PLEX technology. Cell Biol Int. 2008;32:320–5.

32. Lisignoli G, Toneguzzi S, Pozzi C, Piacentini A, Riccio M, Ferruzzi A, Gualtieri G, Facchini A. Proinflammatory cytokines and chemokine production and expression by human osteoblasts isolated from patients with rheumatoid arthritis and osteoarthritis. J Rheumatol. 1999;26:791–9.

33. McGuire DA, Barber FA, Milchgrub S, Wolchok JC. A postmortem examination of poly-L lactic acid interference screws 4 months after implantation during anterior cruciate ligament reconstruction. Arthroscopy. 2001;17:988–92.

34. Martinek V, Seil R, Lattermann C, Watkins SC, Fu FH. The fate of the poly-L-lactic acid interference screw after anterior cruciate ligament reconstruction. Arthroscopy. 2001;17:73–6.

35. Jarvela T, Moisala AS, Paakkala T, Paakkala A. Tunnel enlargement after double-bundle anterior cruciate ligament reconstruction: a prospective, randomized study. Arthroscopy. 2008;24:1349–57.

36. Lee YS, Lee SW, Nam SW, Oh WS, Sim JA, Kwak JH, Lee BK. Analysis of tunnel widening after double-bundle ACL reconstruction. Knee Surg Sports Traumatol Arthrosc. 2012;20:2243–50.

37. Siebold R, Cafaltzis K. Differentiation between intraoperative and postoperative bone tunnel widening and communication in double-bundle anterior cruciate ligament reconstruction: a prospective study. Arthroscopy. 2010;26:1066–73.

38. Lind M, Feller J, Webster KE. Bone tunnel widening after anterior cruciate ligament reconstruction using EndoButton or EndoButton continuous loop. Arthroscopy. 2009;25:1275–80.

39. Hoher J, Moller HD, Fu FH. Bone tunnel enlargement after anterior cruciate ligament reconstruction: fact or fiction? Knee Surg Sports Traumatol Arthrosc. 1998;6:231–40.

2

Comparison of serum markers for muscle damage, surgical blood loss, postoperative recovery, and surgical site pain after extreme lateral interbody fusion with percutaneous pedicle screws or traditional open posterior lumbar interbody fusion

Tetsuro Ohba[*], Shigeto Ebata and Hirotaka Haro

Abstract

Background: The benefits of extreme lateral interbody fusion (XLIF) as a minimally invasive lumbar spinal fusion treatment for lumbar degenerative spondylolisthesis have been unclear. We sought to evaluate the invasiveness and tolerability of XLIF with percutaneous pedicle screws (PPS) compared with traditional open posterior lumbar interbody fusion (PLIF).

Methods: Fifty-six consecutive patients underwent open PLIF and 46 consecutive patients underwent single-staged treatment with XLIF with posterior PPS fixation for degenerative lumbar spondylolisthesis, and were followed up for a minimum of 1 year. We analyzed postoperative serum makers for muscle damage and inflammation, postoperative surgical pain, and performance status. A Roland–Morris Disability Questionnaire (RDQ) and Oswestry Disability Index (ODI) were obtained at the time of hospital admission and 1 year after surgery.

Results: Intraoperative blood loss (51 ± 41 ml in the XLIF/PPS group and 206 ± 191 ml in the PLIF group), postoperative WBC counts and serum CRP levels in the XLIF/PPS group were significantly lower than in the PLIF group. Postoperative serum CK levels were significantly lower in the XLIF/PPS group on postoperative days 4 and 7. Postoperative recovery of performance was significantly greater in the XLIF/PPS group than in the PLIF group from postoperative days 2 to 7. ODI and visual analog scale (VAS) score (lumbar) 1 year after surgery were significantly lower in the XLIF/PPS group compared with the PLIF group.

Conclusions: The XLIF/PPS procedure is advantageous to minimize blood loss and muscle damage, with consequent earlier recovery of daily activities and reduced incidence of low back pain after surgery than with the open PLIF procedure.

Keywords: Lumbar degenerative spondylolisthesis, Extreme lateral interbody fusion, Percutaneous pedicle screws, Minimally invasive surgery, Muscle damage, Low back pain

* Correspondence: tooba@yamanashi.ac.jp
Department of Orthopaedics, University of Yamanashi, 1110 Shimokato, Chuo, Yamanashi 409-3898, Japan

Background

Spinal fusion is a surgical procedure used to fuse two or more vertebrae and to stabilize unstable spine segments. Lumbar spinal fusion surgery has been widely used to manage the pain and neurological symptoms in patients with low back pain (LBP) [1]. Traditional open posterior approaches for fusion and supplemental internal fixation that require extensive dissection of paraspinal musculature can result in permanent erector spinae denervation, loss of function, and late onset of spinal instability [2, 3]. Open lumbar spine surgeries are often accompanied by surgical site pain compared with minimally invasive techniques [4, 5].

Alternatively, more modern, less invasive approaches for lumbar interbody fusion have gained in popularity, one such approach being the mini-open lateral transpsoas approach (XLIF, NuVasive, San Diego, CA, USA) [6]. Benefits of the lateral approach include the preservation of back muscle, and bony and ligamentous structures, and it also allows for the placement of an intervertebral cage. In addition, the current procedure results in correction of spondylolisthesis and rotatory deformity, and indirect nerve decompression by ligamentotaxis force. These advantages may result in less surgical pain and quicker recovery than achieved in traditional approaches [7]. The validity of minimally invasive lumbar interbody fusions with percutaneous pedicle screws (PPS) has been described [8, 9].

By contrast, a comparatively high complication rate of XLIF including postoperative thigh symptoms (range 1–60.1%) has been reported [10]. A recent review concluded there is insufficient evidence for the comparative effectiveness of XLIF compared with traditional posterior lumbar interbody fusion (PLIF) [11, 12]. To evaluate the invasiveness and tolerability of XLIF with PPS compared with PLIF, we evaluated serum markers of muscle damage and inflammation, surgical pain, surgical blood loss, and postoperative recovery of activities of daily living (performance status score) for XLIF with PPS compared with traditional open PLIF surgery.

Methods

Patient group and surgical techniques

Patients were candidates for surgery if fusion was indicated because of degenerative lumbar spondylolisthesis and if a full course of conservative care, in particular, drug and brace treatments, had been exhausted. The following criteria were applied: (1) no history of previous lumbar surgery, (2) severe low back and leg pain, and no improvement with conservative therapy for at least 6 months, (3) fusion length ≤3 intervertebral segments, (4) spondylolytic spondylolisthesis or spinal deformities, or both, were excluded (viz., if the patient had a coronal curve >30°

or a kyphosis >20°). The demographic details of the patients are shown in Table 2.

We included 102 consecutive patients with degenerative spondylolisthesis grade I and II treated at a single institution by two board certified spinal surgeons who have gained expertise in the XLIF procedure before beginning of the study. From April 2012 to March 2014, 56 consecutive patients underwent open PLIF, and from April 2014 to March 2016, 46 consecutive patients underwent single-staged treatment with XLIF, with posterior PPS fixation and intraoperative CT (O-arm) image-guidance navigation as previously described [13] without posterior decompression, and followed up for a minimum of 1 year in the outpatient clinic. Local autologous bone was used in all PLIF PEEK implants and allograft bone was used in all of our XLIF PEEK implants. Resection of rib or iliac bones for bone graft was not performed in the XLIF/PPS group. Patients were allowed to resume activities of daily living the next day depending on their pain from surgery.

Clinical evaluation

Preoperative and postoperative baseline patient health status were evaluated (for pain-related factors) using the Roland–Morris Disability Questionnaire (RDQ), Oswestry Disability Index (ODI) measured on a 50-point scale, Japanese Orthopaedic Association (JOA) score [14], and the visual analog scale (VAS) score for the lumbar spine at the time of hospital admission and 1 year after surgery.

On postoperative days 1, 4, and 7, serum creatine kinase (CK) and C-reactive protein (CRP), and white blood cell (WBC) counts were measured. The postoperative pain regimen for all patients included a daily dose of celecoxib (200 mg) for the duration of admission. Use of any analgesic regimens except celecoxib was an exclusion criterion for this study. On postoperative day 1, all patients were asked to state their level of pain using a 10 cm VAS with 10 cm indicating the worst pain imaginable. Additionally, on postoperative days 2 through 7, all patients were asked to state their level of pain using a numerical rating scale (NRS) ranging from 0 to 10, with 0 indicating no pain and 10 indicating the pain of surgery on the first postoperative day. On postoperative days 1 through 7, a physiotherapist recorded the performance status (PS) for all patients established by the Eastern Cooperative Oncology Group (ECOG). All personnel involved with the study patients during admission, including the nursing staff and physiotherapists, were blinded to the approach used and objectives of the study. All adverse events during and after surgery were reported. The total perioperative blood loss was estimated as the total of the intraoperative record and drainage output.

Radiographic evaluation

Preoperative slip (%) of fused levels was evaluated using lateral X-ray images obtained with the patients in a free-standing posture. Bony fusion was assessed by 2 independent physicians using 3-dimensional computed tomography (CT) at 1 year postoperatively, with the grading of fusion classified according to the system described by Bridwell et al. [15] (Table 1).

Statistical analyses

Data were analyzed using the unpaired T test, Mann–Whitney U test and Fisher exact test to determine significant differences. All statistical calculations were performed using Prism (version 6.0; Graph Pad Software, La Jolla, CA, USA). For all tests, $P < 0.05$ was considered significant.

Results

Comparison of patient demographics

There were no drop out cases and no revision surgery was needed because of implant failures or adjacent segment disease in either group at 1 year follow-up.

Table 2 summarizes the preoperative baseline characteristics of the patients who underwent spinal interbody fusion with XLIF/PPS or open PLIF. There was no significant difference in the mean age, the average body mass index (BMI), preoperative slip (%) of fused level, number of fused levels per patient, or proportion of current smokers between the groups (Table 2). The preoperative lumbar–JOA (L-JOA) scores were 14.1 ± 4.5 and 13.5 ± 3.8 in patients in the XLIF/PPS and PLIF groups, and the preoperative ODI scores were 21.2 ± 6.9 and 19.2 ± 6.5, respectively. The preoperative RDQ scores were similar (Table 2). These findings indicated XLIF/PPS and PILF were performed for patients who had similar pain-related parameters. Surgical time was not significantly different between the groups. Estimated blood loss in patients in the XLIF/PPS group was significantly lower than in the PLIF group (51 ± 41 ml in the XLIF/PPS group and 206 ± 191 ml in the PLIF group; $P < 0.0001$) (Fig. 1).

Table 1 Radiological Evaluation with the Bridwell Anterior Fusion Grading System

Grade	Description
1	Fused with remodeling and trabeculae present
2	Graft intact, not fully remodeled and incorporated, but no lucency present
3	Graft intact, potential lucency present at top and bottom of graft
4	Fusion absent with collapse/resorption of graft

Table 2 Demographics of patients undergoing XLIF with PPS or open PILF

	Intraoperative Technique		P
	XLIF/PPS (n = 46)	PLIF (n = 56)	
Age,* y	71.3 ± 8.6	69.0 ± 9.2	0.19
Sex, female/male	31/15	29/27	0.16
BMI,* kg/m²	23.4 ± 4.1	23.4 ± 4.6	0.98
Preoperative %Slip,* % Number of fused levels,*	1.88 ± 0.7	1.62 ± 0.8	0.1
Current smoking,* n (%)	4 (8.7%)	7 (12.5)	0.75
Preoperative score			
VAS score (lumbar)	4.9 ± 3.2	6.7 ± 2.5	0.37
RDQ score	13.9 ± 5.5	12.8 ± 4.2	0.49
ODI score	21.2 ± 6.9	19.2 ± 6.5	0.17
L-JOA score	14.1 ± 4.5	13.5 ± 3.8	0.41

XLIF = extreme lateral interbody fusion, PPS = percutaneous pedicle screws, PLIF = posterior lumbar interbody fusion, BMI = body mass index, n = number in group, VSA = visual analog scale, RDQ = Roland–Morris Disability Questionnaire, ODI = Oswestry Disability Index, L-JOA = lumbar–Japanese Orthopaedic Association, *Mean ± standard deviation (SD)

Comparison of serum markers for muscle damage and inflammation

The postoperative WBC counts and CRP levels were significantly lower in patients in the XLIF/PPS group on postoperative days 4 and 7 (Fig. 2a and b). The postoperative CK levels reached a maximum on the first postoperative day, and there was no significant difference between groups, being 866 ± 503 U/L in patients in the XLIF/PPS group and 753 ± 482 U/L in patients in the PLIF group. Postoperative CK values were significantly lower in patients in the XLIF/PPS group on postoperative day 4 (296 ± 171 U/L in the XLIF/PPS and 430 ± 367 U/L in the PLIF group; $P = 0.039$) and day 7 (93 ± 46 U/L in the XLIF/PPS group and 151 ± 147 U/L in the PLIF group; $P = 0.025$) (Fig. 2c).

The VAS score and NRS score for surgical pain

The postoperative surgical pain (VAS score) on day 1 was 6.7 ± 2.2 and 6.9 ± 2.3 for the XLIF/PPS and PLIF groups respectively, with no difference between the groups (Fig. 3a). Additionally, there were no significant differences in NRS score for surgical pain between the groups from postoperative day 2 to 7 (Fig. 3b).

Postoperative recovery of activities of daily living

Postoperative PS scores were significantly greater in the XLIF/PPS group than in the PLIF group from postoperative day 2 to day 7 (Fig. 3c).

Complications

The surgery-related complications encountered in our study (8.6%) were minor and acceptable (XLIF/PPS group, 6 patients; PLIF group, 2 patients). There were 5 patients

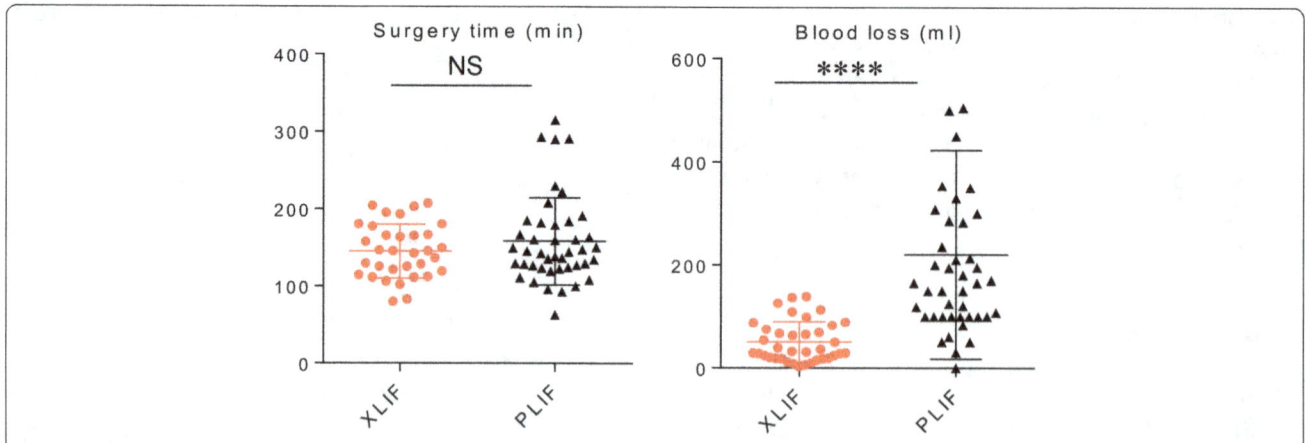

Fig. 1 Surgical time and blood loss between XLIF/PPS and PLIF approaches. ****$P < 0.0001$, NS = not significant. Data were analyzed using the unpaired T test

who showed a temporary thigh sensory change and 4 patients who showed a temporary hip flexion weakness in the XLIF/PPS group. There was 1 patient who showed superficial disturbance of wound healing and 1 patient in the PLIF group required repair for durotomy. None of the patients in either group required reoperation for surgical site infection, inadequate decompression or instability at the operative levels.

Comparison of patient outcomes 1 year after surgery

Table 3 summarizes the 1 year postoperative outcomes of patients who underwent spinal interbody fusion with

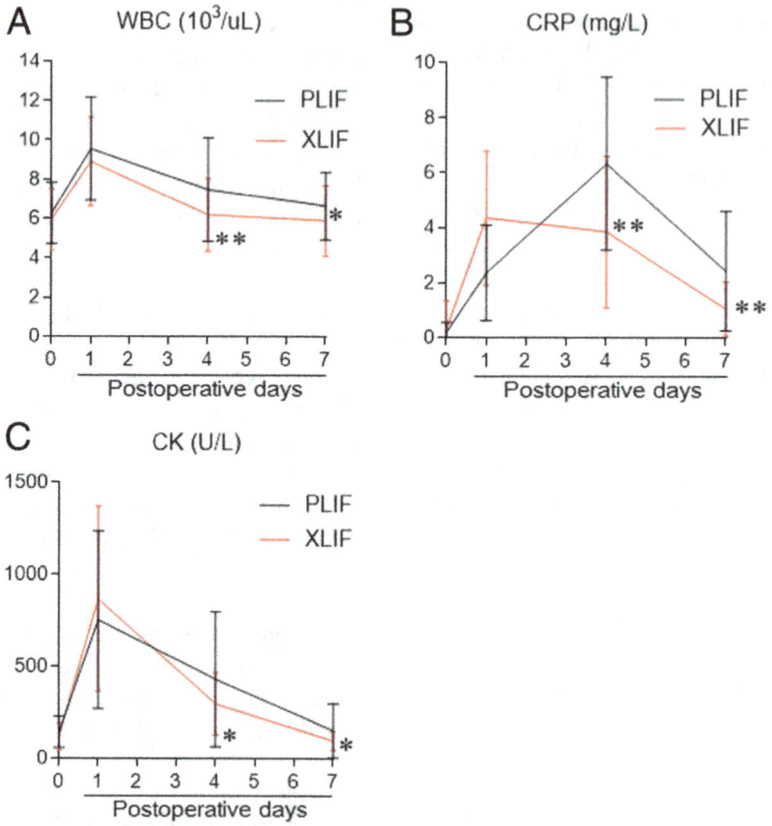

Fig. 2 Postoperative serum levels of **a** white blood cells (WBC), **b** C-reactive protein (CRP), and **c** creatinine kinase (CK). *$P < 0.05$, **$P < 0.005$. Data were analyzed using the unpaired T test

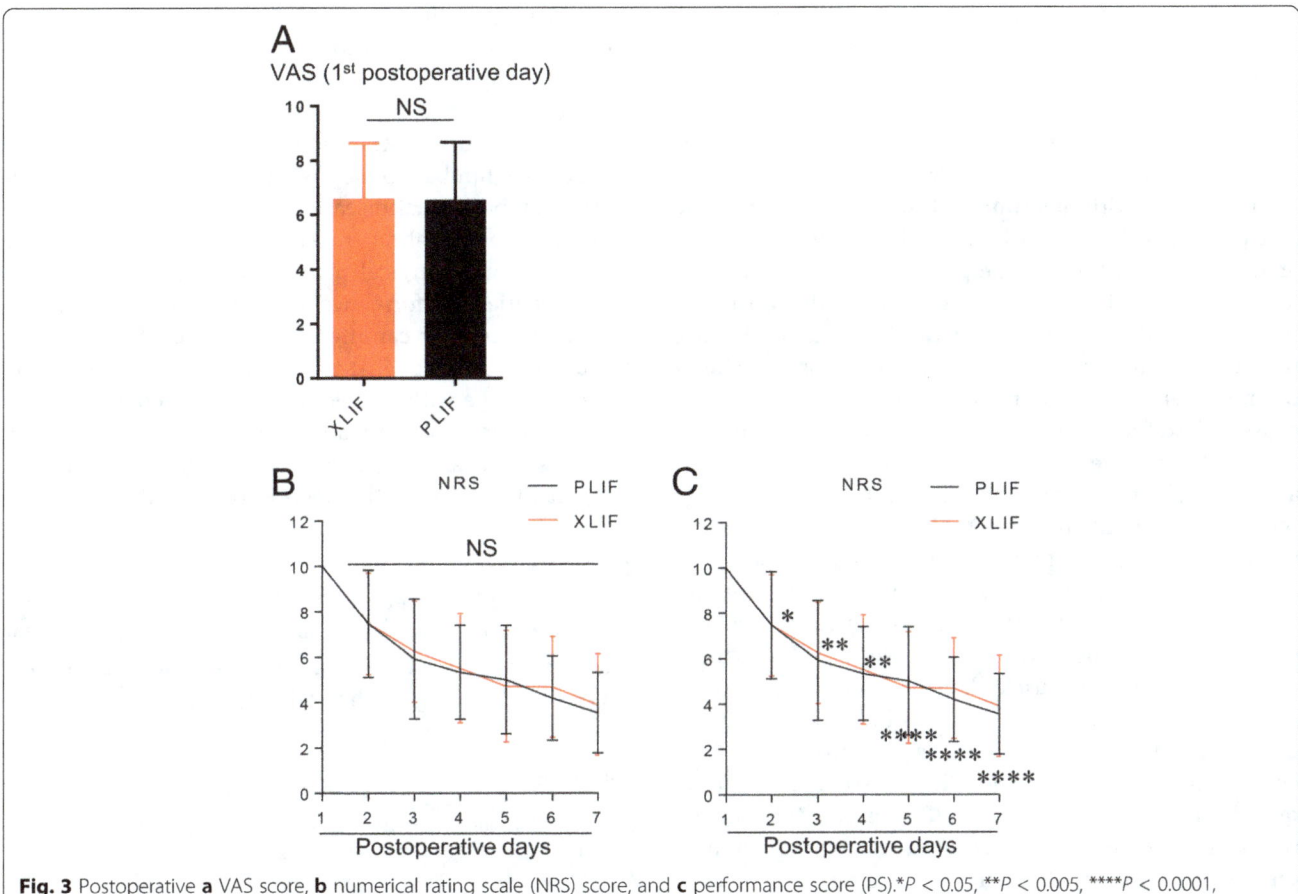

Fig. 3 Postoperative **a** VAS score, **b** numerical rating scale (NRS) score, and **c** performance score (PS).*$P < 0.05$, **$P < 0.005$, ****$P < 0.0001$, NS = not significant. Data were analyzed using the unpaired T test for (**a**). Data were analyzed using Mann–Whitney U test for (**b**) and (**c**)

XLIF/PPS or open PLIF. There was no significant difference in the L-JOA score or RDQ between the groups (Table 3). By contrast, ODI and VAS scores (lumbar) 1 year after surgery were significantly lower in the XLIF/PPS group than in the PLIF group. There were no cases of nonunion (grade 3 or 4) in either group and there were no significant differences in the

Table 3 One-year-postoperative outcomes of patients undergoing XLIF with PPS or open PILF

	Intraoperative Technique		P
	XLIF/PPS ($n = 46$)	PLIF ($n = 56$)	
Length of follow-up (years)	2.2 ± 1.2	4.3 ± 2.2	
VAS score (lumbar)	1.5 ± 2.6	3.7 ± 3.1	**<0.005**
RDQ score	8.2 ± 5.4	8.6 ± 5.9	0.95
ODI score	9.2 ± 7.4	13.5 ± 6.4	**<0.05**
L-JOA score	25.3 ± 3.9	24.1 ± 2.4	0.29
Fusion grade	1.5±0.51	1.5±0.5	0.84

*XLIF = extreme lateral interbody fusion, PPS = percutaneous pedicle screws, PLIF = posterior lumbar interbody fusion, n = number in group, VSA = visual analog scale, RDQ = Roland–Morris Disability Questionnaire, ODI = Oswestry Disability Index, L-JOA = Lumbar–Japanese Orthopaedic Association, *Mean ± standard deviation (SD)

fusion grading between groups using CT at 1 year follow-up (Table 3).

Discussion

Degenerative lumbar spondylolisthesis is one of the disorders most responsive to lumbar fusion. Because of the ability of the interbody fusion technique to correct the listhesis through realignment and stabilization, high rates of improvement on multiple clinical outcome measures after surgery for degenerative lumbar spondylolisthesis have been reported [10]. Recent reports have indicated the effectiveness of XLIF as a surgical treatment for adult spinal deformity, which included greater coronal and sagittal balance correction, and minimized reoperation rate and blood loss [16–18]. By contrast, the benefits of XLIF as a minimally invasive lumbar spinal fusion technique for degenerative lumbar spondylolisthesis remained unclear. Most studies have used comparative approaches focusing simply on complication rates, blood loss, and length of hospital stay as surgical outcomes [11]. Additionally, recent reviews concluded there was insufficient evidence for the effectiveness of XLIF in minimally invasive lumbar spinal fusion and that further studies in support of XLIF in comparison with traditional lumbar interbody fusion approaches are warranted [10, 11]. Therefore, the present study sought to compare XLIF/PPS with traditional open PLIF surgery using multiple outcomes including muscle damage, surgical blood loss, markers of postoperative inflammation, surgical site pain, and postoperative recovery of activities of daily living.

Open PLIF with instrumentation requires extensive soft tissue and back muscle dissection, which is considered to be problematic in the procedure for conventional lumbar fusion [19, 20]. Indeed, a study demonstrated that PPS fixation caused less paraspinal muscle damage than open pedicle screw fixation and had positive effects on postoperative trunk muscle performance [21]. Because it is difficult to quantify blood loss precisely in a minimally invasive procedure, we estimated blood loss as the total of the intraoperative record and drainage output, and found that the XLIF/PPS procedure is extremely advantageous to minimize blood loss. The use of serum markers for inflammation and muscle damage offers objective measures of the invasiveness of the procedure. A postoperative rise in serum CK should indicate the level of muscle damage, and a rise in WBC count and serum CRP levels should indicate the level of inflammation [22]. Our findings showed that WBC counts, and serum CRP and CK levels decreased more quickly in patients in the XLIF/PPS group than in patients in the PLIF group. In accordance with this finding, ODI and VAS score (lumbar) 1 year after surgery were significantly lower in the XLIF/PPS group than in the PLIF group. By contrast, there was no significant difference in the RDQ or L-JOA scores between the groups 1 year after surgery. This finding indicates that although both procedures improved multiple clinical outcome measures compared with PLIF, XLIF/PPS can significantly reduce paraspinal muscle injury which was indicated as less blood loss and lower serum CK level and the incidence of low back pain after surgery.

Unexpectedly, we did not find any difference in postsurgical pain from postoperative days 1 to 7 between the groups in the present study. By contrast, the postoperative recovery of activities of daily living (PS) in patients in the XLIF/PPS group was significantly greater than that in patients in the PLIF group from postoperative days 3 to 7. These findings may result from the difficulty and limitations of accurate self-reported acute pain evaluation using simple pain rating scales [23, 24]. Despite the higher complication rate in the XLIF/PPS group compared with the PLIF group observed in the current study, all of the complications were minor and acceptable. All postoperative thigh symptoms of patients in the XLIF/PPS group were resolved by 1 year after surgery.

This study has limitation that requires further investigation. There was a difference between the two groups in using allograft or autologous bone. This difference

could strongly influence postoperative pain, serum creatine kinase and inflammation markers.

However, to our knowledge, this is the first study to indicate the comparative invasiveness and tolerability of XLIF compared with traditional open PLIF as a minimally invasive lumbar spinal fusion method to treat degenerative lumbar spinal disease; not only by surgical blood loss and complication rates, but also by evaluating muscle damage, surgical pain, postoperative recovery of daily activities (performance status score), and incidence of low back pain 1 year after surgery. The XLIF/PPS procedure is advantageous to minimize blood loss and muscle damage with consequent earlier recovery of daily activities (performance status) and a lower incidence of low back pain after surgery, but does not result in less surgical site pain than the open PLIF procedure.

Conclusions

The XLIF/PPS procedure is advantageous to minimize blood loss and muscle damage, with consequent earlier recovery of daily activities and reduced incidence of low back pain after surgery than with open PLIF.

Abbreviations

CK: Serum creatine kinase; CRP: C-reactive protein; LBP: Low back pain; NRS: Numerical rating scale; ODI: Oswestry Disability Index; PLIF: Posterior lumbar interbody fusion; PPS: Percutaneous pedicle screws; PS: Performance status; RDQ: Roland–Morris Disability Questionnaire; WBC: White blood cell; XLIF: Extreme lateral interbody fusion

Acknowledgements
None

Funding
There is no funding that should be declared.

Authors' contributions
TO substantially analyzed and interpreted the patient data and was a major contributor in drafting the manuscript. SE substantially contributed to the conception and design of the study and contributed to drafting the manuscript. HH substantially contributed to the study design and critically revised the manuscript. All authors read, approved, and take responsibility for the final manuscript.

Competing interests
The authors declare that they have no competing interests.

References
1. Frymoyer JW, Cats-Baril WL. An overview of the incidences and costs of low back pain. Orthop Clin North Am. 1991;22:263–71.
2. Quint U, Wilke HJ, Löer F, Claes L. Laminectomy and functional impairment of the lumbar spine: the importance of muscle forces in flexible and rigid instrumented stabilization – a biomechanical study in vitro. Eur Spine J. 1998;7:229–38.
3. Quint U, Wilke HJ, Shirazi-Adl A, Parnianpour M, Loer F, Claes LE. Importance of the intersegmental trunk muscles for the stability of the lumbar spine. A biomechanical study in vitro. Spine (Phila Pa 1976). 1998;23:1937–45.

4. Sasso RC, Kitchel SH, Dawson EG. A prospective, randomized controlled clinical trial of anterior lumbar interbody fusion using a titanium cylindrical threaded fusion device. Spine (Phila Pa 1976). 2004;29(2):113–22. discussion 121-112

5. O'Toole JE, Eichholz KM, Fessler RG. Surgical site infection rates after minimally invasive spinal surgery. J Neurosurg Spine. 2009;11(4):471–6.

6. Ozgur BM, Aryan HE, Pimenta L, Taylor WR. Extreme Lateral Interbody Fusion (XLIF): a novel surgical technique for anterior lumbar interbody fusion. Spine J. 2006;6(4):435–43.

7. Khajavi K, Shen A, Lagina M, Hutchison A. Comparison of clinical outcomes following minimally invasive lateral interbody fusion stratified by preoperative diagnosis. Eur Spine J. 2015;24(Suppl 3):322–30.

8. Dickerman RD, East JW, Winters K, Tackett J, Hajovsky-Pietla A. Anterior and posterior lumbar interbody fusion with percutaneous pedicle screws: comparison to muscle damage and minimally invasive techniques. Spine (Phila Pa 1976). 2009;34(25):E923–5.

9. Blizzard DJ, Hills CP, Isaacs RE, Brown CR. Extreme lateral interbody fusion with posterior instrumentation for spondylodiscitis. J Clin Neurosci. 2015;22(11):1758–61.

10. Youssef JA, McAfee PC, Patty CA, Raley E, DeBauche S, Shucosky E, Chotikul L. Minimally invasive surgery: lateral approach interbody fusion: results and review. Spine (Phila Pa 1976). 2010;35(26 Suppl):S302–11.

11. Barbagallo GM, Albanese V, Raich AL, Dettori JR, Sherry N, Balsano M. Lumbar Lateral Interbody Fusion (LLIF): comparative effectiveness and safety versus PLIF/TLIF and predictive factors affecting LLIF outcome. Evid Based Spine Care J. 2014;5(1):28–37.

12. Joseph JR, Smith BW, La Marca F, Park P. Comparison of complication rates of minimally invasive transforaminal lumbar interbody fusion and lateral lumbar interbody fusion: a systematic review of the literature. Neurosurg Focus. 2015;39(4):E4.

13. Ohba T, Ebata S, Fujita K, Sato H, Haro H. Percutaneous pedicle screw placements: accuracy and rates of cranial facet joint violation using conventional fluoroscopy compared with intraoperative three-dimensional computed tomography computer navigation. Eur Spine J. 2016;25:1775–80.

14. Fujiwara A, Kobayashi N, Saiki K, Kitagawa T, Tamai K, Saotome K. Association of the Japanese Orthopaedic Association score with the Oswestry disability index, Roland-Morris disability questionnaire, and short-form 36. Spine (Phila Pa 1976). 2003;28(14):1601–7.

15. Bridwell KH, Lenke LG, McEnery KW, Baldus C, Blanke K. Anterior fresh frozen structural allografts in the thoracic and lumbar spine. Do they work if combined with posterior fusion and instrumentation in adult patients with kyphosis or anterior column defects? Spine (Phila Pa 1976). 1995;20(12):1410–8.

16. Berjano P, Lamartina C. Far lateral approaches (XLIF) in adult scoliosis. Eur Spine J. 2013;22(Suppl 2):S242–53.

17. Costanzo G, Zoccali C, Maykowski P, Walter CM, Skoch J, Baaj AA. The role of minimally invasive lateral lumbar interbody fusion in sagittal balance correction and spinal deformity. Eur Spine J. 2014;23(Suppl 6):699–704.

18. Dangelmajer S, Zadnik PL, Rodriguez ST, Gokaslan ZL, Sciubba DM. Minimally invasive spine surgery for adult degenerative lumbar scoliosis. Neurosurg Focus. 2014;36(5):E7.

19. Sihvonen T, Herno A, Paljarvi L, Airaksinen O, Partanen J, Tapaninaho A. Local denervation atrophy of paraspinal muscles in postoperative failed back syndrome. Spine (Phila Pa 1976). 1993;18(5):575–81.

20. Taylor H, McGregor AH, Medhi-Zadeh S, Richards S, Kahn N, Zadeh JA, Hughes SP. The impact of self-retaining retractors on the paraspinal muscles during posterior spinal surgery. Spine (Phila Pa 1976). 2002;27(24):2758–62.

21. Kim DY, Lee SH, Chung SK, Lee HY. Comparison of multifidus muscle atrophy and trunk extension muscle strength: percutaneous versus open pedicle screw fixation. Spine (Phila Pa 1976). 2005;30(1):123–9.

22. Mjaaland KE, Kivle K, Svenningsen S, Pripp AH, Nordsletten L. Comparison of markers for muscle damage, inflammation, and pain using minimally invasive direct anterior versus direct lateral approach in total hip arthroplasty: a prospective, randomized, controlled trial. J Orthop Res. 2015;33:1305–10.

23. de C Williams AC, Davies HT, Chadury Y. Simple pain rating scales hide complex idiosyncratic meanings. Pain. 2000;85(3):457–63.

24. Easton RM, Bendinelli C, Sisak K, Enninghorst N, Regan D, Evans J, Balogh ZJ. Recalled pain scores are not reliable after acute trauma. Injury. 2012;43(7): 1029–32.

3

Comparison of improved range of motion between cam-type femoroacetabular impingement and borderline developmental dysplasia of the hip-evaluation by virtual osteochondroplasty using computer simulation

So Kubota, Yutaka Inaba*, Naomi Kobayashi, Hyonmin Choe, Taro Tezuka and Tomoyuki Saito

Abstract

Background: While cam resection is essential to achieve a good clinical result with respect to femoroacetabular impingement (FAI), it is unclear whether it should also be performed in cases of borderline developmental dysplasia of the hip (DDH) with a cam deformity. The aim of this study was to evaluate improvements in range of motion (ROM) in cases of cam-type FAI and borderline DDH after virtual osteochondroplasty using a computer impingement simulation.

Methods: Thirty-eight symptomatic hips in 31 patients (11male and 20 female) diagnosed with cam-type FAI or borderline DDH were analyzed. There were divided into a cam-type FAI group (cam-FAI group: 15 hips), borderline DDH without cam group (DDH W/O cam group: 12 hips), and borderline DDH with cam group (DDH W/ cam group: 11 hips). The bony impingement point on the femoral head-neck junction at 90° flexion and maximum internal rotation of the hip joint was identified using ZedHip® software. Virtual osteochondroplasty of the impingement point was then performed in all cases. The maximum flexion angle and maximum internal rotation angle at 90° flexion were measured before and after virtual osteochondroplasty at two resection ranges (i.e., slight and sufficient).

Results: The mean improvement in the internal rotation angle in the DDH W/ cam group after slight resection was significantly greater than that in the DDH W/O cam group ($P = 0.046$). Furthermore, the mean improvement in the internal rotation angle in the DDH W/ cam and cam-FAI groups after sufficient resection was significantly greater than that in the DDH W/O cam group (DDH W/ cam vs DDH W/O cam: $P = 0.002$, cam-FAI vs DDH W/O cam: $P = 0.043$).

Conclusion: Virtual osteochondroplasty resulted in a significant improvement in internal rotation angle in DDH W/ cam group but not in DDH W/O cam group. Thus, borderline DDH cases with cam deformity may be better to consider performing osteochondroplasty.

Keywords: Femoroacetabular impingement, Borderline developmental dysplasia of the hip, Impingement simulation, Range of motion

* Correspondence: yute0131@med.yokohama-cu.ac.jp
Department of Orthopaedic Surgery, Yokohama City University, 3-9Fukuura,
Kanazawa-ku, Yokohama, Kanagawa 236-0004, Japan

Background

Femoroacetabular impingement (FAI) is an important cause of hip pain and subsequent osteoarthritis [1]. It is caused by an anatomical abnormality that results in mechanical impingement between the acetabular rim and the femoral head-neck junction during flexion and internal rotation of the hip [2, 3]. A major factor is cam deformity of the femur, which is characterized by an aspherical femoral head and bony bump formation at the femoral head-neck junction, which reduces femoral head-neck offset [2, 3]. FAI causes hip pain during squatting or deep flexion and may therefore reduce range of motion (ROM) at that joint [4]. These morphological abnormalities can be corrected by osteochondroplasty, which releases the bony impingement and improves ROM.

Developmental dysplasia of the hip (DDH) also causes hip pain, and has an etiological factor in the development of hip osteoarthritis [5, 6]. Its essential concept is that a biomechanical abnormality, joint incongruity, or decreased joint contact area may increase mechanical stress at the acetabular rim [6]. Although the basic pathophysiology of DDH is different from that of FAI, there are cases in which borderline DDH co-exists with a cam deformity [7, 8]. While cam resection is essential to achieve a good clinical result with respect to FAI [9, 10], it is unclear whether it should also be performed in cases of borderline DDH. In this regard, computer simulated virtual osteochondroplasty may provide the answer from the point of view of improvement in ROM.

The aim of this study was to investigate improvement in ROM after virtual hip osteochondroplasty using computer impingement simulation models for cam type FAI, borderline DDH with cam deformity, and borderline DDH without cam deformity.

We hypothesized that borderline DDH with cam deformity and cam-type FAI cases would demonstrate similar and significant improvement in ROM after virtual osteochondroplasty.

Methods

This study was approved by the institutional review board at Yokohama City University. In total, 38 symptomatic hips in 31 patients (11 male and 20 female) diagnosed with cam-type FAI or borderline DDH by plain radiography were enrolled. The mean age of the patients was 47.8 ± 13.0 years (range, 21–74 years). The anterior impingement test was positive in all 38 hips. Computed tomography (CT) and radiographic evaluation were performed during the same period (within 3 months) in all cases.

Radiographic evaluation

The lateral center-edge (CE) angle, Tönnis grade and crossover sign were measured on an antero-posterior

(A-P) view of the pelvis. The alpha angle was measured on a cross table lateral view of the hip joint. The measurement procedure was standardized in the picture archiving and communication system.

Definition of cam-type FAI and borderline DDH

Cam-type FAI was defined as an alpha angle $\geq 55°$ [11, 12] and a CE angle $\geq 25°$ [13, 14]. Borderline DDH was defined as a CE angle between 20 and 24° [13, 15]. Borderline DDH with cam deformity was defined as a combination of borderline DDH ($20 \leq CE$ angle $< 25°$) and cam (alpha angle $\geq 55°$). Thus, the 38 hips were assigned to three groups: a cam-type FAI group (cam-FAI group; 15 hips), a borderline DDH without cam deformity group (DDH W/O cam group; 12 hips), and a borderline DDH with cam deformity group (DDH W/ cam group; 11 hips). Pincer-type FAI cases (CE angle $> 40°$) [16], DDH with a CE angle of $< 20°$, or osteoarthritic changes with a Tönnis grade ≥ 2 were excluded.

Computed tomography

CT scans (Sensation16; Siemens AG, Erlangen, Germany) of the pelvis and femurs of all patients were acquired using the following scanner settings: 140 kV and 300 mA; slice thickness, 1.5 mm; pixel resolution, 512×512; voxel size, $0.70 \times 0.70 \times 1.5$ mm.

Computer simulated impingement analysis

ZedHip® (LEXI Co., Ltd., Tokyo, Japan) software was used to perform impingement simulation analysis. Digital imaging and communication in medicine (DICOM) data for each patient were transferred to ZedHip®, and three-dimensional (3D) simulation models of the pelvis and femur were constructed. The functional pelvic plane in a supine position was used as the pelvic plane reference. To set the femoral plane reference, the femoral head center was defined by assigning four reference points. The axis was set using two reference points: the head center and the mid-point between the medial and lateral epicondyles. Then, the pelvis and femur were segmented. The bony impingement point on the femoral head-neck junction at 90° flexion and maximum internal rotation of the hip joint was then identified (Fig. 1). The bony impingement was contact point between the acetabular rim and the femoral head-neck junction at the terminal point of the impingement simulation. If the impingement point appeared below 90° of flexion, the case was excluded. The impingement region of interests was defined into 2 regions (i.e., proximal region and distal region) in A-P view of the hip joint [17], and difference in the distribution of the impingement point was evaluated between cam-FAI and DDH W/ cam groups.

Virtual resection of the impingement point was then performed by the same investigator using ZedHip®. The

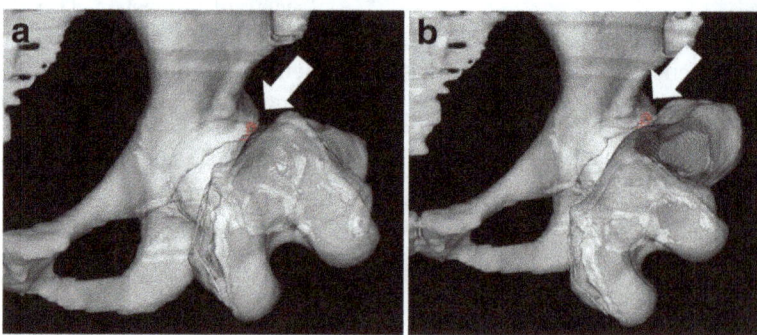

Fig. 1 Pre- and postoperative 3D images of the impingement simulation Impingement points are identified by arrows. The impingement point at the femoral head-neck junction at 90° flexion and maximum internal rotation of the hip joint is shown preoperatively (**a**) and postoperatively (**b**)

center of resection area was decided based on the impingement point by ZedHip®. Figure 2 shows the defined area of resection based on each impingement point. Because the resection depth for cam deformity would typically be 4–8 mm [18], two different versions were modeled: slight resection at a depth of 4 mm and sufficient resection at a depth of 8 mm. The width of the resected area in a horizontal slice was modeled as slight (8 mm) and sufficient (16 mm). The length of the resection was standardized at 15 mm (1.5 mm slice × 10 slices) in each axial image [19]. The edge of each resection area was trimmed smoothly to simulate clinical situation.

The maximum flexion angle and maximum internal rotation angle at 90° flexion was measured both before and after virtual osteochondroplasty using ZedHip® using each resection model (i.e., slight resection and sufficient resection) for cam-type FAI, borderline DDH with cam deformity, and borderline DDH without cam deformity cases.

Statistical analysis

The demographic data and imaging study results for all groups were evaluated using one-way factorial analysis of variance, as were the maximum flexion angle and maximum internal rotation angle at 90° flexion before virtual osteochondroplasty and improvements in the angle of maximum flexion angle and maximum internal rotation at 90° flexion. Difference in the distribution of the impingement point was evaluated using contingency table. Intraobserver reliability was calculated using intraclass correlation coefficients and their 95% confidence intervals (CIs) to assess the reliability of the improvement in the internal rotation angle at each resection models. P values < 0.05 were considered statistically significant. All statistical analyses were performed using dedicated statistical analysis software (SPSS 16.0; IBM Corp., Armonk, NY, USA).

Results

The demographic data for the three groups are presented in the Table 1. The mean body mass index (BMI) in the cam-FAI group was significantly higher than that in the DDH W/O cam group ($P = 0.012$). positive crossover sign was seen in 9 hips out of 38 hips, and it was seen most in cam-type FAI group.

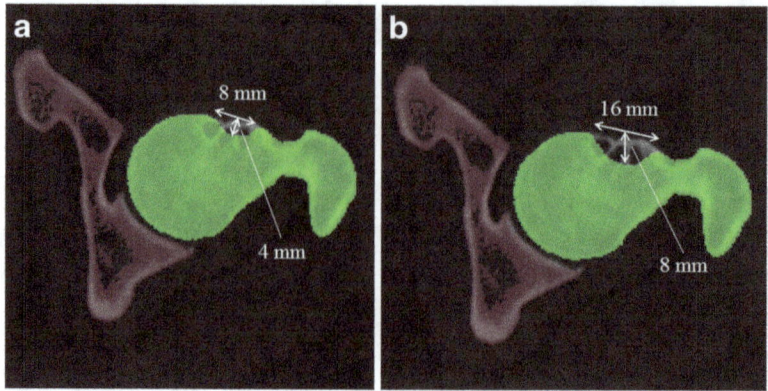

Fig. 2 The virtual resection of the impingement point The depth and width of the resection in the horizontal slice and the vertical resection length around the impingement point were standardized (i.e., slight resection (**a**), sufficient resection (**b**))

Table 1 Demographic data for the cam-FAI, DDH W/ cam, and DDH W/O cam groups

	Cam-FAI (n = 15)	DDH W/ cam (n = 11)	DDH W/O cam (n = 12)
Sex (male / female)	11 / 4	1 / 10	1 / 11
Age (mean ± SD)	48.7 ± 12.5	49.9 ± 11.9	44.8 ± 15.1
BMI (mean ± SD)	23.5 ± 3.2	22.1 ± 2.5	20.4 ± 2.2
CE angle (mean ± SD)	32.3 ± 4.2	22.0 ± 1.5	21.7 ± 1.7
alpha angle (mean ± SD)	65.7 ± 7.6	63.6 ± 6.1	49.5 ± 3.6
Tönnis grade (0 / 1)	10 / 5	7 / 4	10 / 2
Crossover sign (positive/ negative)	6 / 9	2 / 9	1 / 11

BMI body mass index, *CE* center-edge, *SD* standard deviation

The differences in the maximum flexion angle prior to virtual osteochondroplasty are shown in Fig. 3. The mean maximum flexion angle in the cam-FAI group was 113.1 ± 6.9°, whereas that in the DDH W/ cam and DDH W/O cam groups was 122.5 ± 14.7° and 132.8 ± 9.0°, respectively. The mean maximum flexion angle in the DDH W/O cam group was significantly greater than that in the cam-FAI group ($P = 0.001$). Differences in the maximum internal rotation angle prior to virtual osteochondroplasty are shown in Fig. 4. The mean maximum internal rotation angle in the cam-FAI group was 25.8 ± 11.8°, whereas that in the DDH W/ cam and DDH W/O cam groups was 38.9 ± 19.9° and 62.4 ± 15.0°, respectively. The mean maximum internal rotation angle in the DDH W/O cam group was significantly greater than that in the cam-FAI ($P = 0.001$) and DDH W/ cam groups ($P = 0.002$).

The impingement region in the cam-FAI group was distributed to 9 hips in the proximal region, and 6 hips in the distal region. The impingement region in the DDH W/ cam group was distributed to 8 hips in the proximal region, and 3 hips in the distal region. There was no significant difference in the distribution of the impingement point between cam-FAI and DDH W/ cam groups ($P = 0.68$).

The mean improvement in the flexion angle in the cam-FAI group after slight resection was 0.3 ± 1.0°, whereas that in the DDH W/ cam and DDH W/O cam groups was 0.6 ± 1.3° and 0.0 ± 0.0°, respectively. The mean improvement in the flexion angle in the cam-FAI group after sufficient resection was 0.4 ± 1.5°, whereas that in the DDH W/ cam and DDH W/O cam groups was 1.2 ± 2.0° and 0.2 ± 0.6°, respectively. There was no significant difference in any of these values between the three groups, regardless of resection type. The mean improvement in the internal rotation angle in each of the three groups after virtual resection is shown in Fig. 5. The improvement in the cam-FAI group after slight resection was 3.3 ± 2.1°, whereas that in the DDH W/ cam and DDH W/O cam groups was 4.7 ± 5.3° and 1.4 ± 1.3°, respectively. The mean improvement in the internal rotation angle after slight resection was significantly greater in the DDH W/ cam group than in the DDH W/O cam group ($P = 0.046$); however, there was no significant difference between the cam-FAI and DDH W/O cam groups. The mean improvement in the internal rotation angle in the cam-FAI group after sufficient resection was 7.4 ± 3.9°, whereas that in the DDH W/ cam group and DDH W/O cam groups was 10.0 ± 5.9° and

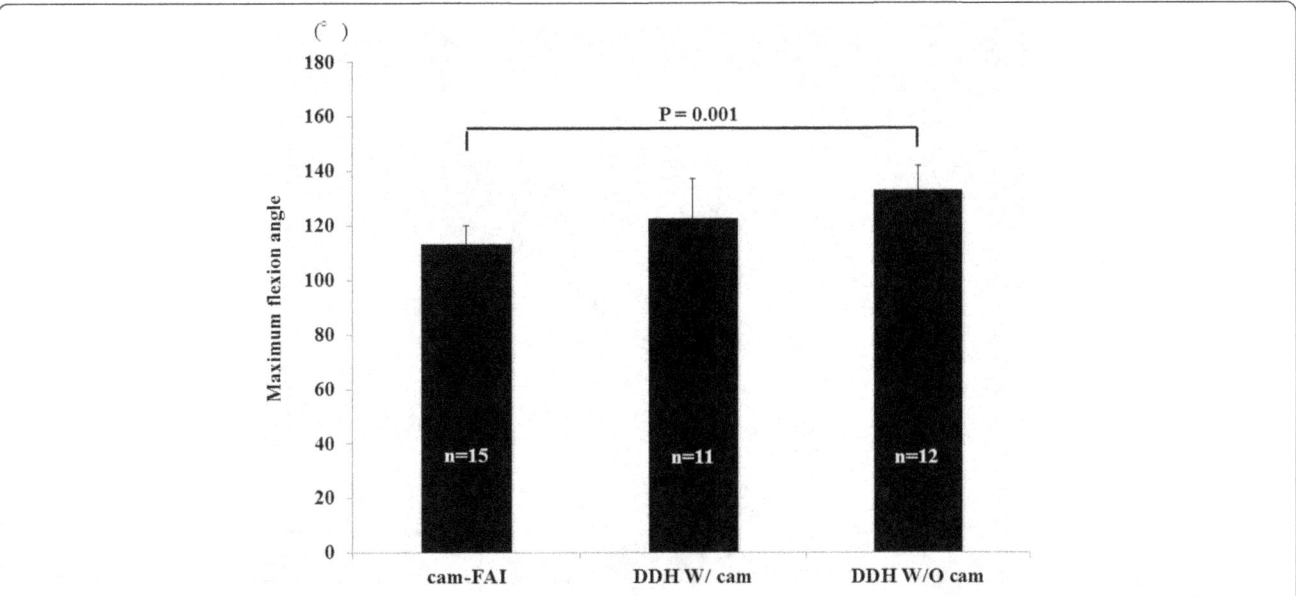

Fig. 3 Maximum flexion angle in the three groups before virtual osteochondroplasty The mean maximum flexion angle in the DDH W/O cam group was significantly greater than that in the cam-FAI FAI group ($P = 0.001$)

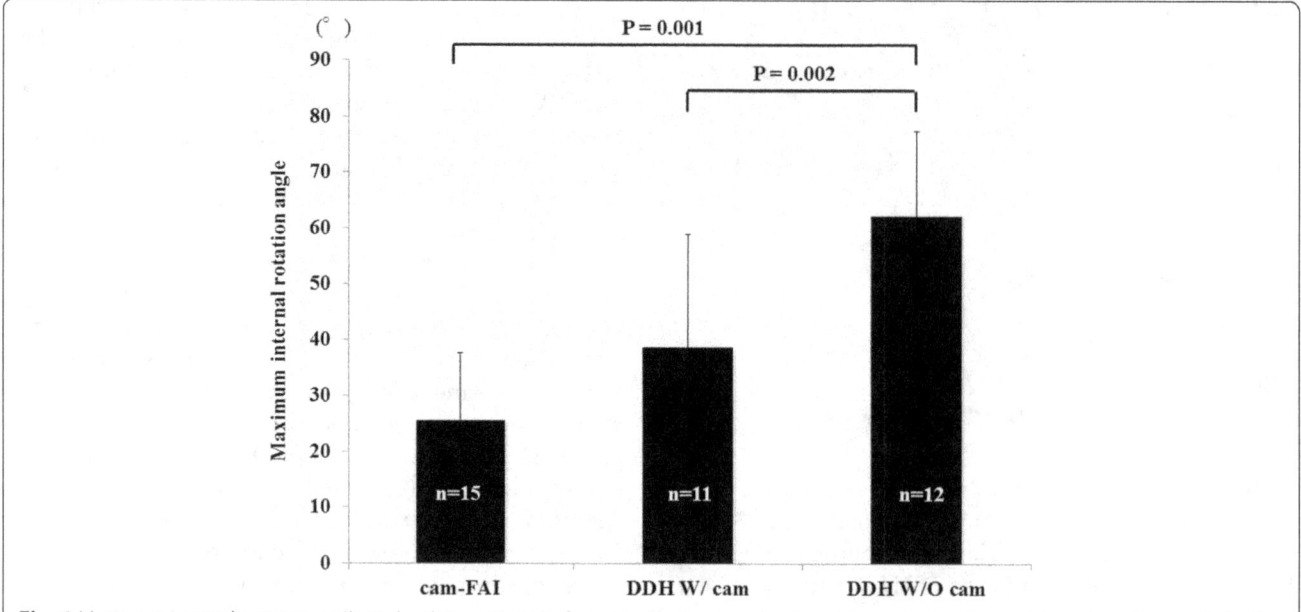

Fig. 4 Maximum internal rotation angle in the three groups before virtual osteochondroplasty The mean maximum internal rotation angle in the DDH W/O cam group was significantly greater than that in the cam-FAI (*P* = 0.001) and DDH W/ cam groups (*P* = 0.002)

3.3 ± 2.5°, respectively. The mean improvement in the internal rotation angle in the DDH W/ cam group after sufficient resection was significantly greater than that in the DDH W/O cam group (*P* = 0.002), as was that in the cam-FAI group (*P* = 0.043). There was no significant difference between the cam-FAI and DDH W/ cam groups in the improved internal rotation angle regardless of resection type, however, that in the DDH W/ cam group was tended to show more improvement than cam-FAI group for both slight and sufficient resections (Fig. 6).

In assessing the reliability of measuring the improvement in the internal rotation angle by computer simulation, intraobserver reliability was 0.917 (95% CIs, 0.792–0.969) at slight resection, and that was 0.828 (95% CIs, 0.594–0.933) at sufficient resection, both showing good reliability.

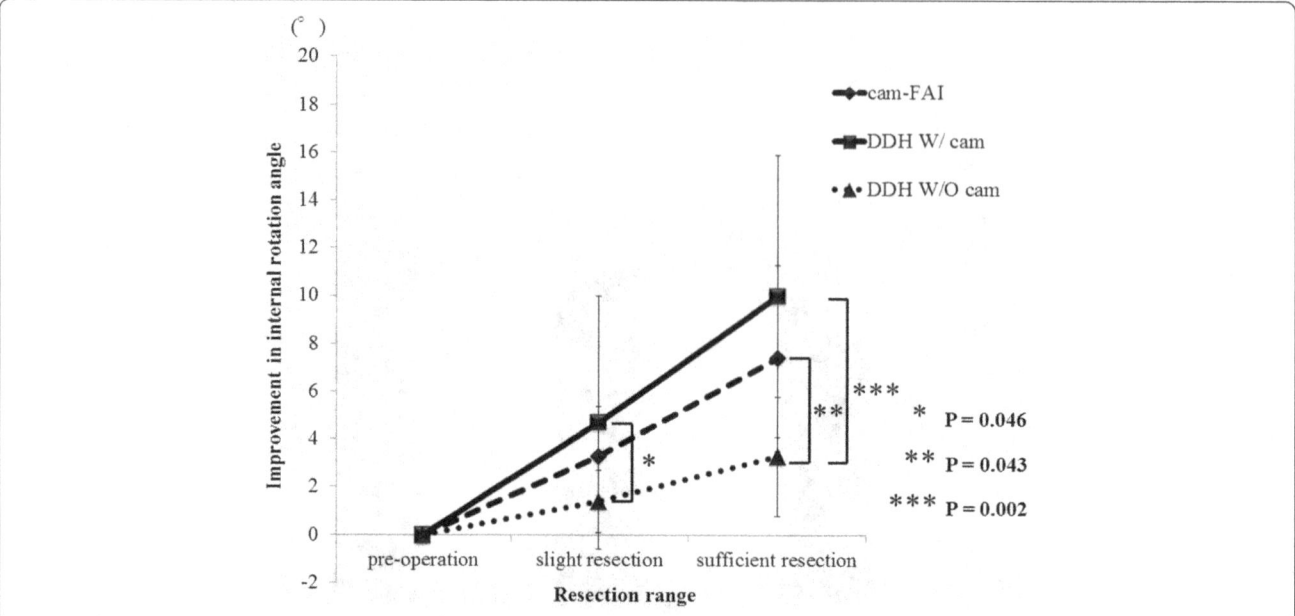

Fig. 5 Improvement in the internal rotation angle after each type of resection The mean improvement in the internal rotation angle in the DDH W/ cam group after slight resection was significantly greater than that in the DDH W/O cam group (*P* = 0.046), as was that after sufficient resection (*P* = 0.002). The improvement in the cam-FAI group was significantly greater than that in the DDH W/O cam group (*P* = 0.043)

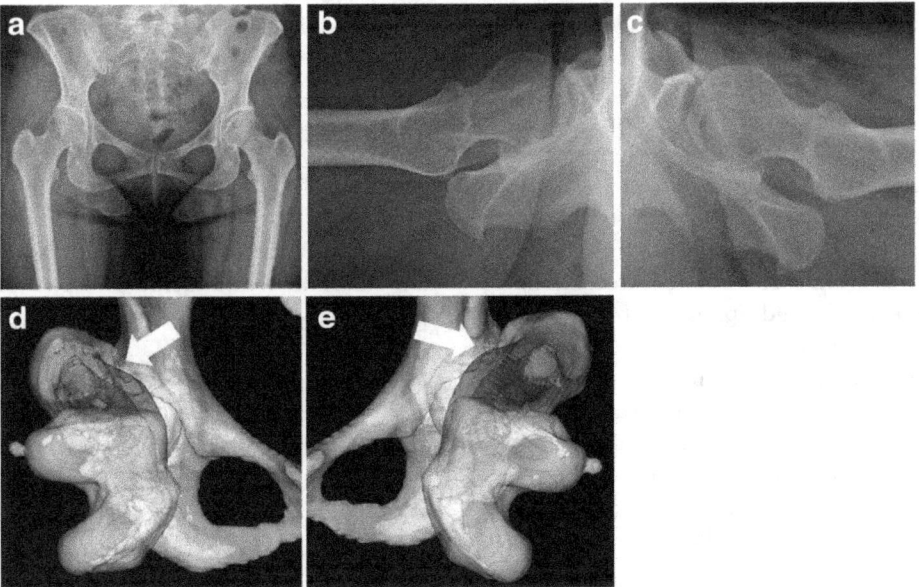

Fig. 6 A representative case of borderline DDH These images are of a 47-year-old woman with borderline DDH with cam deformity in the right hip and borderline DDH without cam deformity in the left hip. The CE angle in the right hip was 21° and that in the left was 24° (**a**). The alpha angle in the right hip was 67° (**b**) and that in the left was 51° (**c**). Impingement points are identified by arrows (**d, e**). The preoperative maximum internal rotation angle for both hip joints was 49°. The internal rotation angle in the right hip after slight resection was 53°, whereas that after sufficient resection was 65° (**d**). The final improvement in the internal rotation angle of the right hip joint was 16°. However, the internal rotation angle in the left hip after sufficient resection was 52° (**e**). Thus, the final improvement in the internal rotation angle of the left hip joint was 3°

Discussion

Here, we demonstrated that patients with borderline DDH with cam and cam-type FAI showed similar and significant improvement in the internal rotation angle after virtual osteochondroplasty; however, the procedure was not effective for those with borderline DDH without cam. The clinical implication is that it may be better to consider performing osteochodroplasty even in borderline DDH with cam deformity. This is the first study to use computer simulation analysis to examine the effect of cam osteochondroplasty in cases of borderline DDH with cam deformity. In fact, there was no significant difference of pre-operative internal rotation angle between cam-FAI and DDH W/ cam groups. Although preoperative internal rotation angle between DDH W/ cam group seems to be good enough to avoid impingement, the virtual osteochondroplasty resulted in the most improvement in three groups.

Several studies have performed virtual resection of cam lesions using 3D finite element models and computer simulations. Alonso-Rasgado et al. [18] reported that, to reduce the risk of femoral neck fracture, the resection depth should be < 10 mm or 1/3 the diameter of the neck, whereas Rothenfluh et al. [19] reported that the depth of the resection should be no more than 20% of the diameter of the femoral neck, and that the resection length should be no more than 20 mm. The main aim of these studies was to use 3D finite element

analysis to measure mechanical strength after virtual osteochondroplasty. Bedi et al. [20] used computer simulation models to examine improvements in ROM after performing virtual cam and pincer resection for FAI. While virtual osteochondroplasty at defined regions of impingement resulted in a significant improvement in both hip flexion and internal rotation angle in the eight FAI cases examined, no patients with borderline DDH were included. Nevertheless, these previous simulation studies using virtual osteochondroplasty showed that computer simulation methods have an important role to play in predicting surgical outcome. We believe that the novelty of the present study is the finding of differences in surgical outcome, i.e., improved ROM after virtual osteochondroplasty, for patients with one of three different conditions: cam-type FAI, borderline DDH, and especially borderline DDH with cam deformity.

Previous studies examined clinical results after hip arthroscopy in cases of DDH [13, 21–23]. Byrd et al. [13] and Jayasekera N et al. [22] reported satisfactory results, even in the presence of dysplasia. Similarly, Fukui et al. [21] reported that arthroscopy of the hip can be successful in young patients with mild to moderate DDH or FAI. However, Uchida et al. [23] reported a clinical failure rate of 32.1% when treating patients with DDH. Ida et al. [7] reported that 40% of patients with DDH showed radiographic evidence of cam deformity, and that significantly more patients in the DDH with cam deformity group than in the DDH alone group had a positive preoperative anterior impingement test. Paliobeis et al. [8] reported that 47% of patients with FAI showed radiographic evidence of dysplasia. Thus, co-existence of borderline DDH with cam deformity appears certain. Based on the results presented herein, cam osteochondroplasty may be an effective treatment for cases of borderline DDH with cam deformity, even if they undergo only slight resection, whereas cases of cam-type FAI should undergo sufficient resection. By contrast, the procedure would appear to be ineffective for those with borderline DDH cases without cam deformity. Thus, it is essential to establish the co-existence of cam deformity, especially in cases of borderline DDH. In actual surgery, the joint capsule must be released to expose femoral head-neck junction to perform cam resection. In that case, the plication of the capsule after cam resection is essential. These procedures are relatively complicated and needs certain invasion. If there is no need to perform the cam resection, capsular release could be minimized. Therefore, it is important to predict whether the cam resection is effective or not preoperatively by virtual osteochondroplasty. While hip arthroscopy for severe DDH cases should be cautious [21, 23], performing the computer simulation of virtual osteochondroplasty may provide the positive reason for the cam resection in borderline DDH with cam deformity cases.

One of the limitations of this study is that we were unsure whether our models of osteochondroplasty were optimized for cam deformity in terms of resection depth, width, and length of the femoral head-neck junction. Several studies reported "reasonable" resection areas for the femoral neck that would minimize the risk of femoral neck fracture; therefore, we were guided by these studies [18, 19]. While the clinical validity of this resection model needs to be considered, it was essential that we used standardized models of osteochondroplasty for computer simulation. Another limitation is that the influence of soft tissues, including the labrum, ligaments, and joint capsule, was not considered in the computer simulation. Further, the clinical important issue is that we could not measure actual clinical outcome after osteochodroplasty in all cases. The relationship between actual clinical outcomes and virtual surgery should be investigated. Regarding this point, we should note that it is impossible to argue the clinical outcomes only by improvement of ROM. However, Kemp et al. [24] reported that greater hip ROM was independently associated with better scores in several clinical outcomes including quality of life. Thus, the improvement of ROM should be one of the positive factors for getting satisfactory clinical outcomes.

Conclusion

In conclusion, virtual osteochondroplasty resulted in a significant improvement in internal rotation angle in cases of borderline DDH with cam deformity but not in cases of borderline DDH without cam deformity. Thus, careful consideration should be given to cam resection in cases of borderline DDH with cam deformity using computer simulation. Further studies are needed to validate the clinical outcome of patients with borderline DDH with cam deformity that undergo osteochondroplasty.

Abbreviations
3D: Three-dimensional; A-P: Antero-posterior; BMI: Body mass index; CE: Center-edge; CIs: Confidence intervals; CT: Computed tomography; DDH: Developmental dysplasia of the hip; DICOM: Digital imaging and communication in medicine; FAI: Femoroacetabular impingement; ROM: Range of motion

Acknowledgments
We thank Dr. Yohei Yukizawa, Dr. Hiroyuki Ike, Dr. Masaki Kawamura, Dr. Yoko Matsuda, and Dr. Takuma Naka for their valuable contributions to the current study.

Funding
There was no funding source.

Authors' contributions
SK performed study design, acquisition of data, analysis and interpretation of data, preparation of manuscript. YI review the paper and revised the draft version. NK performed study design, analysis and interpretation of data, review the paper. HC and TT performed analysis and interpretation of data. TS review and revised final version of manuscript. All authors confirmed to approve of the final manuscript.

Competing interests
The authors declare that they have no competing interests.

References
1. Ganz R, Parvizi J, Beck M, Leunig M, Notzli H, Siebenrock KA. Femoroacetabular impingement: a cause for osteoarthritis of the hip. Clin Orthop Relat Res. 2003;417:112–20.
2. Beall DP, Sweet CF, Martin HD, Lastine CL, Grayson DE, Ly JQ, Fish JR. Imaging findings of femoroacetabular impingement syndrome. Skelet Radiol. 2005;34(11):691–701.
3. Beck M, Kalhor M, Leunig M, Ganz R. Hip morphology influences the pattern of damage to the acetabular cartilage: femoroacetabular impingement as a cause of early osteoarthritis of the hip. J Bone Joint Surg Br. 2005;87(7): 1012–8.
4. Philippon MJ, Maxwell RB, Johnston TL, Schenker M, Briggs KK. Clinical presentation of femoroacetabular impingement. Knee Surg Sports Traumatol Arthrosc. 2007;15(8):1041–7.
5. Jacobsen S, Sonne-Holm S, Soballe K, Gebuhr P, Lund B. Hip dysplasia and osteoarthrosis: a survey of 4151 subjects from the Osteoarthrosis substudy of the Copenhagen City heart study. Acta Orthop. 2005;76(2):149–58.
6. Reijman M, Hazes JM, Pols HA, Koes BW, Bierma-Zeinstra SM. Acetabular dysplasia predicts incident osteoarthritis of the hip: the Rotterdam study. Arthritis Rheum. 2005;52(3):787–93.
7. Ida T, Nakamura Y, Hagio T, Naito M. Prevalence and characteristics of cam-type femoroacetabular deformity in 100 hips with symptomatic acetabular dysplasia: a case control study. J Orthop Surg Res. 2014;9:93. doi: 10.1186/s13018-014-0093-4.
8. Paliobeis CP, Villar RN. The prevalence of dysplasia in femoroacetabular impingement. Hip Int. 2011;21(2):141–5.

9. Hufeland M, Kruger D, Haas NP, Perka C, Schroder JH. Arthroscopic treatment of femoroacetabular impingement shows persistent clinical improvement in the mid-term. Arch Orthop Trauma Surg. 2016;136(5):687–91.

10. Palmer DH, Ganesh V, Comfort T, Tatman P. Midterm outcomes in patients with cam femoroacetabular impingement treated arthroscopically. Arthroscopy. 2012;28(11):1671–81.

11. Domayer SE, Ziebarth K, Chan J, Bixby S, Mamisch TC, Kim YJ. Femoroacetabular cam-type impingement: diagnostic sensitivity and specificity of radiographic views compared to radial MRI. Eur J Radiol. 2011; 80(3):805–10.

12. Lohan DG, Seeger LL, Motamedi K, Hame S, Sayre J. Cam-type femoral-acetabular impingement: is the alpha angle the best MR arthrography has to offer? Skelet Radiol. 2009;38(9):855–62.

13. Byrd JW, Jones KS. Hip arthroscopy in the presence of dysplasia. Arthroscopy. 2003;19(10):1055–60.

14. Notzli HP, Wyss TF, Stoecklin CH, Schmid MR, Treiber K, Hodler J. The contour of the femoral head-neck junction as a predictor for the risk of anterior impingement. J Bone Joint Surg Br. 2002;84(4):556–60.

15. Domb BG, Stake CE, Lindner D, El-Bitar Y, Jackson TJ. Arthroscopic capsular plication and labral preservation in borderline hip dysplasia: two-year clinical outcomes of a surgical approach to a challenging problem. Am J Sports Med. 2013;41(11):2591–8.

16. Kutty S, Schneider P, Faris P, Kiefer G, Frizzell B, Park R, Powell JN. Reliability and predictability of the centre-edge angle in the assessment of pincer femoroacetabular impingement. Int Orthop. 2012;36(3):505–10.

17. Kobayashi N, Inaba Y, Kubota S, Nakamura S, Tezuka T, Yukizawa Y, Choe H, Saito T. The distribution of impingement region in cam-type femoroacetabular impingement and borderline dysplasia of the hip with or without cam deformity: a computer simulation study. Arthroscopy. 2017; 33(2):329–34.

18. Alonso-Rasgado T, Jimenez-Cruz D, Bailey CG, Mandal P, Board T. Changes in the stress in the femoral head neck junction after osteochondroplasty for hip impingement: a finite element study. J Orthop Res. 2012;30(12):1999–2006.

19. Rothenfluh E, Zingg P, Dora C, Snedeker JG, Favre P. Influence of resection geometry on fracture risk in the treatment of femoroacetabular impingement: a finite element study. Am J Sports Med. 2012;40(9):2002–8.

20. Bedi A, Dolan M, Magennis E, Lipman J, Buly R, Kelly BT. Computer-assisted modeling of osseous impingement and resection in femoroacetabular impingement. Arthroscopy 2012;28(2):204-210.

21. Fukui K, Trindade CA, Briggs KK, Philippon MJ. Arthroscopy of the hip for patients with mild to moderate developmental dysplasia of the hip and femoroacetabular impingement: outcomes following hip arthroscopy for treatment of chondrolabral damage. Bone Joint J. 2015;97-b(10):1316–21.

22. Jayasekera N, Aprato A, Villar RN. Hip arthroscopy in the presence of Acetabular dysplasia. Open Orthop J. 2015;9:185–7.

23. Uchida S, Utsunomiya H, Mori T, Taketa T, Nishikino S, Nakamura T, Sakai A. Clinical and radiographic predictors for worsened clinical outcomes after hip arthroscopic Labral preservation and capsular closure in developmental dysplasia of the hip. Am J Sports Med. 2016;44(1):28–38.

24. Kemp JL, Makdissi M, Schache AG, Finch CF, Pritchard MG, Crossley KM. Is quality of life following hip arthroscopy in patients with chondrolabral pathology associated with impairments in hip strength or range of motion? Knee Surg Sports Traumatol Arthrosc. 2015;24(12):3955–61.

4

Open subpectoral biceps tenodesis in patients over 65 does not result in an increased rate of complications

Andreas Voss[1,2*†], Simone Cerciello[3,4†], Jessica DiVenere[1], Olga Solovyova[5], Felix Dyrna[1], John Apostolakos[1], David Lam[1], Mark P. Cote[1], Knut Beitzel[2] and Augustus D. Mazzocca[1]

Abstract

Background: Long head biceps tendon pathology is a common cause of anterior shoulder pain and is often associated with other shoulder conditions, such as rotator cuff tears and osteoarthritis. It is well accepted that older patients are at increased risk for major and minor peri- and postoperative complications.

The purpose of this study is to investigate patients over 65 years old who underwent subpectoral biceps tenodesis and compare the complication rates of this group to those of patients younger than 65 years old. The hypothesis is, that there would be no difference in complication rates and that clinical outcome scores for patients over 65 were satisfying and showed improvements over time.

Methods: There were 337 patients who underwent open subpectoral biceps tenodesis, between January 2005 and June 2015, 23 were identified as being over the age of 65 with a minimum follow up of 12 months. All patients over the age of 65 were evaluated pre- and postoperatively using Simple Shoulder Test (SST), American Shoulder and Elbow Surgeons (ASES), Constant-Murley (CM) and Single Assessment Numeric Evaluation (SANE). Intraoperative and postoperative adverse events (fracture, infection, wound opening, rupture/failure and neurovascular injuries) related to the tenodesis procedure and to the surgery itself were collected from all 337 patients in a routine postoperative follow-up.

Results: The under 65 group (range 27–64 years) at an average follow up (FU) of 30 months (range 12–91 months) showed a 5.4% (17 out of 314) post-operative complication rate related to the subpectoral tenodesis, whereas the group over 65 (range 65–77 years) at an average follow up of 33 months (range 12–79 months) showed an 8.7% (2 out of 23) complication rate.

Conclusion: This study demonstrates that in patients over the age of 65, biceps tenodesis is a successful procedure when performed for biceps tendinopathy and concomitantly with other surgical procedures of the shoulder, and does not result in an increased rate of complications when compared to a group of patients under the age of 65.

Keywords: Shoulder, Subpectoral, Biceps, Tenodesis, Open tenodesis, Over 65

* Correspondence: a.voss@tum.de
†Equal contributors
[1]Department of Orthopaedic Surgery, University of Connecticut Health Center, Farmington, CT, USA
[2]Department of Orthopaedic Sports Medicine, Technical University of Munich, Munich, Germany
Full list of author information is available at the end of the article

Background

Long head biceps tendon (LHB) pathology is a common cause of anterior shoulder pain and is often associated with other shoulder conditions [1–4]. Therefore, biceps tenodesis is a common and well accepted procedure. The main purpose is to restore the physiological shape of the upper limp and to avoid postoperative cramping of the biceps muscle, as a known symptom after tenotomy. According to Giphart et al. [5] there is no significant difference in motion after a tenotomy compared to intact biceps tendon.

It is well accepted that patients over the age of 65 are at increased risk for major and minor peri- and postoperative complications [6–11]. Although there are no studies that correlate the rate of complications in biceps tenodesis to age, based on the above mentioned data, it seems reasonable to infer that this procedure may have a greater rate of complications with increasing age as well. Risks of fracture during drilling and insertion of the interference screw, wound complications, and venous thromboembolic disease are of particular concern.

Though the evidence is mixed a greater incidence of wound infections in older patients has been described in the literature [12–15], as well as several case reports describing proximal humerus fracture during subpectoral biceps tenodesis [16, 17]. Due to the concern regarding increased rates of complications in older patients, some surgeons elect to perform only biceps tenotomies in these patients. The limited evidence in the literature, reports comparable outcomes for biceps tenodesis versus tenotomy [18–23], though studies show that patients treated with tenotomies have greater incidence of postoperative cramping and cosmetic deformity [18–21, 23].

To our knowledge, there is no published literature evaluating the complications and outcomes of biceps tenodesis in patients older than 65. Therefore, the purpose of this study was to retrospectively evaluate prospectively collected clinical outcomes data in patients over 65 years old who underwent subpectoral biceps tenodesis, to report their clinical outcome data and to compare the complication rates to those of patients younger than 65 years old who had the same procedure performed. Our hypothesis is that there would be no difference in adverse events among patients over 65. Furthermore, we hypothesized, that clinical outcome scores were satisfying and showed improvements over time.

Methods

This is a retrospective case series of prospectively collected data of all patients 65 or older who underwent open subpectoral biceps tenodesis with an interference screw fixation, between 2005 and June 2015, in a singles surgeon's practice (n = 380). Patients were identified through an outcome registry query (IRB# IE-13-151-1). Patients undergoing concomitant arthroplasty, resurfacing procedure, or revision procedures were excluded (n.43).

All patients were included in the decision process of the surgical procedure regarding tenotomy vs. tenodesis and the patient made the final decision. Indication for tenodesis in patients over 65 years old include: Chronic atrophic changes in the LHBT, painful and therapy resistant tenosynovitis, symptomatic intra-articular partial tears (>25%) of the LHBT, additional treatment during rotator cuff repair surgery, pulley lesion with biceps instability (subluxation and luxation), SLAP lesion in elderly patients, painful and hyperthrophic LHBT with secondary impingement and subpectoral biceps pain. Contraindications for subpectoral biceps tenodesis were: obesity, diabetes, highly osteoporotic bone, increased cardio vascular morbidity, tumor at the proximal humerus and patient with implants (e.g.: plates and nails). Obesity was defined according to the WHO (BMI ≥ 30). Patients who presented with documented back pain, caused by a fractured or collapsed vertebra, loss of height over time, a bone fracture from standing height or a diagnosed osteoporosis through bone mineral density measurements were not eligible for subpectoral biceps tenodesis.

Outcome measures including the Simple Shoulder Test (SST), American Shoulder and Elbow Surgeons (ASES), Constant-Murley (CM) and Single Assessment Numeric Evaluation (SANE) were prospectively collected preoperatively and postoperatively in all patients over the age of 65, including adverse events and postoperative complications. All patients below 65 have been seen and evaluated on a regular basis to determine if any adverse event or postoperative complications occurred, but complete postoperative outcome data (SST, ASES, CM and SANE) was not obtained for all patients. Adverse events including death, venous thromboembolic disease, intraoperative and/or postoperative fracture, intraoperative nerve or vessel damage, superficial and deep surgical site infections, wound dehiscence, repair failure and large postoperative hematoma. Additional information abstracted from the medical record included indications for primary procedure, e.g. persistent pain and shoulder stiffness.

Surgical technique [24]

After arthroscopic tenotomy of the LHBT, the skin incision is followed by a safe blunt dissection of the pectoralis major tendon until the bicipital groove and the long head of the biceps tendon are exposed. The LHBT is then stitched starting 2 cm from the musculotendinous junction for 2 cm. A guide pin is used to drill a unicortical hole in the ventral aspect of the cortex within the bicipital groove, followed by an 8-mm unicortical reamer. After unicortical drilling an 8-mm tap is used to prepare the cortex. One of the stiches end is then loaded through the biceps tenodesis screwdriver, the other end is left free. An 8-mm screw is deployed along with the tendon into the previously drilled 8 mm hole till the screw is flush with the humeral cortex. The two ends of the suture are then tied over the screw securing the screw in place.

Statistical analysis

Descriptive statistics to characterize the study group were calculated using means and standard deviation or frequency and proportion where appropriate. No power analysis has been performed because this study is a sample of convenience. Difference between the pre- and postoperative outcome scores in patients ≥65 years of age were compared with a paired t test. Rates of adverse events were compared between patients ≥65 and <65 years of age with Fischer's exact test. The alpha level for all comparisons was set at 0.05 using Stata 12 (StataCorp. 2011. Stata Statistical Software: Release 12. College Station, TX: StataCorp LP).

Results

This search resulted in 337 patients of whom 314 patients were included in the under 65 years group and 23 in the over 65 group. The study group consisted of 23 patients (Table 1). The average age at time of surgery was 69.7 years (range 65–77) and the average length of follow-up was 33 months (range 12–79). Biceps tenodesis was associated with a concomitant procedure in all cases (Fig. 1). Two patients (8.7%) had biceps related complications including one biceps tendonitis and one LHB rupture. Three patients (13%) had postoperative complications not strictly related to the tenodesis itself. One developed a wound infection related to the rotator cuff repair, which required arthroscopic irrigation and debridement and antibiotics; the infection resolved, and the patient went on to have no

further sequelae and excellent outcomes. Two patients developed a postoperative adhesive capsulitis, related to rotator cuff repair, which resolved with appropriate physical therapy (Table 2). There were no incidences of death, intraoperative fracture, intraoperative nerve or vessel damage, repair failure, or persistent pain.

In the under 65 cohort ($n = 314$) the average age at the time of surgery was 50 years (range 29–64) and the average FU was 30 months (range 12–91 months). Biceps tenodesis was performed as an isolated procedure in 5 cases or in association with other procedures in 309 cases (see flowchart diagram). Seventeen patients (5.4%) had complications related to the tenodesis itself (hematoma, granuloma, infection, rupture, pain over the tenodesis). Thirty-eight patients (12.1%) had persistent pain (variable location), 48 (15.3%) had complications related to the cuff repair (adhesive capsulitis, weakness, failure), and 12 (3.8%) had various complications (tingling, post traumatic fracture) (Tab. 2). There were no incidences of death, intraoperative fracture, or intraoperative nerve or vessel damage. The difference in complication rates between the under and over 65 years groups was not statistically significant ($p = 0.23$).

Pre- and postoperative outcomes in the older than 65 group were assessed. The mean pre- and postoperative ASES scores were 45.1 (±19.9) and 90.8 (±16.2), respectively. The SST score increased from 5.6 (±3.1) to 10.6 (±2.2), the CM increased from 37.0 (±13.8) to 89.2 (±9.0) and the post-operative SANE score showed good results with a mean of 89.6 (±15.3). All of these improvements were statistically significant ($p < 0.001$).

Discussion

The most important finding of the present study is the comparable specific complication rate of subpectoral tenodesis in patients older (8.7%) and younger (5.4%) than 65 years. The general rate of complications was 21.7% in the over 65 years cohort and 36.6% in the under 65 years group. Moreover, the functional outcomes are encouraging with significant improvement in all examined tools (ASES, SST, CM and SANE). The outcomes are comparable to those reported in recent studies on younger patients with persistent pain having been reported in up to 50% of patients. [25, 26].

These findings are particularly interesting since they may help change the management of biceps pathology in this older cohort of patients. In fact, it is well established that pathology of the LHB either traumatic or degenerative is a common cause of anterior shoulder pain [27], and operative treatment options include tenotomy or tenodesis. Historically biceps tenotomy has been proposed in older patients (over 65 years) or in case of low-demanding activities [20, 28]. This approach had two explanations. From one side the orthopaedic literature highlighted that increasing age, increased the risk of morbidity and

Table 1 Descriptive data of included study population with additional clinical scores for patients over the age of 65

	Over 65 yrs	Under 65 yrs	P value
Number of patients	23	314	
Average age	69.7	50	
Average lenght of FU (months)	33	30	
% of complications related to the tenodesis itself	8.3%	5.4%	ns
% of complications not related to the tenodesis itself	12.5%	31.2%	
Increase in ASES score	45.6	na	$p < 0.001$
Increase in Constant score	52.2	na	$p < 0.001$
Increase in SST	5.0	na	$p < 0.001$

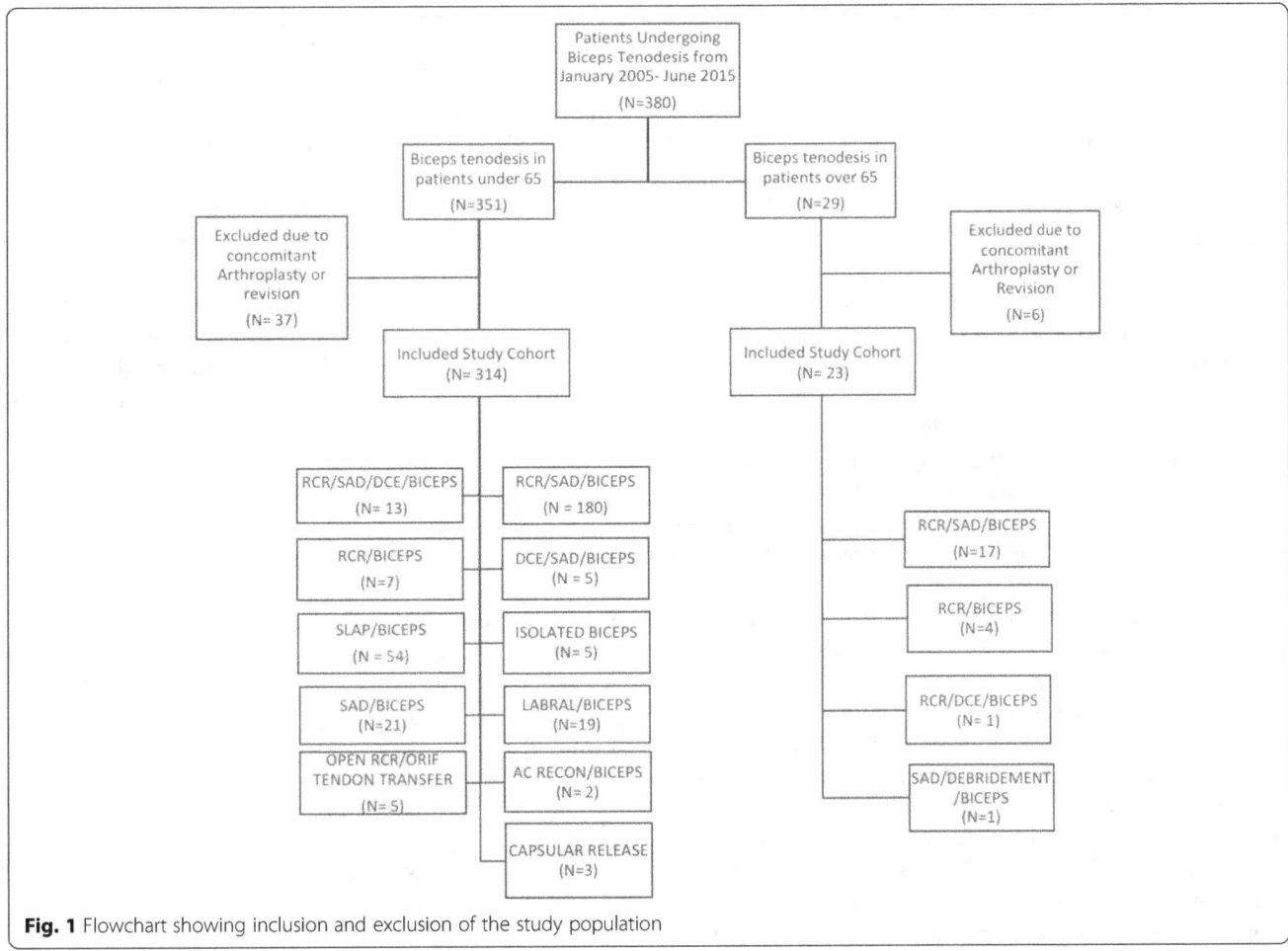

Fig. 1 Flowchart showing inclusion and exclusion of the study population

mortality in operated patients, particularly that of fracture, wound infection, and venous thromboembolic disease [1, 6–15, 29–32]. From the other, it is well established that tenotomy requires reduced immobilization with reduced adverse side effects and postoperative rehabilitation with decreased risk of postoperative stiffness. However, the drawback of this option is the increased incidence of postoperative cramping and poor cosmesis [18–21, 23, 27]. Conversely, tenodesis has been generally performed in younger and more active subjects. Subpectoral fixation has been initially described [33] to reduce the rate of

postoperative pain traditionally associated with arthroscopic techniques [34]. This seems related to the more distal tenodesis site achievable with subpectoral tenodesis [35].

Unfortunately, a variable spectrum of complications has been described including failure or re-rupture of the tendon, hematoma, infection, persistent pain, reaction to a fixation device, nerve injury, cosmetic deformity, and fracture [36, 37]. Humeral fractures have been observed with cortical screws [16, 17] as a consequence of the reduced bone resistance when a hole is drilled [38]. Euler et al. have demonstrated a correlation with laterally eccentric

Table 2 Overview of complications related to the subpectoral tenodesis in both over and under 65 years

	Over 65 yrs			Under 65 yrs		
Patients	23			314		
Complications related to the tenodesis	n.2 (8.7%)	LHB tendonitis	n.1 (4.3%)	n.17 (5.4%)	hematoma, granuloma, infection, rupture, pain over the tenodesis	n.17 (5.4%)
		LHB rupture	n.1 (4.3%)			
Complications not related to the tenodesis	n.3 (13%)	Adhesive capsulitis	n.2 (8.7%)	n.98 (31.2%)	Persistent pain	n.38 (12.1%)
		Wound infection	n.1 (4.3%)		adhesive capsulitis, weakness, failure	n.48 (15.3%)
					tingling, post traumatic fracture	n.12 (3.8%)

screws [39]. This risk is even higher in old patients with reduced bone mineral density (BMD). According to these evidences, the best treatment option of pathologic LHB is still debated, especially in older patients. This study is comparing the complications rates of LHB subpectoral tenodesis with screw fixation in patients with more than 65 years and less than 65 years. In addition, functional outcomes in the over 65 years cohort were reported. All patients had the same surgical technique performed by the same senior surgeon. In addition, although the analysis of the data was retrospective they were prospectively collected by an independent surgeon. The difference in rates of complications strictly related to LHB tenodesis between the two groups (8.7% in the older group vs 5.4% in the younger group was not statistically significant (p = 0.23). This data is however higher than what has been reported by Rios et al. (3%) [40], and Nho et al. (2%) [41]. General complications rate was higher in both groups with the majority of them being persistent pain or complications related to concomitant procedures such as cuff repair (adhesive capsulitis, weakness, failure of the repair. However major adverse effects such as deaths, intraoperative fractures, intraoperative nerve or vessel damage were not observed. The reasonable for his difference might be multifarious and related the accompanied primary surgical rotator cuff repair. Therefore, a greater degree of tendon retraction, the surgical reconstruction of massive cuff tears compared to single tendon ruptures or the general morbidity of the population presented in our department might influence the rate. In addition to complications, clinical outcomes in the older patient group were evaluated. Statistically significant improvement across all outcome measures collected was observed with final ASES being 90.8 ($\pm$16.2), SST score 10.6 ($\pm$2.2) and CM increased 89.6 ($\pm$9.0). In addition, the mean postoperative SANE was 89.9 ($\pm$15.3)., indicating a high level of satisfaction with the outcome of the procedure. These data were similar to those reported in previous series on isolated subpectoral tenodesis [42, 43]. In the series by Mazzocca et al. at an average FU of 29 months, mean Constant-Murley score was 90.2, ASES score was 89.2, SST score 10.6, and SANE score 86.9% [43]. Werner et al. reported similar results at an average FU of 3.3 years with a mean Constant-Murley score of 91.8, ASES score of 88.4, SST score of 10.6, and SANE score of 86.8% [42]. Though many surgeons believe that a patient age over 65 is a contraindication to biceps tenodesis, the present study did not show an increased incidence of complications in this specific patient population whereas confirm the satisfactory outcomes previously reported in younger patients.

Several limitations were identified during the course of this study. Firstly, the retrospective design has inherent limitations due to the inability to randomize the sample and manipulate the independent variable. Secondly there

are unequal sample sizes between the group of interest and the younger age group. This was due to the distribution of the patients see in our clinic and operated on. Thirdly, the cohort of patients over the age of 65 is relatively small. As there are little reports on outcomes and complications in this patient population, we believe that this is a meaningful contribution to the literature. Finally, as the biceps tenodesis procedure was a concomitant procedure in most cases, it is impossible to distinguish the amount of clinical improvement that can be attributed to the biceps procedure. However, we believe that if patients continued to have pain or limitations due to their biceps tendon, it would be reflected in their postoperative clinical outcomes.

Conclusion

This study demonstrates that in patients over the age of 65, biceps tenodesis is a successful procedure when performed for biceps tendinopathy and concomitantly with other surgical procedures of the shoulder, and does not result in an increased rate of complications when compared to a group of patients under the age of 65. In addition, the functional outcomes are comparable to those reported in recent studies on younger cohorts.

Abbreviations

ASES: American shoulder and elbow surgeons; BMD: Bone mineral density; CM: Constant-Murley; FU: Follow up; IRB: Institutional review board; LHB: Long head biceps tendon; SANE: Single assessment numeric evaluation; SST: Simple shoulder test

Acknowledgements

None.

Funding

The University of Connecticut Health Center/UConn Musculoskeletal Institute has received research funding for this study from Arthrex Inc. (Naples. Fl). The company had no influence on study design, data collection, interpretation of the results, or the final manuscript. This work was supported by the German Research Foundation (DFG) and the Technische Universität München within the funding programme Open Access Publishing.

Authors' contributions

AV Principle investigator, data analysis, substantial contributions to the conception or design of the work, SC Substantial contributions to the conception or design of the work, major contribution to discussion. JD Data analysis, patient record management (paper files), OS Data analysis, patient record management (online files), FD Revising the work critically for important intellectual content. JA Data analysis, patient record management (online files), native language corrections. DL Data analysis, patient record management (paper files), MC Independent data analysis to verify the result from principle investigator. KB Revising the work critically for important intellectual content, data analysis. ADM Final approval of the version to be published. The authors attest that the manuscript has been read and a proved by all authors, and each author believes that the manuscript represents honest work. All authors read and approved the final manuscript.

Competing interests

The following authors declare that they have no competing interests: SC, JD, OS, FD, JA, DL, MC. The following authors declare that they have competing interests: AV received finical support from the German Research Foundation (DFG) and the Technische Universität München for publication of this manuscript (processing fee). KB, ADM are consultants for Arthrex Inc., (Naples, Fl, USA), ADM received research funding from Arthrex Inc., (Naples, Fl, USA). None of the authors have non-financial competing interests.

Author details

[1]Department of Orthopaedic Surgery, University of Connecticut Health Center, Farmington, CT, USA. [2]Department of Orthopaedic Sports Medicine, Technical University of Munich, Munich, Germany. [3]Department of Orthopaedic Surgery, Casa di Cura Villa Betania, Rome, Italy. [4]Department of Orthopaedic Surgery, Marrelli Hospital, Crotone, Italy. [5]Department of Orthopaedic Surgery, NYU Hospital for Joint Disesases, New York, NY, USA.

References

1. Della Rocca GJ, Leung KS, Pape HC. Periprosthetic fractures: epidemiology and future projections. J Orthop Trauma. 2(25 Suppl):S66–70.
2. Gill TJ, McIrvin E, Mair SD, Hawkins RJ. Results of biceps tenotomy for treatment of pathology of the long head of the biceps brachii. J Shoulder Elb Surg. 2001;10:247–9.
3. Ide J, Maeda S, Takagi KA. Comparison of arthroscopic and open rotator cuff repair. Arthroscopy. 2005;21:1090–8.
4. Scheibel M, Schroder RJ, Chen J, Bartsch M. Arthroscopic soft tissue tenodesis versus bony fixation anchor tenodesis of the long head of the biceps tendon. Am J Sports Med. 2011;39:1046–52.
5. Giphart JE, Elser F, Dewing CB, Torry MR, Millett PJ. The long head of the biceps tendon has minimal effect on in vivo glenohumeral kinematics: a biplane fluoroscopy study. Am J Sports Med. 2012;40:202–12.
6. Acosta FLJ, McClendon JJ, O'Shaughnessy BA, et al. Morbidity and mortality after spinal deformity surgery in patients 75 years and older: complications and predictive factors. J Neurosurg Spine. 15:667–74.
7. Daubs MD, Lenke LG, Cheh G, Stobbs G, Bridwell KH. Adult spinal deformity surgery: complications and outcomes in patients over age 60. Spine (Phila Pa 1976). 2007;32:2238–44.
8. Easterlin MC, Chang DG, Talamini M, Chang DC. Older age increases short-term surgical complications after primary knee arthroplasty. Clin Orthop Relat Res.
9. Schoenfeld AJ, Carey PA, Cleveland AW 3rd, Bader JO, Bono CM. Patient factors, comorbidities, and surgical characteristics that increase mortality and complication risk after spinal arthrodesis: a prognostic study based on 5,887 patients. Spine J.
10. Schoenfeld AJ, Ochoa LM, Bader JO, Belmont PJJ. Risk factors for immediate postoperative complications and mortality following spine surgery: a study of 3475 patients from the National Surgical Quality Improvement Program. J Bone Joint Surg Am. 93:1577–82.
11. Lindahl H, Malchau H, Oden A, Garellick G. Risk factors for failure after treatment of a periprosthetic fracture of the femur. J Bone Joint Surg Br. 2006;88:26–30.
12. Carroll K, Dowsey M, Choong P, Peel T. Risk factors for superficial wound complications in hip and knee arthroplasty. Clin Microbiol Infect.
13. Dale H, Skramm I, Lower HL, et al. Infection after primary hip arthroplasty: a comparison of 3 Norwegian health registers. Acta Orthop. 82:646–54.
14. Veeravagu A, Patil CG, Lad SP, Boakye M. Risk factors for postoperative spinal wound infections after spinal decompression and fusion surgeries. Spine (Phila Pa 1976). 2009;34:1869–72.
15. Ridgeway S, Wilson J, Charlet A, Kafatos G, Pearson A, Coello R. Infection of the surgical site after arthroplasty of the hip. J Bone Joint Surg Br. 2005;87:844–50.
16. Reiff SN, Nho SJ, Romeo AA. Proximal humerus fracture after keyhole biceps tenodesis. Am J Orthop (Belle Mead NJ). 39:E61–3.
17. Sears BW, Spencer EE, Getz CL. Humeral fracture following subpectoral biceps tenodesis in 2 active, healthy patients. J Shoulder Elb Surg. 20:e7–11.
18. Boileau P, Baque F, Valerio L, Ahrens P, Chuinard C, Trojani C. Isolated arthroscopic biceps tenotomy or tenodesis improves symptoms in patients with massive irreparable rotator cuff tears. J Bone Joint Surg Am. 2007;89:747–57.
19. Delle Rose G, Borroni M, Silvestro A, et al. The long head of biceps as a source of pain in active population: tenotomy or tenodesis? A comparison of 2 case series with isolated lesions. Musculoskelet Surg. 1(96 Suppl):S47–52.
20. Frost A, Zafar MS, Maffulli N. Tenotomy versus tenodesis in the management of pathologic lesions of the tendon of the long head of the biceps brachii. Am J Sports Med. 2009;37:828–33.
21. Hsu AR, Ghodadra NS, Provencher MT, Lewis PB, Bach BR. Biceps tenotomy versus tenodesis: a review of clinical outcomes and biomechanical results. J Shoulder Elb Surg. 20:326–32.
22. Osbahr DC, Diamond AB, Speer KP. The cosmetic appearance of the biceps muscle after long-head tenotomy versus tenodesis. Arthroscopy. 2002;18:483–7.
23. Slenker NR, Lawson K, Ciccotti MG, Dodson CC, Cohen SB. Biceps tenotomy versus tenodesis: clinical outcomes. Arthroscopy. 28:576–82.
24. Voss A, Cerciello S, Yang J, Beitzel K, Cote MP, Mazzocca AD. Open subpectoral Tenodesis of the proximal biceps. Clin Sports Med. 2016;35:137–52.
25. Friedman JL, FitzPatrick JL, Rylander LS, Bennett C, Vidal AF, McCarty EC. Biceps Tenotomy versus Tenodesis in active patients younger than 55 years: is there a difference in strength and outcomes? Orthop J Sports Med. 2015; 3:2325967115570848.
26. Gombera MM, Kahlenberg CA, Nair R, Saltzman MD, Terry MA. All-arthroscopic suprapectoral versus open subpectoral tenodesis of the long head of the biceps brachii. Am J Sports Med. 2015;43:1077–83.
27. Friedman DJ, Dunn JC, Higgins LD, Warner JJ. Proximal biceps tendon: injuries and management. Sports Med Arthrosc Rev. 2008;16:162–9.
28. Slenker NR, Lawson K, Ciccotti MG, Dodson CC, Cohen SB. Biceps tenotomy versus tenodesis: clinical outcomes. Arthroscopy. 2012;28:576–82.
29. Lubbeke A, Roussos C, Barea C, Kohnlein W, Hoffmeyer P. Revision total hip arthroplasty in patients 80 years or older. J Arthroplast. 27:1041–6.
30. Meek RM, Norwood T, Smith R, Brenkel IJ, Howie CR. The risk of peri-prosthetic fracture after primary and revision total hip and knee replacement. J Bone Joint Surg Br. 93:96–101.
31. Singh JA, Jensen MR, Harmsen SW, Lewallen DG. Are gender, comorbidity, and obesity risk factors for postoperative periprosthetic fractures after primary total hip arthroplasty? J Arthroplasty. 28:126-131 e121–122
32. CC W, MK A, SS W, Lin LC. Risk factors for postoperative femoral fracture in cementless hip arthroplasty. J Formos Med Assoc. 1999;98:190–4.
33. Mazzocca AD, Rios CG, Romeo AA, Arciero RA. Subpectoral biceps tenodesis with interference screw fixation. Arthroscopy. 2005;21:896.
34. Lutton DM, Gruson KI, Harrison AK, Gladstone JN, Flatow EL. Where to tenodese the biceps: proximal or distal? Clin Orthop Relat Res. 2011;469:1050–5.
35. Johannsen AM, Macalena JA, Carson EW, Tompkins M. Anatomic and radiographic comparison of arthroscopic suprapectoral and open subpectoral biceps tenodesis sites. Am J Sports Med. 2013;41:2919–24.
36. Mazzocca AD, Bicos J, Santangelo S, Romeo AA, Arciero RA. The biomechanical evaluation of four fixation techniques for proximal biceps tenodesis. Arthroscopy. 2005;21:1296–306.
37. Provencher MT, LeClere LE, Romeo AA. Subpectoral biceps tenodesis. Sports Med Arthrosc Rev. 2008;16:170–6.
38. Ho KW, Gilbody J, Jameson T, Miles AW. The effect of 4 mm bicortical drill hole defect on bone strength in a pig femur model. Arch Orthop Trauma Surg. 2010;130:797–802.
39. Euler SA, Smith SD, Williams BT, Dornan GJ, Millett PJ, Wijdicks CA. Biomechanical analysis of subpectoral biceps tenodesis: effect of screw malpositioning on proximal humeral strength. Am J Sports Med. 2015;43:69–74.
40. Rios D MgF, Horan MP, Millett PJ. Complications following subpectoral biceps tenodesis with interference screw fixation. J Shoulder Elb Surg. 2013;22:e26.
41. Nho SJ, Reiff SN, Verma NN, Slabaugh MA, Mazzocca AD, Romeo AA. Complications associated with subpectoral biceps tenodesis: low rates of incidence following surgery. J Shoulder Elbow Surg. 2010;19:764–8.
42. Werner BC, Evans CL, Holzgrefe RE, et al. Arthroscopic suprapectoral and open subpectoral biceps tenodesis: a comparison of minimum 2-year clinical outcomes. Am J Sports Med. 2014;42:2583–90.
43. Mazzocca AD, Cote MP, Arciero CL, Romeo AA, Arciero RA. Clinical outcomes after subpectoral biceps tenodesis with an interference screw. Am J Sports Med. 2008;36:1922–9.

5

An evaluation of the potential consequences of drilling titanium and tantalum implants during surgery

Paweł Skowronek[1], Paweł Olszewski[1], Wojciech Święszkowski[2], Marcin Sibiński[3], Marek Synder[3] and Michał Polguj[4*] (iD)

Abstract

Background: The aim of the study was to evaluate the potential consequences of drilling titanium alloy (Ti) and tantalum (Ta) implants.

Methods: During an in vitro study, four holes were made in each of two spatially porous trabecular implants: one Ta and the other Ti alloy (Ti-6Al-7Nb). The weight and the volume of particles produced during the drilling were then measured using a Radwag XA 110/2X (USA) laboratory balance.

Results: The loss of mass of the Ti and Ta implants was respectively 1.26 g and 2.48 g, and the volume of free particles was respectively 280 mm^3 and 149 mm^3. The particles were recovered after each stage. Despite the use of 5 μm filters, around 0.6% of the total implant mass from both implants was not recovered after drilling (roughly 2% of the mass of the particles created).

Conclusion: It is technically difficult to make holes in Ti and Ta implants using standard surgical tools, and the process creates a significant amount of metal particles which cannot be removed, despite intensive flushing. This may have a potentially adverse influence on the survival of the implant and result in negative systemic consequences.

Keywords: Hip arthroplasty, Knee arthroplasty, Augments, Revision, Loosening, Drilling

Background

The reconstruction of joints with revision augments is gaining popularity as a method of enabling the replacement of bone tissue through the metal elements, thus allowing osteointegration of the bone tissue with the implant. Currently, orthopaedic surgery employs implants which use various methods of maintaining a porous outer structure; the most common being hydroxyapatite coatings and trabecular metal implants, which have a spatially porous architecture that allows bone tissue to heal within the implant. The most commonly used implants are made from such materials as tantalum or titanium and its alloys [1–9].

At the macroscopic level, various kinds of spatial elements can be used to permit the partial alignment of bone defects. Such elements can be combined with each other and with bone tissue. Most have already been provided with holes for titanium screws to allow primary stabilization. These elements are usually connected to each other using polymethyl methacrylate (PMMA), a bone cement, or they can be joined mechanically using screws [2, 3, 10]. This porous tantalum biomaterial has shown to have very good characteristics for bone ingrowth [10, 11]. Unfortunately, the creation of standardized holes does not always offer full potential stability for the implant in bone tissue; this requires the creation of additional holes in the implant or risks damage to the metal structure of the implant while testing the mechanical stability of two or more metal elements. During procedures performed in our own surgical practice,

* Correspondence: michal.polguj@umed.lodz.pl
[4]Department of Angiology, Medical University of Łódź, ul. Narutowicza 60, 90-136 Łódź, Poland
Full list of author information is available at the end of the article

difficulties have often been encountered in creating stable external augments with standard holes, even with good pre-operative planning. Hence, the question arises whether drilling porous titanium or tantalum augments is safe for the patient and may potentially compromise implant stability.

During the mechanical production of the implant, many small metal particles are created; these may have a significant impact on the survival rate of the implant and its secondary stabilization, hasten its wearing and may loosen the node elements of the tribological endoprosthesis. The release of macroscopic and microscopic particles can also ultimately lead to osteolysis and metalosis of the tissues. In vitro studies have also reported necrotic effects to be associated with the fibroblast [12, 13].

The aim of the study was to evaluate the potential consequences of drilling titanium alloy (Ti) and tantalum (Ta) implants. No similar studies were identified by a review of extant literature.

Methods

This in vitro study used two trabecular implants made from spatially porous materials, one from tantalum, and the second from titanium alloy (Ti-6Al-7Nb) (Zimmer, USA). The tantalum implant has a consistent 3D tantalum structure similar to cancellous bone and up to 80% porosity. Its average pore size is of 440 μm, has low modus of elasticity and a 0.98 coefficient of friction for net shape parts. The titanium implant also has a 3D structure. Its porosity is 67% and strength (extendibility) < 40 MPa [14]. The standard orthopaedic titanium and tantalum samples had a height of 10 mm. In each material sample, four holes were made to the full depth of the twist drill with a diameter of 4.5 mm. (BBrown Aesculap, Germany Tuttlingen). This drill diameter is one of the standard drill diameters used in orthopaedic surgical procedures of the knee.

Before the holes were made, the volume of the individual implants was measured as well as their mass. Initial attempts were made using a standard drill used for bone tissue. A drill press was used to make the holes. Unfortunately, after a 10 min drilling period, with the hole being cooled with 0.9% NaCl aqueous solution, only holes of 2 mm depth were obtained in each implant material, without the possibility of drilling all the way through. Using this technique, more than 200 ml of fluid with metal elements was obtained, which under in vivo conditions, may remain in the bone tissue and surrounding soft tissues.

After changing drill bits for one with a sharp cobalt carbide bit, it was possible to make through-holes in the samples of both implant materials. The use of a bit tipped with carbide cobalt shortened the time to drill each hole to approximately 25 s, and this time was similar for both materials.

Next, the volume and weight of the particles created in the drilling process were measured. During the drilling operation, saline was used to cool the drill bit. After all the holes were created, all material derived from the drilling process was collected. Then, any additional material remaining within the 3D structure of the Ti alloy and Ta implants was collected by further washing with distilled water using an ultrasonic bath. The volume and weight of the individual sizes of the metal particles were obtained by filtration, by running both the saline and distilled water through filter papers with reducing pore sizes. All samples were weighed using Radwag XA 110/2X (USA) laboratory scales with an accuracy of 0.01 mg. The volume of the obtained "fines" was measured by titration using a 10 mm^3 measurement system.

The study had been approved by the Bioethical Committee of the Medical University of Łódź, Poland and followed the rules of the Declaration of Helsinki.

Results

The loss of mass of the implants was measured, as was the volume and size of the particles obtained while drilling the through-holes. The loss of mass of the titanium implant (1.26 g) was approximately half that of tantalum (2.48 g) (Fig. 1). However, the volume of free particles created by the drilling of the titanium implant (280 mm3) was nearly twice that of the tantalum implant (149 mm3) (Fig. 2).

The first evaluation of the proportion of free particles was obtained from the NaCl solution used as a cooling fluid during drilling; both macroscopic and microscopic particles were present in the fluid. In this transfer stage, an ultrasonic system was used with a filter diameter of 200 μm. In total, 67.83% (titanium alloy) and 68.43% (tantalum) of all particles produced as a result of drilling were obtained from the fluid.

The second wash in distilled water using an ultrasonic bath recovered an additional 29.20% of the entire volume of implant particles for titanium alloy and 13.91% for tantalum. In this stage, the filter diameter was

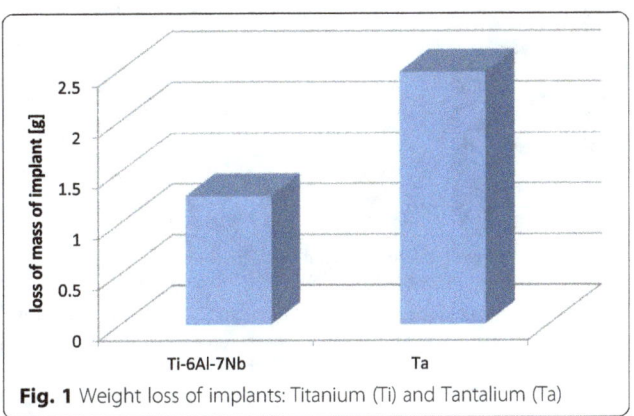

Fig. 1 Weight loss of implants: Titanium (Ti) and Tantalium (Ta)

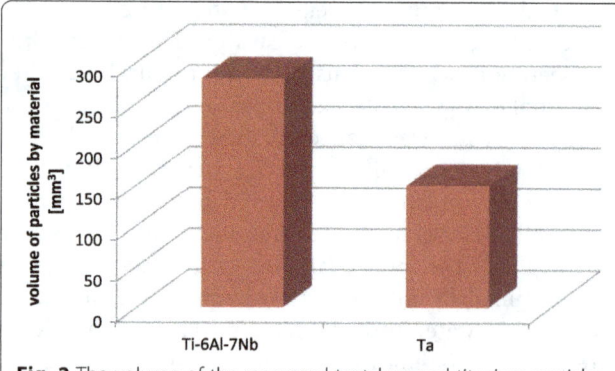

Fig. 2 The volume of the recovered tantalum and titanium particles from drilling the titanium (Ti), and tantalum (Ta) implants

50 μm. Finally, after the implant was cooled, the smallest filter with the diameter of 5 μm was used. An additional 0.4% of total particle volume was obtained from the titanium alloy and 9.32% from the filtrate after rinsing the implant, and 0.56% of the volume of particles of titanium alloy and 6.37% loss in volume of implants for tantalum material particles (Fig. 3). About 0.6% of the entire weight of the implants before drilling (about 2% by weight of the particles created by drilling) was not recovered after drilling, despite the use of 5 μm filters.

Discussion

Highly porous tantalum designs are known to have good mechanical properties and have been shown to exhibit superior stability to traditional cementless acetabular implants [2]. The greater potential for bone and fibrous ingrowth demonstrated by tantalum may be related to its porosity, which is approximately two to three times greater than that of cobalt, chromium or titanium mesh [10, 11]. Those implants have several additional advantages: the modulus of elasticity of porous tantalum is similar to that of subchondral bone, allowing greater

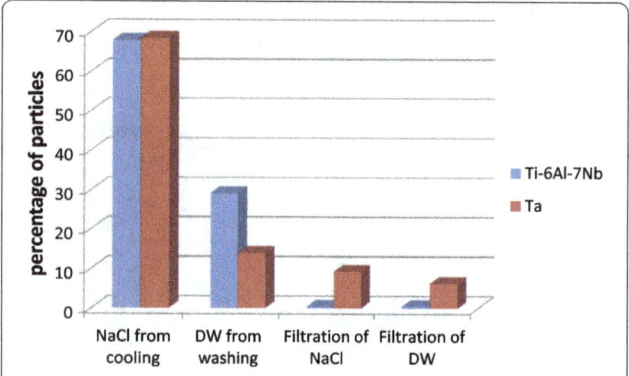

Fig. 3 The percentages of recovered titanium (Ty), and tantalum (Ta) after drilling implants and the use of measurements for the different stages of the recovery of the particles with saline (NaCl) and distilled water (DW)

physiological transfer of load to the host bone; in addition, they are stronger than structural allografts, and have a higher coefficient of friction than traditional cementless designs, resulting in better stability [1–3]. These properties allow these implants to be used in modern orthopaedics in difficult primary and revision hip and knee arthroplasties, foot and ankle surgery or dental implants [4–8]. Trabecular metal implants have also been awarded higher scores in selected arthroplasties than conventional components [9].

The aim of the present study was to identify the potential consequences of drilling holes in Ti alloy and Ta implants. In addition to the difficulties associated with creating holes in the tested implant materials, there is a high risk of leaving particles of implant material in the living tissue. Despite intensive washing under laboratory conditions, it was not possible to remove all the free particles created while drilling the material and avoid damage to the implant. The effectiveness of the removal of metal particles would arguably be much less when performed in the operating room, resulting in even more particles remaining in the tissues of the patient. Twice the volume of particles were left by the titanium alloy implant than the tantalum implant. Also, a greater amount of the smallest particles were left behind when tantalum was used, with an associated greater risk of them entering the blood vessels.

Hence, intraoperative interference with the structure of both tantalum and titanium implants may be detrimental to the patient [12, 13, 15]. It can also shorten the biofunctionality of the prosthesis and lead to systemic effects. Leaving particles of titanium alloy or tantalum behind after drilling can increase the risk of faster wear of the surface polymer or ceramic inserts and the tribological head node of the prosthesis, and can increase the risk of bone disease, especially around the cup, consequently shortening the functional lifetime of the prosthesis [15]. Furthermore, small particles of metal particles including Ti and Ta particles has been shown to cause fibroblast necrosis in in vitro studies [12, 13]. Mostardi et al. found cell death to occur equally for both metals, and that its degree was related to the size and concentration of the particles produced rather than the type of metal tested [13]. Small metal particles can pass through the cell plasma membrane and enter the blood stream mainly by diffusion or endocytosis [16]. Diffusion can occur directly or through membrane channels, and conveys metal nanoparticles measuring 200 nm or smaller, with a preference for those of 50 nm [16, 17]. Larger fragments are taken up by phagocytic processes of specialized cells such as macrophages [18].

An additional problem may be associated with the increase in biotoxicity associated with released particles of niobium, vanadium and aluminum present in the titanium alloy implants. It seems that despite leaving behind a greater mass of metal shavings in the patient, the Ta implants may in fact be less harmful, insofar that they do not subject the patent to any elevated risk of biotoxicity, type I or IV allergy or risk of accumulating rare metals in the CNS [19, 20]. In the case of the titanium implants, twice the number of metal ions remained, particularly vanadium and niobium, which results in a greater risk of negative biological impact. Despite intensive rinsing it was not possible to fully remove the remaining metal particles created while drilling the holes. In the case of tantalum, a greater number of smaller particles were left in the operating field, with a greater risk of absorption into the blood. Regarding the use of tantalum without the use of niobium or aluminum, the toxicity of the remaining tantalum ions should be less than with Ti-Al-Ni or Ti-Al-V alloys [19–21]. Therefore we predict that interoperative drilling in the implant of the structure, particularly those constructed from of alloys of different metals, may have detrimental effects for the patient: it can result in increased chance of nephrotoxicity, ion accumulation in the central nervous system and the possibility of allergy. This mainly applies to alloys with vanadium and niobium [19–21].

In our opinion, it is not recommended that additional holes be created in Ta and Ta augments in everyday surgical practise. It is impossible to remove drilling products by passive and pressure washing in a laboratory setting, and in the operating area it would be not possible even with the use of lavage systems. In addition, it is impossible to drill holes in the implants with standard bone drills, and carbide drill bits that could be used for medical purposes are rarely available in operative surgery: no suitable supplier could be found in our country.

As similar articles could not be found in the literature, it is difficult to compare the results of our study with others. This is intended as a pilot study which will be continued in the future to gain results that will be suitable for statistical analysis.

Conclusions

The creation of openings in Ti alloy and Ta implants is a technically difficult operation when performed using standard surgical tools, and results in the creation of a significant amount of metal particles, which cannot be removed, despite intensive flushing. This may have a potential adverse influence on the survival of the endoprosthesis and have negative systemic consequences.

Abbreviations

PMMA: Polymethyl methacrylate; Ta: Tantalum implant; Ti: Titanium implant

Acknowledgements

The authors thank mgr. Edward Lowczowski, an English native, for his revision of the manuscript.

Funding

Authors have no financial or personal relationship with a third party whose interests could be positively or negatively influenced by the article's content. This research did not receive any specific grant from funding agencies in the public, commercial, or not-for-profit sectors.

Authors' contributions

PS, MŚ - conceived the study and write the manuscript; PS - fund collection; PS, PO, WŚ - participated in the data collection and analyses, MP - helped to draft the manuscript and review of literature; MS, MŚ, MP - participated in manuscript design and coordination; MS - supervision and interpretation of data. All authors have read and approved the final manuscript.

Competing interests

The authors declare that they have no competing interests.

Author details

[1]Clinic of Orthopedic and Traumatology, Regional Hospital and Kochanowski Medical University, Kielce, Poland. [2]Faculty of Materials Science and Engineering, Warsaw University of Technology, Warsaw, Poland. [3]Clinic of Orthopedics and Pediatric Orthopedics, Medical University of Lodz, Lodz, Poland. [4]Department of Angiology, Medical University of Łódź, ul. Narutowicza 60, 90-136 Łódź, Poland.

References

1. Meneghini RM, Ford KS, CH MC, Hahssen AD, Lewallen DG. Bone remodeling around porous metal cementless acetabular components. J Arthroplast. 2010;25:741–7.
2. Meneghini RM, Meyer C, Buckley CA, Hanssen AD, Lewallen DG. Mechanical stability of novel highly porous metal acetabular components in revision total hip arthroplasty. J Arthroplast. 2010;25:337–41.
3. Levine BR, Sporer S, Poggie RA, Delia Valle CJ, Jacobs JJ. Experimental and clinical performance of porous tantalum in orthopedic surgery. Biomaterials. 2006;27:4671–81.
4. Kamada T, Mashima N, Nakashima Y, Imai H, Takeba J, Miura H. Mid-term clinical and radiographic outcomes of porous tantalum modular acetabular components for hip dysplasia. J Arthroplast. 2015;30:607–10.
5. Papadelis EA, Karampinas PK, Kavroudakis E, Vlamis J, Polizois VD, Pneumaticos SG. Isolated Subtalar distraction Arthrodesis using porous tantalum: a pilot study. Foot Ankle Int. 2015; [Epub ahead of print]
6. Papi P, Jamshir S, Brauner E, Di Carlo S, Ceci A, Piccoli L, Pompa G. Clinical evaluation with 18 months follow-up of new PTTM enhanced dental implants in maxillo-facial post-oncological patients. Ann Stomatol (Roma). 2015;5:136–41.
7. Sagherian BH, Claridge RJ. Salvage of failed total ankle replacement using tantalum trabecular metal: case series. Foot Ankle Int. 2015;36:318–24.
8. Boureau F, Putman S, Arnould A, Dereudre G, Migaud H, Pasquier G. Tantalum cones and bone defects in revision total knee arthroplasty. Orthop Traumatol Surg Res. 2015;101:251–5.
9. Fernandez-Fairen M, Hernández-Vaquero D, Murcia A, Torres A, Llopis R. Trabecular metal in total knee arthroplasty associated with higher knee scores: a randomized controlled trial. Clin Orthop Relat Res. 2013;471:3543–53.
10. Bobyn JD, Stackpool GJ, Hacking SA, Tanzer M, Krygier JJ. Characteristics of bone ingrowth and interface mechanics of a new porous tantalum biomaterial. J Bone Joint Surg Br. 1999;81:907–14.
11. Hacking SA, Bobyn JD, Toh K, Tänzer M, Krygier JJ. Fibrous tissue ingrowth and attachment to porous tantalum. J Biomed Mater Res. 2000;52:631–8.

12. Mostardi RA, Pentello A, Kovacik MW, Askew MJ. Prosthetic metals have a variable necrotic threshold in human fibroblasts: an in vitro study. J Biomed Mater Res. 2002;59(4):605–10.

13. Mostardi RA, Meerbaum SO, Kovacik MW, Gradisar IA Jr. Response of human fibroblasts to tantalum and titanium in cell culture. Biomed Sci Instrum. 1997;33:514–8.

14. Grohowski J. Praxis technology: taking the next step in the commercialisation of high performance TiMIM alloys. Powder Injection Moulding International. 2016;10(2):63–9.

15. Lehmann I, Sack U, Lehmann J. Metal ions affecting the immune system. Met Ions Life Sci. 2011;8:157–85.

16. Billi F, Campbell P. Nanotoxicology of metal wear particles in total joint arthroplasty: a review of current concepts. J Appl Biomater Biomech. 2010;8:1–6.

17. Gratton SE, Ropp PA, Pohlhaus PD, Luft JC, Madden VJ, Napier ME, DeSimone JM. The effect of particle design on cellular internalization pathways. Proc Natl Acad Sci U S A. 2008;105(33):11613–8.

18. Papageorgiou I, Yin Z, Ladon D, et al. Genotoxic effects of particles of surgical cobalt chrome alloy on human cells of different age in vitro. Mutat Res. 2007;619:45–58.

19. Madden EF, Fowler BA. Mechanisms of nephrotoxicity from metal combinations: a review. Drug Chem Toxicol. 2000;23(1):1–12.

20. Evrard L, Waroquier D, Parent D. Allergies to dental metals. Titanium: a new allergen. Rev Med Brux. 2010;31(1):44–9.

21. Goutam M, Giriyapura C, Mishra SK, Gupta S. Titanium allergy: a literature review. Indian J Dermatol. 2014;59(6):630.

6

Prevalence of musculoskeletal disorders among school teachers from urban and rural areas in Chuquisaca, Bolivia

María Teresa Solis-Soto[1,2*], Anabel Schön[2], Angel Solis-Soto[3], Manuel Parra[2] and Katja Radon[2]

Abstract

Background: Musculoskeletal disorders (MSD) are important health problems in working populations. The study aimed to determine the prevalence of MSD among school teachers from urban and rural areas in Chuquisaca, Bolivia.

Methods: A cross-sectional study was conducted in 60 randomly selected schools. In total, 1062 teachers were invited to participate (response 58%). The Spanish version of the Standardized Nordic questionnaire was used assessing the 12-months and 7-days prevalence of MSD as well as the 12-months prevalence of work limiting pain. Prevalence were calculated for the different parts of the body; as summary measures, MSD in any part of the body and in ≥3 parts of the body were assessed. Crude and adjusted odds ratios with 95% confidence intervals were calculated using logistic regression models adjusting for age, sex, teaching level and school type.

Results: Prevalence of MSD in any part of the body was 86% during the last 12 months, 63% during the last 7 days and 15% for work limiting pain. MSD was most common in the neck (12-months prevalence 47%) and least common in the wrist/hands (26%). In the adjusted model, teachers working in rural areas presented significantly higher odds than teachers from urban schools for work-limiting pain during the last 12-months considering any part of the body (aOR 2.2; 95% CI 1.1–4.1), and for ≥3 parts of the body (aOR 3.7; 95% CI 1.3–10.6).

Conclusion: The prevalence of MSD is high in School teachers, even more in teachers working in rural areas. It is needed to identify risk factors for MSD in teachers in order to propose appropriate strategies to control and reduce it.

Keywords: Musculoskeletal disorders, Nordic questionnaire, Rural, Schools teachers, Urban

Background

Musculoskeletal disorders (MSD) have been reported as one of the most common and important health problems in working populations, generating social and economic implications [1]. In teachers, prevalence of MSD was found to range between 39% and 95% [2]. In general, they reported more frequently back, neck and upper limbs problems although there have been marked differences between the type of teacher and the body part affected.

Teachers working conditions in rural schools face greater challenges than in urban areas, such as social and geographic isolation, poor working conditions, poor remuneration, limited opportunities for professional improvement, lack of adequate resources, careless buildings, cultural differences and poor community involvement [3, 4]. Additionally educational system in many countries has no adequate strategies to attract and retain competent and qualified teachers [5], impacting on working conditions with greater limitations in rural schools.

Some studies reported that physical factors such as prolonged standing, sitting and uncomfortable posture are known to be associated with increased prevalence of MSD [6]. In addition, several studies suggest that psychosocial factors including high workload and demands,

* Correspondence: maritesolissoto@gmail.com
[1]Universidad San Francisco Xavier de Chuquisaca, Estudiantes, 96 Sucre, Bolivia
[2]Institute for Occupational, Social and Environmental Medicine, Occupational and Environmental Epidemiology & Net Teaching Unit, University Hospital Munich (LMU), Munich. Ziemssenstr. 1, 80336 Munich, Germany
Full list of author information is available at the end of the article

high perceived stress levels, low social support, low job control, low job satisfaction and monotonous work are associated with MSD among school teachers [7]. In this sense, it is possible that teachers in rural areas may be more exposed to develop musculoskeletal disorders.

In Bolivia, teachers and administrative staff working in the educational sector represent the largest public workforce (around 100,000 workers) [8]. According to the World Bank, expenditure of the Bolivian Government on education increased from 5.7% in 1999, to 6.4 in 2012 [9]. Chuquisaca, one of the nine departments (regions) in Bolivia, is located in the south part of the country. It has an estimated population of 616,073 inhabitants from which 50.2% are living in rural areas [10]. Illiteracy rate in Chuquisaca is around 8 to 37%, school attendance between 69 to 89% and coverage for primary education 86.2%, lower than the national coverage (92%) [11]. As in other Latin American countries, educational indicators in Bolivia and in Chuquisaca show big differences between urban and rural areas with lower educational levels and more unfavorable working conditions in rural areas [11–13].

Working and health conditions in Latin-American and especially in Bolivian teachers have been scarcely explored. In the same way, there are few reports exploring health conditions in teachers working in rural areas. Therefore the objectives in our study were to determine the prevalence of musculoskeletal disorders considering the whole body and to compare differences between schools teachers working in rural and urban areas of Chuquisaca, Bolivia.

Methods

A cross-sectional study was conducted in Chuquisaca, Bolivia from August to November 2015.

Participants

The Bolivian educational system is organized in alternative education (adult, permanent and special education) and regular education which includes preschool, primary, secondary and higher education in public, private and semi-public schools (Public using private infrastructure). Teachers working in regular education in Chuquisaca region were the target group for this study comprising a total of 8954 teachers working in 1284 schools (Regional Education Direction Register 2014), 57% of them in rural areas.

In order to sample the teachers, a simple one-stage cluster sampling was performed including all 626 geographically accessible schools with at least 5 teachers. These schools employed about 86% of all teachers in Chuquisaca. Of these, we randomly selected 27 schools located in urban areas and 33 located in rural areas as primary sampling unit and invited all teachers working

in those schools (1062) to participate in the questionnaire study.

Sample size was calculated using StatCalc-EpiInfo. An estimated prevalence for 12-months MSD of 50% was considered. In order to reach a statistical power of 80% to detect differences of 5% in the prevalence of MSD between urban and rural areas, 240 teachers in both urban and rural areas were needed.

Instruments

Validated questions to explore sociodemographic variables and working conditions at school were used from the VI National Survey of Working Conditions and Health (Spain) [14] and from the Working Conditions and Health Teaching Study published by the Regional Office of Education of UNESCO for Latin America and the Caribbean, OREALC/ UNESCO respectively [15]. For the assessment of musculoskeletal disorders the Spanish version of the Standardized Nordic questionnaire was used [16]. It explores the 12-months, 7-days prevalence of musculoskeletal disorders or discomfort in neck, wrist or hands, shoulders, upper and low back, hips or thighs, knees and ankles or feet as well as the 12-months prevalence of work limiting pain in the same body areas. This questionnaire has been reported to be a reliable and valid screening and surveillance tool for musculoskeletal disorders (MSD) [17]. An English version of the questionnaire is available in Additional file 1.

Sociodemographic information included: age (categorized into 4 groups: < 30 years, 30–39, 40–49 and ≥ 50 years), gender (male and female), and school location (rural and urban). Teaching level was grouped in exclusive primary teachers, exclusive secondary teachers and teachers working at primary and secondary level. Type of school was categorized in Public and Private (including public school with private infrastructure) considering the type of school administration where the teacher was working most hours.

To define the outcome, the following definitions were used:

12-months musculoskeletal disorder (MSD): was considered present if self-reported ache, pain or discomfort in neck, wrist or hands, shoulders, upper and low back, hips or thighs, knees and ankles or feet during the last 12 months was reported (Separately for each part of the body)

7-days MSD: was defined as 7-days prevalence of MSD.

12-months work limiting pain was defined as work impediment in the last 12 months prior to survey because of MSD.

Any MSD was considered when the teacher reported 12-months MSD in any part of the body (neck, wrist or hands, shoulders, upper and low back, hips or thighs, knees and ankles or feet) respectively. If no disorder was present in the last 12-months than also no disorder can be present in the last 7 days nor can the pain be work-limiting. The choice of the time frames was determined based in previous studies in order to explore past pain (during the last 12 months) and also current but chronic or recurrent pain (disorder reported during the last 12 months and during the last 7 days) [16, 18].

The number of the parts of the body affected was computed adding up the number of places that were reported with discomfort. The range was between 0 (no body parts affected) to 8 (all body parts affected). The median value of this sum was used as cut off (≥ 3).

Procedure

The selected schools were contacted to explain the research objectives and coordinate visits. For every teacher, every school received an envelope with the questionnaire, information sheet and informed consent form. Two boxes were set up in each school, the first one to deposit the full questionnaire (in a sealed envelope), and the second one to deposit the signed informed consent form. The ID number on the questionnaire was not written on the informed consent form in order to ensure anonymity of the study. Teachers were told to note down their personal ID so that they could withdraw participation at any time.

Data analysis

As quality control a double-entry of data and congruence checking was performed EpiInfo v. 7 for Windows. Data was exported to SPSS v.17 for further analysis.

In order to check for the potential dependence of samples due to the cluster sampling, intraclass correlation coefficients (ICC) were computed to analyze the correlation of responses within the clusters (schools) for each of the outcomes [19]. ICC was less than 0.001 for all definitions of MSD. For that reason the analyses were not adjusted for cluster sampling.

The number of cases and period prevalence of the MSD outcomes were calculated for a general description of the study population comparing the distribution in rural and urban areas. In addition, crude (OR) and adjusted odds ratios (aOR) as well as their corresponding 95% confidence intervals (95%CI) were calculated using bivariate and multivariate logistic regression models. The models were adjusted for sociodemographic and working conditions variables which were statistically significant associated with exposure and outcome (p value ≤0.05) in the bivariate analysis (Table 1).

Results

A total of 620 teachers returned the complete questionnaire reaching response of 58% (57% in urban and 59% in rural schools). For analysis, 103 questionnaires were

Table 1 Description of the study population ($N = 517$)

		Urban n (%)	Rural n (%)	P value*
Age (years)	< 30	25 (11.6)	67 (22.6)	< 0.01
	30–39	49 (22.7)	120 (40.5)	
	40–49	61 (28.2)	65 (22.0)	
	≥ 50	81 (37.5)	44 (14.9)	
Gender	Female	166 (76.5)	201 (68.4)	0.04
	Male	51 (23.5)	93 (31.6)	
Teaching level	Primary	120 (55.6)	124 (42.2)	< 0.01
	Secondary	60 (27.8)	134 (45.6)	
	Primary and secondary	36 (16.7)	36 (12.2)	
Type of school	Public	133 (62.7)	276 (93.2)	< 0.01
	Private	79 (37.3)	20 (6.8)	

Some percentages do not add up to 100% due to rounding
*Chi square Test

excluded because participants were administrative staff ($N = 19$) or did only complete the questionnaire partially ($N = 84$). There were no statistically significant differences in descriptive variables between included and excluded teachers.

In rural areas compared to urban areas, teachers were statistically significantly younger, more likely to be male, to work at the secondary level and to work at a public school (Table 1).

The period prevalence of MSD in any region was 86%, 63% and 15% for the last 12-months, 7-days and 12-months prevalence of work limiting pain respectively and 48%, 26% and 5% for musculoskeletal disorders in three or more parts of the body (Table 2). In general, rural area showed a higher prevalence of MSD although the difference was not statistically significant for all outcome definitions.

The 12-months prevalence of musculoskeletal disorders ranged from 26% for wrist/hands to 47% for neck. Only for neck and knee disorders the prevalence was higher in urban areas. Following the same pattern, 7-day prevalence ranged from 14% for disorders in wrist/hands to 31% for neck disorders. For work limiting pain during last 12-months it ranged from 3% for wrist/hands to 6% for neck (Table 2).

The adjusted logistic regression models basically confirmed the bivariate analyses: teachers working in rural areas reported statistically significantly higher odds than teachers from urban schools for any work limiting musculoskeletal pain during the last 12-months prior to survey (aOR 2.2; 95% CI 1.1–4.1) and for work limiting pain in at least 3 parts of the body (aOR 3.7; 95% CI 1.3–10.6) (Table 3). For specific parts of the body, work-limiting pain in ankles or feet was higher in rural than in urban teachers (aOR 4.4; 95% CI 1.4–13.7). No statistically significant differences were seen for the 12-months nor

Table 2 Prevalence of musculoskeletal disorders (MSD) in school teachers from urban and rural areas in Chuquisaca, Bolivia (N = 517)

N missing = 7	12-months prevalence			7-days prevalence			12-months prevalence of work limiting pain		
	Total n (%)	Urban n (%)	Rural n (%)	Total n (%)	Urban n (%)	Rural n (%)	Total n (%)	Urban n (%)	Rural n (%)
Neck/Upper extremities									
Neck	244 (47.2)	106 (48.2)	138 (46.5)	158 (30.6)	62 (28.2)	96 (32.3)	31 (6.0)	6 (2.7)	25 (8.4)
Shoulders	179 (34.6)	69 (31.4)	110 (37.0)	92 (17.8)	30 (13.6)	62 (20.9)	18 (3.5)	3 (1.4)	15 (5.1)
Wrist/Hands	133 (25.7)	47 (21.4)	86 (29.0)	72 (13.9)	24 (10.9)	48 (16.2)	14 (2.7)	4 (1.8)	10 (3.4)
Any MSD in upper extremities	325 (63.7)	134 (62.0)	191 (65.0)	214 (42.0)	81 (37.5)	133 (45.2)	42 (8.2)	8 (3.7)	34 (11.6)
Back									
Upper back	185 (35.8)	68 (30.9)	117 (39.4)	101 (19.5)	37 (16.8)	64 (21.5)	28 (5.4)	8 (3.6)	20 (6.7)
Low back	171 (33.1)	73 (33.2)	98 (33.0)	110 (21.3)	42 (19.1)	68 (22.9)	27 (5.2)	7 (3.2)	20 (6.7)
Any back disorder	238 (46.7)	95 (44.0)	143 (48.6)	142 (27.8)	56 (25.9)	86 (29.3)	37 (7.3)	10 (4.6)	27 (9.2)
Lower extremities									
Hips/Thighs[a]	165 (31.9)	65 (29.5)	100 (33.7)	101 (19.5)	41 (18.6)	60 (20.2)	19 (3.7)	4 (1.8)	15 (5.1)
Knees[a]	194 (37.5)	86 (39.1)	108 (36.4)	117 (22.6)	46 (20.9)	71 (23.9)	25 (4.8)	8 (3.6)	17 (5.7)
Ankles/Feet[a]	157 (30.4)	51 (23.2)	106 (35.7)	100 (19.3)	36 (16.4)	64 (21.5)	19 (3.7)	5 (2.3)	14 (4.7)
Any disorder in lower extremities	312 (61.2)	127 (58.8)	185 (62.9)	190 (37.3)	78 (36.1)	112 (38.1)	39 (7.6)	10 (4.6)	29 (9.9)
Summary measures: Any part of the body									
Any MSD[b]	442 (85.5)	186 (84.5)	256 (86.2)	328 (63.4)	134 (60.9)	194 (65.3)	77 (14.9)	19 (8.6)	58 (19.5)
MSD in ≥ 3 parts of the body	247 (47.8)	98 (44.5)	149 (50.2)	132 (25.5)	50 (22.7)	82 (27.6)	25 (4.8)	6 (2.7)	19 (6.4)

[a]One or both
[b]MSD in neck, shoulders, wrist, hands, upper or lower back, hips, thighs, knees, ankles or feet

Table 3 Unadjusted and adjusted odds ratios comparing the prevalence of musculoskeletal disorders (MSD) in Bolivian school teachers from urban and rural areas (N = 517)

N missing = 23	12-months prevalence		7-days prevalence		12-months work limiting pain prevalence	
	Crude OR[a] (95% CI)	Adjusted OR[a,b] (95% CI)	Crude OR[a] (95% CI)	Adjusted OR[a,b] (95% CI)	Crude OR[a] (95% CI)	Adjusted OR[a,b] (95% CI)
Neck/Upper extremities						
Neck	0.93 (0.7–1.3)	0.65 (0.4–1.0)	1.22 (0.8–1.8)	0.84 (0.5–1.3)	3.28 (1.3–8.1)	2.59 (0.9–7.5)
Shoulders	1.29 (0.9–1.9)	1.23 (0.8–1.9)	1.67 (1.0–2.7)	1.81 (1.0–3.2)	3.85 (1.1–13.5)	3.59 (0.9–14.8)
Wrist/Hands	1.50 (1.0–2.3)	1.36 (0.8–2.2)	1.58 (0.9–2.7)	1.29 (0.7–2.4)	1.88 (0.6–6.1)	1.83 (0.4–7.5)
Any MSD in upper extremities	1.14 (0.8–1.6)	0.87 (0.6–1.4)	1.38 (1.0–2.0)	1.15 (0.7–1.8)	3.40 (1.5–7.5)	2.51 (1.0–6.3)
Back						
Upper back	1.45 (1.0–2.1)	1.15 (0.7–1.8)	1.36 (0.9–2.1)	1.02 (0.6–1.7)	1.90 (0.8–4.4)	2.26 (0.8–6.1)
Low back	0.99 (0.7–1.4)	0.77 (0.5–1.2)	1.26 (0.8–1.9)	0.77 (0.5–1.3)	2.20 (0.9–5.3)	1.63 (0.6–4.6)
Any back disorder	1.21 (0.8–1.7)	1.08 (0.7–1.6)	1.18 (0.8–1.8)	0.87 (0.5–1.4)	2.08 (1.0–4.4)	2.06 (0.9–4.9)
Lower extremities						
Hips/Thighs (One or both)	1.21 (0.8–1.8)	0.96 (0.6–1.5)	1.11 (0.7–1.7)	0.84 (0.5–1.4)	2.87 (0.9–8.8)	2.64 (0.8–9.2)
Knees (One or both)	0.89 (0.6–1.3)	1.07 (0.7–1.6)	1.19 (0.8–1.8)	1.21 (0.7–2.0)	1.60 (0.7–3.8)	2.04 (0.8–5.3)
Ankles/Feet (One or both)	1.84 (1.2–2.7)	2.25 (1.4–3.6)	1.40 (0.9–2.2)	1.60 (0.9–2.7)	2.13 (0.8–6.0)	4.35 (1.4–13.7)
Any MSD in lower extremities	1.18 (0.8–1.7)	1.27 (0.8–1.9)	1.09 (0.8–1.6)	0.95 (0.6–1.5)	2.25 (1.1–4.7)	2.17 (0.9–5.0)
Summary measures: Any part of the body						
Any MSD	1.14 (0.7–1.9)	1.14 (0.6–2.1)	1.21 (0.8–1.7)	0.96 (0.6–1.5)	2.57 (1.5–4.5)	2.16 (1.1–4.1)
MSD in ≥ 3 body places	1.25 (0.8–1.8)	1.00 (0.7–1.5)	1.30 (0.9–1.9)	0.95 (0.6–1.5)	2.44 (1.0–6.2)	3.69 (1.3–10.6)

[a]Reference category: Urban area (OR = 1)
[b]Adjusted by age, sex, teaching level and school type

the 7-days prevalence of symptoms regardless of body part in these adjusted models.

Discussion

This study aimed to explore self-reported musculoskeletal disorders (MSD) considering 12-months and 7-days prevalence as well as the 12-months prevalence of work limiting pain comparing teachers from urban and rural schools. Prevalence of MSD was high and especially work-limiting pain was more common in teachers employed at rural than in those working in urban schools.

Our results showed considerable prevalence of MSD affecting several parts of the body maybe due to the variety of activities that teachers perform each day at work. Almost half of the participants reported MSD in ≥ 3 parts of the body during the last 12-months and 26% during the last 7-days. It is relatively high if we compare with Brazilian teachers, where 7-days prevalence (≥ 3 parts of the body) was 15.9% in 2011 [20]. This could be explained due to differences in geographic context. Brazilian study comprised metropolitan area with high Municipal Human Development Index (0.717) than the region studied in Bolivia (0.563) [21], and probably working and living conditions are different.

In agreement with previous studies, we found considerable prevalence of disorders reported in the neck and upper extremities but also in back and lower extremities [2]. Although the main focus of the present study is to compare the prevalence of musculoskeletal disorder in urban and rural areas, a major limitation of the study is the lack of inclusion of risk factors that explain these differences. Individual factors, as well as working conditions under which the teachers perform their work could explain the presence of specific musculoskeletal disorders for each region of the body. MSD in neck and upper extremities can be a consequence of the significant use of uncomfortable physical activities, like 'head down' posture, during reading, writing on a blackboard or marking of assignments for several hours [22, 23]; but also back and lower extremities could be affected due to long hours standing while teaching [24], postural overloads in the classroom, uncomfortable back support while seated, recurrent twisting, and prolonged static postures [25]. Additionally teachers face every day social and psychological demands inside and outside the school [26, 27], and have reported less time for rest after work, because of extra work at home [28], which could lead in chronic and disabling musculoskeletal disorders [29]. Little information is available about work limiting pain prevalence in teachers. Our results reported a prevalence around 15% for any musculoskeletal disorder, lower than previously reported. One study in Brazilian public school teachers found a prevalence of work-limiting pain in any part of the body of 47.4% [30], also Converso et al. reported a prevalence of 42.9% suffering moderate to severe limiting musculoskeletal pain in nursery school and kindergarten teachers in Italy [31]; In the same way staff at special schools in Germany reported a prevalence of chronic back pain of 27.6% [32]. This difference could be explained, because those studies explored MSD mainly in teachers from special schools, where physical demands as frequently carrying and lifting heavy loads must be taken into consideration.

This is the first study comparing working and health conditions in teachers working in urban and rural areas in Bolivia. Our study showed higher MSD prevalence in rural areas, especially for work-limiting pain independently to age, sex, teaching level and school type. Living and working conditions in rural areas of Bolivia, represents a great challenge for professionals, especially because limited geographic access, bad road conditions, distancing from the family and poor social support between peers, limited access to technology (including internet), language and cultural issues and poor academic support of parents [4]. Additionally the perceived role of the teacher in the rural areas implies a closer work with the community which could demand more physical and psychological demands in the daily work [33]. This situation often leads to the concentration of professionals in urban areas impacting on the quality of education and increasing inequalities between these two areas [34].

Most of the studies explored musculoskeletal disorders through self-reported questionnaires. Although this could have its limitations, Nordic Questionnaire has shown to be a good screening tool, especially in occupational settings. A study found a sensitivity of 100% and specificity of 88% to detect subjects with chronic or recurring low back pain for this questionnaire [17]. Additionally information about pain or discomfort during the last seven days could provide more reliable information minimizing memory recall bias. In this sense we may assume that this situation is not different in our study because teachers were able to understand these questions through their level of education, and fill it in a reliable way due to the anonymous report in the study.

Even though our study had 58% of response, it is within the expected percentage considering studies which focused in musculoskeletal disorders in schools teachers [2]. Nevertheless it is possible that teachers who did not want to participate in the study were those with greater workload and possibly those who may have presented less muscular disorders. Due to feasible reasons, we had to exclude schools with very difficult geographic access or with very few students, mainly located in the rural area (less than 15% from the total). Working conditions and in particular psychosocial factors at work could be a challenge for teachers working in those schools because perception of social, cultural, and professional isolation reported in teacher working in rural areas [35]. For that reason it is possible that the differences between rural and urban areas could be underestimated in our study.

Conclusions

Although prevalence of musculoskeletal disorders is considerable in school teachers in Chuquisaca, it is within the range reported previously. Teachers working in rural areas reported higher prevalence and more severe symptoms than teachers working in urban areas. It is needed to explore in-depth risk factors related to musculoskeletal disorders in this occupational group in order to propose appropriate strategies to control and reduce it. In the same way, it is important to consider surveillance systems in working conditions which include musculoskeletal disorders in teachers.

Abbreviations

95%CI: 95% Confidence intervals; aOR: Adjusted odds ratio; ICC: Intraclass correlation coefficients; MSD: Musculoskeletal disorders; OR: Odds ratio; OREALC: Regional Bureau of Education for Latin America and the Caribbean; UNESCO: United Nations Educational, Scientific and Cultural Organization

Acknowledgements

The authors would like to express special gratitude to all the study participants for their cooperation and to the Center for International Health of the University Hospital Munich (LMU) for the financial support.

Funding

This study was supported by the Network Funds 2015 through the Center for International Health of the University Hospital Munich (LMU) within the Higher Education Excellence in Development Cooperation (Exceed) program of the German Academic Exchange Service (DAAD) and the Federal Ministry for Economic Cooperation and Development (BMZ) – Germany.

Authors' contributions

MTSS participated in the design of the study, data collection, performed the statistical analysis and wrote the paper. AS and ASS participated in data collection. KR and MP conceived of the study, and participated in its design and coordination and helped to draft the manuscript. All authors revised the manuscript critically for important intellectual content, and approved the final manuscript.

Competing interests

The authors declare that they have no competing interests.

Author details

^{1}Universidad San Francisco Xavier de Chuquisaca, Estudiantes, 96 Sucre, Bolivia. ^{2}Institute for Occupational, Social and Environmental Medicine, Occupational and Environmental Epidemiology & Net Teaching Unit, University Hospital Munich (LMU), Munich. Ziemssenstr. 1, 80336 Munich, Germany. ^{3}Centro de Diagnóstico Neurológico, Urriolagoitia, 354 Sucre, Bolivia.

References

1. Summers K, Jinnett K, Bevan S. Musculoskeletal disorders, workforce health and productivity in the United States. The center for workforced health and performance. London: Lancaster university; 2015.
2. Erick PN, Smith DRA. Systematic review of musculoskeletal disorders among school teachers. BMC Musculoskelet Disord. 2011;12:260.
3. Adedeji SO, Olaniyan O. Improving the conditions of teachers and teaching in rural schools across African countries. Ethiopia: UNESCO-IICBA Addis Ababa; 2011.
4. Villarroel Rosende G, Sánchez SX. Relación familia y escuela: Un estudio comparativo en la ruralidad. Estudios pedagógicos (Valdivia). 2002;(28):123–41.
5. Alcalde DEV. Atraer y retener buenos profesionales en la profesión docente: políticas en Latinoamérica. Revista de Educación. 2006;340:117–40.
6. Mohan V, Justine M, Jagannathan M, Bt Aminudin S, Bt Johari SH. Preliminary study of the patterns and physical risk factors of work-related musculoskeletal disorders among academicians in a higher learning institute. J Orthop Sci. 2015;20(2):410–7.
7. Erick P, Smith D. Musculoskeletal disorder risk factors in the teaching profession: a critical review. OA Musculoskelet Med. 2013;1(3):29.
8. United Nations Educational SaCOU. World data on education - Bolivia. 2010.
9. Bank W. Government expenditure on education, total (% of GDP) [Internet]. 2012 [updated 2016; cited 2017 January, 3]. Available from: http://data. worldbank.org/indicator/SE.XPD.TOTL.GD.ZS.
10. National Institute of Statistics (INE). Population projections by department and municipality, 2012–2020 [Internet]. 2016 [cited 2016 October, 7]. Available from: http://www.ine.gob.bo/.
11. National Institute of Statistics Bolivia. Socioeconomic statistics of the department of Chuquisaca [Internet]. 2011 [cited 2017 January, 8]. Available from: http://www.ine.gob.bo/index.php/prensa/publicaciones.
12. Lopez N, Pereyra A, Sourrouille F. Disparidades urbanas y rurales en América Latina. Algunas de sus implicancias en el acceso a la educación. Buenos Aires, Argentina: United Nations Educational, Scientific and Cultural Organization; 2007.
13. La YM. educación rural en Chuquisaca. Elementos para futuras investigaciones. La Paz, Bolivia: Programa de Investigación Estratégica en Bolivia; 2011.
14. Almodóvar A, Pinilla F. VI National Survey of working conditions (ENCT). España: National Institute of Safety and Health at Work (INSHT; 2007.
15. Robalino M, Körner A. Condiciones de trabajo y salud docente. Estudios de casos en Argentina, Chile, Ecuador, México, Perú y Uruguay. Santiago, Chile: Oficina Regional de Educación de la UNESCO para América Latina y el Caribe, OREALC/UNESCO; 2005.
16. Kuorinka I, Jonsson B, Kilbom A, Vinterberg H, Biering-Sorensen F, Andersson G, et al. Standardised Nordic questionnaires for the analysis of musculoskeletal symptoms. Appl Ergon. 1987;18(3):233–7.
17. Takekawa KS, Goncalves JS, Moriguchi CS, Coury HJ, Sato Tde O. Can a self-administered questionnaire identify workers with chronic or recurring low back pain? Ind Health. 2015;53(4):340–5.
18. Hoy D, Brooks P, Blyth F, Buchbinder R. The epidemiology of low back pain. Best Pract Res Clin Rheumatol. 2010;24(6):769–81.
19. Killip S, Mahfoud Z, Pearce K. What is an intracluster correlation coefficient? Crucial concepts for primary care researchers. Ann Fam Med. 2004;2(3):204–8.
20. de Ceballos AG, Santos GB. Factors associated with musculoskeletal pain among teachers: sociodemographics aspects, general health and well-being at work. Rev Bras Epidemiol. 2015;18(3):702–15.
21. Programa de las Naciones Unidas para el Desarrollo – PNUD. Índice de Desarrollo Humano en los Municipios de Bolivia. Informe Nacional de Desarrollo Humano 2004. La Paz, Bolivia; 2004.
22. Bogaert I, De Martelaer K, Beutels M, De Ridder K, Zinzen E. Posture analysis among Flemish secondary school teachers: difference between the use of chalkboards and electronic school boards during classroom teaching. Ergonomics. 2016;59(11):1487–93.
23. Chiu TT, Lam PK. The prevalence of and risk factors for neck pain and upper limb pain among secondary school teachers in Hong Kong. J Occup Rehabil. 2007;17(1):19–32.
24. Abdulmonem A, Hanan A, Elaf A, Haneen T, Jenan A. The prevalence of musculoskeletal pain & its associated factors among female Saudi school teachers. Pak J Med Sci. 2014;30(6):1191–6.
25. Yue P, Liu F, Li L. Neck/shoulder pain and low back pain among school teachers in China, prevalence and risk factors. BMC Public Health. 2012;12:789.
26. Arvidsson I, Hakansson C, Karlson B, Bjork J, Persson R. Burnout among Swedish school teachers - a cross-sectional analysis. BMC Public Health. 2016;16(1):823.

27. Agai-Demjaha T, Minov J, Stoleski S, Zafirova B. Stress causing factors among teachers in elementary schools and their relationship with demographic and job characteristics. Open Access Maced J Med Sci. 2015;3(3):493–9.

28. Shimizu M, Wada K, Wang G, Kawashima M, Yoshino Y, Sakaguchi H, et al. Factors of working conditions and prolonged fatigue among teachers at public elementary and junior high schools. Ind Health. 2011;49(4):434–42.

29. Vignoli M, Guglielmi D, Balducci C, Bonfiglioli R. Workplace bullying as a risk factor for musculoskeletal disorders: the mediating role of job-related psychological strain. Biomed Res Int. 2015;2015:712642.

30. Fernandes MH, da Rocha VM, Costa-Oliveira d. AG. [factors associated with teachers' osteomuscular symptom prevalence]. Revista de salud publica (Bogota, Colombia). 2009;11(2):256–67.

31. Converso D, Viotti S, Sottimano I, Cascio V, Guidetti G. Work ability, psycho-physical health, burnout, and age among nursery school and kindergarten teachers: a cross-sectional study. La Medicina del lavoro. 2015;106(2):91–108.

32. Claus M, Kimbel R, Spahn D, Dudenhoffer S, Rose DM, Letzel S. Prevalence and influencing factors of chronic back pain among staff at special schools with multiple and severely handicapped children in Germany: results of a cross-sectional study. BMC Musculoskelet Disord. 2014;15:55.

33. Vera Bachmann D, Osses S, Schiefelbein FE. Las Creencias de los profesores rurales: una tarea pendiente para la investigación educativa. Estudios pedagógicos (Valdivia). 2012;38(1):297–310.

34. Blanes J. Bolivia: las áreas metropolitanas en perspectiva de desarrollo regional. EURE (Santiago). 2006;32(95):21–36.

35. Goodpaster KP, Adedokun OA, Weaver GC. Teachers' perceptions of rural STEM teaching: implications for rural teacher retention. Rural Educ. 2012;33(3):9–22.

36. World Health organization. Standards and operational guidance for ethics review of health-related research with human participants. Geneva, Switzerland: WHO Document Production Services; 2011.

7

Impaired contractile function of the supraspinatus in the acute period following a rotator cuff tear

Ana P. Valencia[1,2], Shama R. Iyer[1], Espen E. Spangenburg[3], Mohit N. Gilotra[1] and Richard M. Lovering[1*]

Abstract

Background: Rotator cuff (RTC) tears are a common clinical problem resulting in adverse changes to the muscle, but there is limited information comparing histopathology to contractile function. This study assessed supraspinatus force and susceptibility to injury in the rat model of RTC tear, and compared these functional changes to histopathology of the muscle.

Methods: Unilateral RTC tears were induced in male rats via tenotomy of the supraspinatus and infraspinatus. Maximal tetanic force and susceptibility to injury of the supraspinatus muscle were measured in vivo at day 2 and day 15 after tenotomy. Supraspinatus muscles were weighed and harvested for histologic analysis of the neuromuscular junction (NMJ), intramuscular lipid, and collagen.

Results: Tenotomy resulted in eventual atrophy and weakness. Despite no loss in muscle mass at day 2 there was a 30% reduction in contractile force, and a decrease in NMJ continuity and size. Reduced force persisted at day 15, a time point when muscle atrophy was evident but NMJ morphology was restored. At day 15, torn muscles had decreased collagen-packing density and were also more susceptible to contraction-induced injury.

Conclusion: Muscle size and histopathology are not direct indicators of overall RTC contractile health. Changes in NMJ morphology and collagen organization were associated with changes in contractile function and thus may play a role in response to injury. Although our findings are limited to the acute phase after a RTC tear, the most salient finding is that RTC tenotomy results in increased susceptibility to injury of the supraspinatus.

Keywords: Contractility, Muscle force, Rat, Eccentric injury, Neuromuscular junction, Collagen organization

Background

Rotator cuff (RTC) tears, particularly in the supraspinatus muscle, are a common orthopedic problem resulting in shoulder dysfunction and can result in disability [17, 41, 73, 76]. Despite substantial biologic tendon healing after a RTC repair, persistent problems include high re-tear rates and long-term functional deficits of the muscle-tendon unit that may persist even in the absence of a recurrent tendon tear [6].

In RTC tears, loss of tendon continuity is clearly the initial, paramount problem, but associated changes in the muscle are a major obstacle to full recovery. Large

RTC tears can lead to irreversible muscle atrophy and fatty infiltration, especially in older patients [22, 39]. Muscle weakness can result in gleno-humeral instability and poor shoulder function [29, 70, 72, 78], but it is unclear how RTC tendon tears specifically impact strength of the RTC muscles. Much of the available data has been ascertained from studies on animals, which provide control over many variables (i.e. age, gender, history, etc.) and other advantages, such as a means to use identical injuries to study underlying mechanisms.

Previous work has suggested that the RTC muscles respond differently to injury from muscles in the hind limb [13], and that damaged RTC muscles have fewer satellite cells [31] with decreased proliferative capacity [46], all of which may help explain the poor outcomes observed after RTC tears compared to other muscle-

---
* Correspondence: rlovering@som.umaryland.edu
[1]Department of Orthopaedics, University of Maryland School of Medicine, AHB, Rm 540, 100 Penn St., Baltimore, MD 21201, USA
Full list of author information is available at the end of the article

tendon tears [25, 27, 75]. To the best of our knowledge, susceptibility to eccentric contraction-induced injury of torn RTC muscles has never been assessed, even though eccentric movement of the RTC is necessary for activities of daily living [51], and is recommended for shoulder rehabilitation [12, 32, 33, 80]. The overall aim of this work was to assess contractile function in the rat supraspinatus after a two-tendon RTC tear, and to compare such changes to biological markers such as atrophy, NMJ morphology, lipid content, and fibrosis. A second aim was to assess supraspinatus muscle susceptibility to eccentric injury after RTC tear. Such information on contractility and susceptibility to injury could help with decision making in the period leading up to repair and post-repair rehabilitation.

Methods

All protocols were approved by the University of Maryland Institutional Animal Care & Use Committee. We used male rats (Sprague-Dawley, body weight 242 ± 11 g, Charles River Laboratories, Germantown, MD) at approximately 3 months of age. Rats were randomly assigned to three groups (Control, 2D, or 15D). Twenty rats underwent tenotomy 15 days (15D, $N = 10$) or 2 days (2D, N = 10) prior to muscle testing, and ten rats were used as weight-matched controls (CTRL, N = 10). Rats from each group were tested on the same day. Before each experiment, the animal was anesthetized (~ 4-5% isoflurane in an induction chamber, then ~ 2% isoflurane via a nosecone for maintenance) using a precision vaporizer (cat # 91103, Vet Equip, Inc., Pleasanton, CA). During the procedure, the animal was kept warm by use of a heat lamp. To avoid possible findings in histology, protein analysis, or imaging that might be due to muscle testing and/or eccentric injury, weight-matched rats (CTRL, 2D, and 15D, $N = 6$ each group) that did not undergo contractile testing were used.

Tenotomy

Since the histopathology of the rat supraspinatus better mimics the human condition of RTC tear when the supraspinatus and infraspinatus tendons are cut [24, 36, 43, 61], both of these tendons were surgically released. Unilateral dual tenotomy of the supraspinatus and infraspinatus tendons were performed after induction of anesthesia. After shaving and cleaning the skin, a small longitudinal incision was made over the acromion and deltoid. The deltoid muscle was split to expose the superior aspect of the RTC. The supraspinatus and infraspinatus tendons were transected as distally as possible, both to mimic the typical location of a tear and to provide sufficient tendon for attachment to the load cell for testing at later time points. Incisions were closed using sterile Vicryl 4.0 silk suture (Johnson & Johnson, New

Brunswick, NJ). All animals were monitored until recovery from the inhalation anesthesia, and buprenorpophine was administered (0.05 mg/kg) subcutaneously as needed.

In vivo contractile function and susceptibility to injury

Contractile function of the supraspinatus muscle was measured in vivo as described previously [74]. Briefly, in the anesthetized animal, the scapula was immobilized in a custom designed rig as described previously [74] and the tendon of the supraspinatus muscle was released and attached to a load cell (FT03, Grass Instruments, Warwick, RI & QWLC-8 M, Honeywell, Morris Plains, NJ). The suprascapular nerve was stimulated via subcutaneous needle electrodes (36BTP, Jari Electrode Supply, Gilroy, CA) placed at the suprascapular notch. Single twitches (1 ms, S48 square pulse stimulator, Grass Instruments, West Warwick, RI) were applied at different muscle lengths to determine the optimal length (resting length, L_o). At L_o, a force-frequency plot was obtained by progressively increasing the frequency of pulses during a 200 ms pulse train.

For muscle injury, a custom program on commercial software (Labview version 8.5, National Instruments, Austin, TX) was used to synchronize contractile activation and the onset of forced lengthening. A stepper motor (model T8904, NMB Technologies, Chatsworth, CA) was used to induce muscle lengthening. Injury resulted from 30 forced lengthening contractions superimposed onto maximal isometric contractions spaced 0.5 min apart (CTRL $N = 5$, 2D $N = 4$, and 15D N = 4). The moment arm of the supraspinatus relative to the axis of rotation was ~3.7 mm, a 30° angular displacement represents a strain approximating 15% L_0 of the supraspinatus muscle, which is within the physiological range of supraspinatus lengthening. Maximal isometric force was obtained after 2 min rest and it was compared to the maximal isometric force recorded before injury protocol.

Assessment of NMJ morphology

Supraspinatus muscles were dissected and stored in 4% paraformaldehyde until stained with α-bungarotoxin (α-BTX) conjugated to Alexa-488 (Molecular Probes B13423, Eugene, OR). A total of 80 NMJs were imaged (30 CTRL, 25 2D, 25 15D) and analyzed as described previously [54–56]. Labeling was performed on tissue whole mounts harvested from the mid-belly, the point at which the nerve enters the muscle. Whole mounts were sampled from at least 3 animals in each group. Digital images of NMJs from whole mount tissue preparations were obtained with a Zeiss 510 confocal laser-scanning microscope with pinhole set at 1.0 Airy unit. A maximum intensity flat plane projection was made from Z-stacked images in ImageJ software (NIH) to account for the depth of the NMJ. Only NMJs in a complete *en face* view were selected for analysis. After background was subtracted and noise despeckled, a Gaussian Blur filter with σ = 2.00 was applied. Binary images were then generated from which total area and total perimeter were quantified using tracing tools for the total NMJ endplate. Dispersion index (DI) was calculated as total stained area / total area * 100, describing NMJ density. To quantify continuity and branching of the NMJ, binary images were skeletonized and histograms describing the connectivity for each pixel were generated as previously described [56]. Histogram bins correspond to the number of neighboring pixels for each pixel. One neighbor implies a terminal pixel, two neighbors imply a pixel along a single branch, and 3 or more neighbors indicate that a pixel exists at a branch node. Thus, discontinuities (terminal pixel) or branching (3+ neighbors) may be quantified within the motor endplate [38].

Lipid droplet staining

Muscles (> 3 sections per muscle) were sectioned in the mid-belly at a thickness of 10 μm and were stained with BODIPY-493/503 (Invitrogen, Carlsbad, CA) at 1:200 dilution for 1 hour to identify neutral lipid in muscle (N = 6 per group). Sections were mounted in Vectashield. Sections were visualized using a confocal microscope (Zeiss 510), and fluorescence of ~600 muscle fibers per group was quantified using ImageJ software (NIH, Bethesda, MD) as previously described [48]. Briefly, the integrated density, mean gray value, and area were measured for individual muscle fibers (~100 myofibers per animal), along with several background readings. The fluorescence for each muscle fiber was calculated by the following equation: Integrated density − (area of muscle fiber × mean fluorescence of background readings) × 100.

Western blotting

Samples (N = 4 per group) from the mid-belly of supraspinatus muscles (50 mg) were homogenized in tissue-TEK lysis buffer (Invitrogen), and protein concentration was measured using BCA protein assay (Thermo Fisher Scientific). In a 4–15% gradient gel, 20 μg of protein were loaded, and separated proteins were transferred to a nitrocellulose membrane. Membranes were stained with Ponceau red (Sigma) to confirm successful transfer of protein and equal loading of lanes. Membranes were then blocked in 5% milk and incubated overnight in primary Anti-Ubiquitin antibody (Sigma, cat number U0508) at a 1:500 dilution. Membranes were visualized after incubation with HRP-conjugated goat antibodies and ECL substrate (Thermo Fisher Scientific). Bands

were quantified using ImageJ software and normalized to total protein.

Sirius red staining

Sections were stained for 1 h with Sirius red (0.1% Direct Red saturated in aqueous picric acid, Sigma), and rinsed with acidified water (5% acetic acid). Samples (N = 6 per group) from the mid-belly of the muscle (>3 sections per muscle) were mounted and imaged under brightfield microscopy followed by polarized light microscopy (Nikon). Pictures were taken under the same conditions and exposure time. Birefringent collagen was then analyzed as previously described [65]. Briefly, we determined the number of pixels with 8-bit hue thresholds for red, orange, yellow, and green using ImageJ. The proportion of each hue was calculated by dividing the pixels for each hue to the sum of total colored pixels.

MRI imaging

Small animal in vivo magnetic resonance imaging (MRI) was performed as described [49, 57, 71]. High-resolution dual-echo proton density and T2-weighted rapid acquisition relaxation-enhanced (RARE) MR images (TR/TEeff/ NA, 1500.00 ms/12.94 ms/4) were on a 7 Tesla Bruker Biospec 7 T/30 MR system (Biospec 7 T/30; Bruker Biospin, Billerica, Massachusetts) with a four-channel phased array surface coil. T2-weighted images with and without fat-suppression were acquired for one animal at day 2 and day 15 after tenotomy to evaluate the fat content in supraspinatus muscle. Contralateral shoulder was used as a control. For ex vivo imaging, harvested supraspinatus muscles from each group were fixed in 4% paraformaldehyde, patted dry, and placed in a conical tube with Fluorinert FC-40 solution (Sigma). High-resolution T2-weighted RARE MR images (TR/TEeff/ NA, 2500.00 ms/30 ms/1) with and without fat-suppression were acquired (2.5 h scan).

Statistical analysis

Normality and homogeneity of variance were verified for all data before analysis (SigmaStat, San Rafael, CA). To evaluate potential differences between the three groups a One-Way ANOVA was used. Post-hoc Holm-Sidak test was performed to identify differences compared to the control group. Significance was set at p 0.05 and data are represented as mean ± standard deviation.

Results

Tendon transection resulted in supraspinatus muscle retraction of approximately 5 mm (Fig. 1a) by day 2, or almost 20% of resting muscle length in the rat supraspinatus [74]. There was no further change in muscle shortening over time, but the tendon scarred down by day 15, in such a way that the space between the tendon

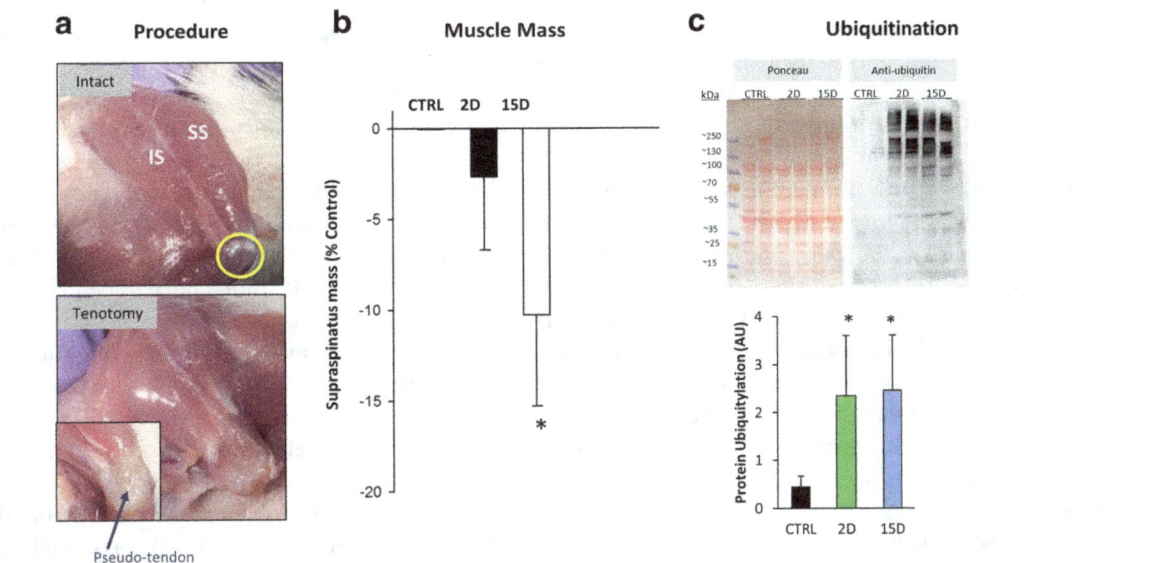

Fig. 1 Supraspinatus tendon in a model of a RTC tear. **a** *Top panel.* Normal anatomy of the rat RTC (used as control) is shown, with the supraspinatus muscle (SS) and infraspinatus muscle (IS), including attachment of their tendons to the greater tubercle of the humerus (yellow circle). RTC tear was surgically induced by tenotomizing the supraspinatus and infraspinatus tendons. *Bottom panel.* After 2 days (2D), the RTC tear results in retraction of the tendons. Fifteen days after RTC tear (15D), the space between the muscle tendon and insertion site is filled by a fibrous-connective tissue (arrow) that reattaches the supraspinatus to the humeral head (inset). **b** As expected, supraspinatus muscle mass was slightly altered after tenotomy and significantly reduced by day 15. **c** Western blot analysis was used to detect ubiquitinated proteins in total protein extracts of supraspinatus muscles. Equal amounts of protein were loaded and confirmed with Ponceau and probed with anti-ubiquitin antibody. Total protein ubiquitination was upregulated at 2 and 15 days after tenotomy in supraspinatus muscle compared to control (CTRL). All data are presented as mean ± SD, $p < 0.05$. *, indicates statistical significance compared to control

and insertion site was filled by a fibrous-connective tissue, forming an ill-defined "pseudo-tendon" that reattaches the muscle to the humeral head (Fig. 1a, inset) [4, 77]. As expected and shown by others [23, 43, 77], there was a loss of muscle mass 15 days after supraspinatus tenotomy ($P = 0.04$ Fig. 1b). The progressive decrease in muscle mass after tenotomy was preceded by increased conjugation of ubiquitin to muscle proteins in total cell lysate from muscles at day 2 ($P = 0.01$); and remained elevated at day 15 ($P = 0.01$;

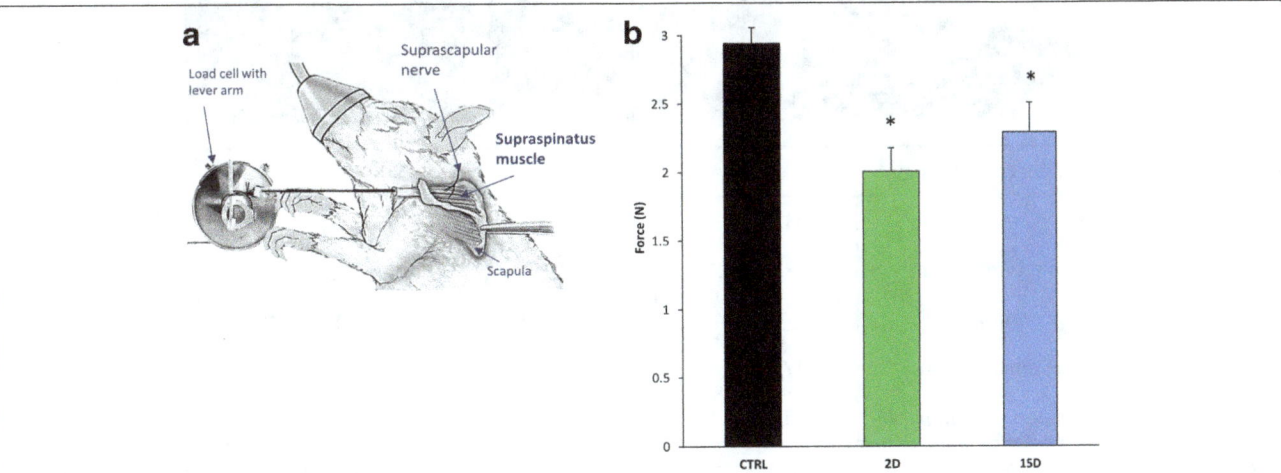

Fig. 2 Maximal isometric force is lower in tenotomized supraspinatus at 2D and 15D. **a** Apparatus to measure muscle in vivo contractility and susceptibility to injury in the supraspinatus muscle. The insertion of the supraspinatus was released and the tendon tied to a load cell. The suprascapular nerve was stimulated via subcutaneous needle electrodes to activate the supraspinatus maximally. A series of maximal twitches was used to determine optimal length (L_o) and the force-frequency relationship was determined to obtain maximal isometric force. **b** When compared to control, the mean of maximal isometric force per group was 30% lower at 2D and 20% lower at 15D. Maximal force was not different between the tenotomized groups. All data are presented as mean ± SD, $p < 0.05$. *, indicates statistical significance compared to control

Fig. 1c), suggesting higher protein degradation via the ubiquitin-proteasome pathway [8].

By day 15, there was a 10% decrease in muscle mass and a 20% reduction in muscle force compared to control ($P = 0.007$; Fig. 2, blue bar). However, at day 2 there was a 30% decline in isometric force ($P = 0.0002$; Fig. 2, green bar) despite no significant loss in muscle mass ($P = 0.31$; Fig. 1b). Our findings suggest that mechanisms beyond simple atrophy influence contractile force 2 days after tenotomy. Since there is a strong structure-function relationship for the NMJ, and its disruption likely results in altered excitation-contraction coupling [54], i.e. muscle activation, we assessed NMJ morphology. At the 2-day time point, NMJs exhibited significant reductions in area, perimeter, and altered continuity, compared to the control ($P = 0.007$) and 15-day group ($P = 0.004$; Fig. 3).

We have used small animal magnetic resonance imaging (MRI) previously to assess the overall structure of hindlimb muscles [44, 45, 49, 53, 57, 79]. Here, we applied this modality in vivo and ex vivo to detect fat in the supraspinatus muscle. We compared T2-weighted images with fat-suppression to T2-weighted images without fat-suppression. Although the technique was effective to visualize subcutaneous fat (Fig. 4a, red arrows), *intramuscular* fat was not detected at any time point after RTC tear (not all time points shown). This was consistent with absence of any increases in intramyocellular lipid content with histological staining ($P = 0.602$; Fig. 4b-c).

There are conflicting results regarding fibrosis in the rat supraspinatus after RTC tear, with some investigators reporting fibrosis [23, 43] while others do not [62, 68]. We did not find an increase in the percent area of interstitial collagen staining ($P = 0.492$; Fig. 5a). However, based on the birefringent properties of collagen stained with Picosirius red under polarized light [1, 50, 65] (see Methods), there was a change in collagen organization at day 15. Collagen birefringence in control muscles had a greater proportion of pixels closer to the red spectrum ($P = 0.007$; Fig. 5b) when analyzed as a proportion of total colored pixels. However, supraspinatus muscles at 15D had a greater proportion of yellow and green pixels compared to control ($P = 0.017$, $P = 0.007$) indicating altered collagen organization (i.e. reduced collagen packing density, thin collagen) [65]. No differences were evident at 2D compared to control.

The screenshot in Fig. 6a shows an example of a lengthening contraction of the supraspinatus (closed arrow) superimposed onto a maximal isometric contraction (open arrow). We used a protocol of 30 eccentric contractions to the supraspinatus to induce injury and examined the loss in maximal isometric force. Fig. 6b illustrates the loss in isometric force after each eccentric

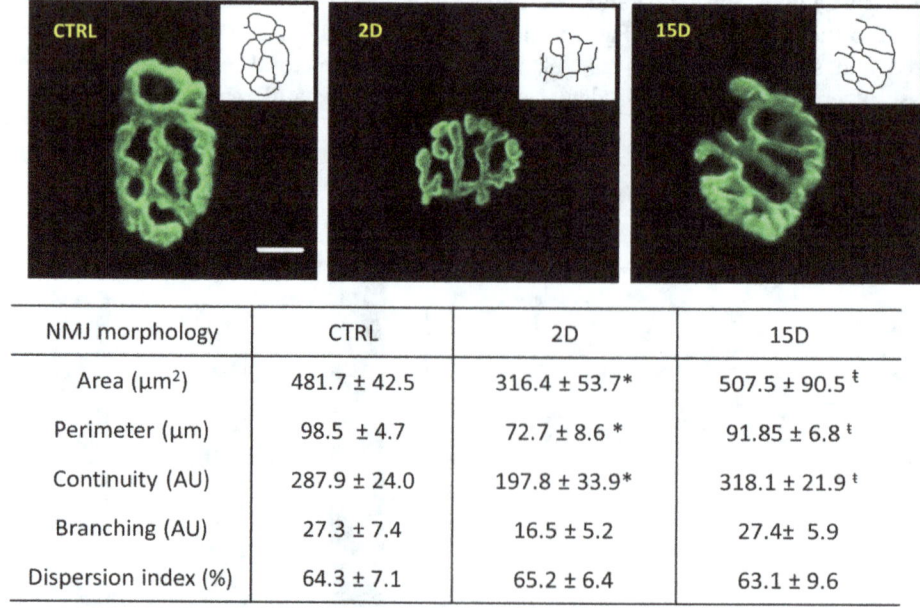

NMJ morphology	CTRL	2D	15D
Area (μm^2)	481.7 ± 42.5	316.4 ± 53.7*	507.5 ± 90.5 ^{t}
Perimeter (μm)	98.5 ± 4.7	72.7 ± 8.6 *	91.85 ± 6.8 ^{t}
Continuity (AU)	287.9 ± 24.0	197.8 ± 33.9*	318.1 ± 21.9 ^{t}
Branching (AU)	27.3 ± 7.4	16.5 ± 5.2	27.4± 5.9
Dispersion index (%)	64.3 ± 7.1	65.2 ± 6.4	63.1 ± 9.6

Fig. 3 NMJ morphology is altered in tenotomized supraspinatus at 2D, but recovers at 15D. Neuromuscular junctions (NMJs) of at least three supraspinatus muscles per group were fluorescently stained with an acetylcholine receptor binding neurotoxin (α-Bungarotoxin, BTX, green) and imaged using confocal microscopy. Z-stacked images were analyzed and quantified using ImageJ software. Skeletonized images are shown in the white panel for each NMJ to further illustrate continuity and branching of NMJs. At 2D, NMJs were smaller and morphology was altered, as evidenced by decreased continuity of NMJ branches. No significant differences were seen in NMJ morphology compared to control at 15D. Scale bar represents 10 μm. All data are presented as mean ± SD, $p < 0.05$. *, indicates statistical significance compared to control, and t indicates statistical significance compared to 2D

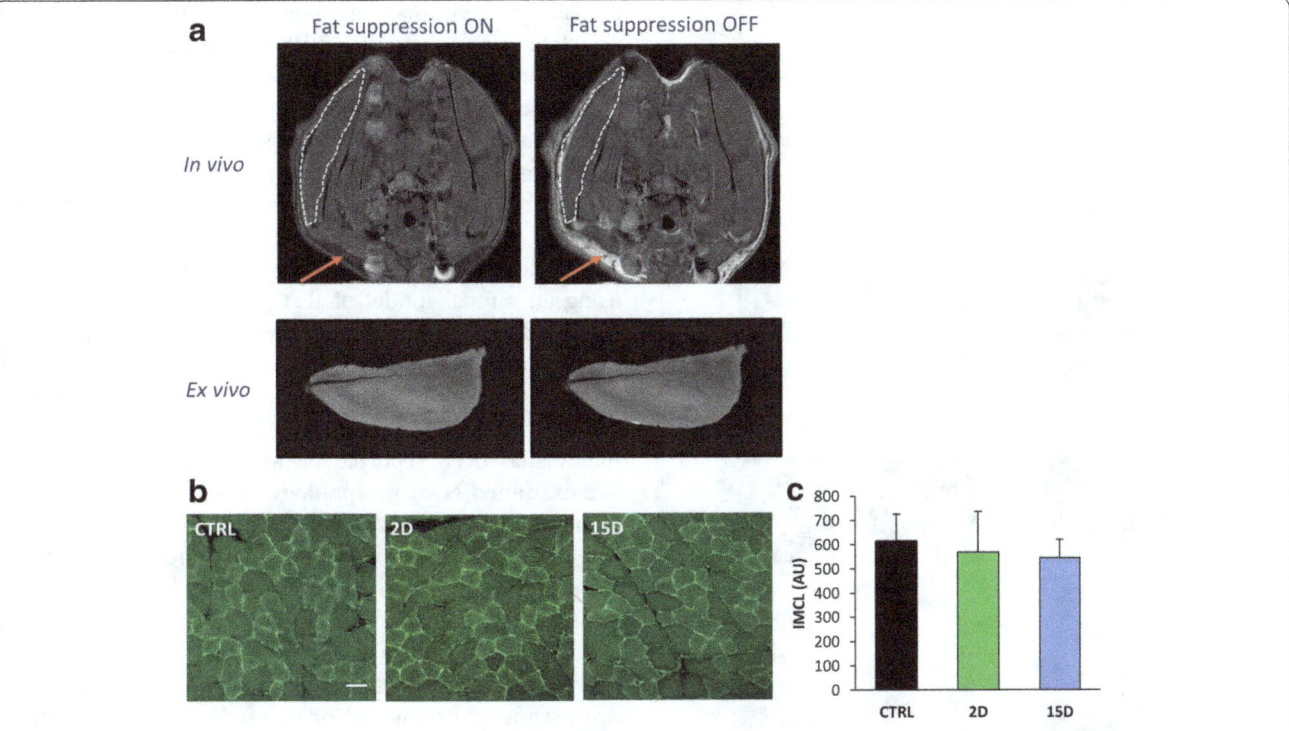

Fig. 4 Lipid content is not altered in tenotomized supraspinatus at 2D or 15D. **a** Axial sections of in vivo magnetic resonance imaging (MRI) of a rat 15 days after unilateral RTC tear. When fat suppression is turned off, the white signal represents fat (note the obvious white signal from subcutaneous fat, red arrow). Fat was not detected in any axial sections in the torn supraspinatus (outlined by white dotted line). A longer (> 2 h), more detailed MRI scan of supraspinatus muscles ex vivo corroborated this finding. **b** Neutral lipids were stained in cross-sections from the mid-belly of the supraspinatus using Bodipy-493/503 and quantified (**c**) using ImageJ. No differences in intramyocellular lipid at 2D and 15D were found compared to controls. Scale bar represents 50 μm. All data are presented as mean ± SD, $p < 0.05$

contraction for a representative animal from each group. Supraspinatus muscles at 15D were more susceptible to injury evidenced by a greater drop in isometric force followed by a short recovery period after injury ($P = 0.009$; Fig. 6c). Absolute force before and after injury was 2.47 N ± 0.80 and 1.41 N ± 0.42 for control, 2.11 N ± 1.11 and 1.16 ± 0.59 for 2D, and 2.22 N ± 0.69 and 1.06 N ± 0.23 for 15D respectively.

Discussion

RTC tears result in measurable histological changes to the RTC muscles [43, 61] but none of these indirect biological markers can account for the changes in contractile function [26, 66, 67]. Muscle contractile function is therefore considered the most valid and comprehensive measure of muscle health [10]. Our findings suggest that muscles become weaker and susceptible to injury after a simple tenotomy, even without direct trauma to the muscle fibers.

Given the high rate of poor outcomes after shoulder surgery, understanding the mechanisms leading to insufficient function is critical to develop effective treatments. Similar to other studies, we found a significant loss in muscle mass of RTC muscles 2 weeks following RTC

tear [34, 42, 77]. While the ubiquitin-proteasome pathway is the main protein degradation pathway of skeletal muscle, previous studies show no changes in expression of key ubiquitin ligases, e.g. muscle RING-finger protein-1 (MuRF)1 and muscle atrophy F-box (MAFbx), after RTC tear [23, 42], as their expression can be transient as atrophy progresses [16]. Given our finding of acute increased protein ubiquitination (a downstream process of ubiquitin ligase expression) preceding significant loss in supraspinatus mass after tenotomy, the ubiquitin-proteasome system may play a more significant role in muscle atrophy induced by RTC tear than previously suggested [23, 34]. It is possible for ubiquitin ligases to be more active during the acute phase of injury, rather than later time points. Furthermore, additional ubiquitin ligases have been identified to regulate muscle mass [7] that have not been assessed in torn RTC muscles. We cannot rule out the possibility that the lack of changes in muscle mass at 2D was due to swelling, as inflammation and water content were not analyzed.

Although muscle atrophy could be a contributing factor to the decrease in contractile function, the initial drop in contractile force was evident before a significant

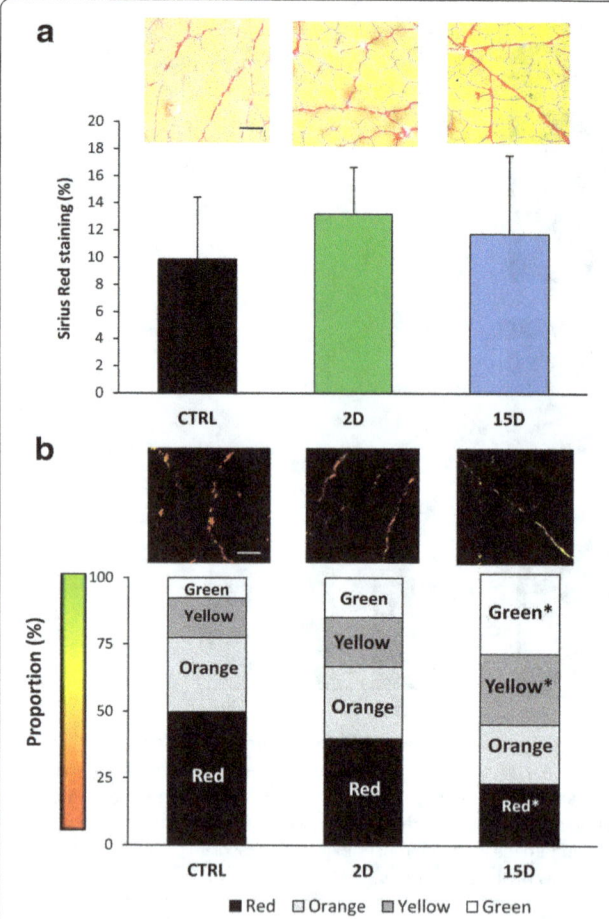

Fig. 5 Collagen organization is altered in tenotomized supraspinatus at 15D. **a** Representative images from the mid-belly of muscle cross-sections stained with Picosirius red viewed under brightfield microscopy. Collagen content was visualized using Picosirius red staining, and quantified using a threshold on ImageJ to calculate the percentage of pixels stained per area. No differences in total collagen content are evident between groups. **b** Collagen organization was assessed using Picosirius red-stained sections viewed under polarized light. Red represents more densely packed collagen that is perpendicular to muscle fibers, and green represents loosely packed collagen that is parallel to the fibers. When analyzed as a proportion to total colored pixels, supraspinatus muscle at 15D has a lower proportion of red pixels and greater proportion of yellow and green pixels compared to control, indicating altered collagen organization (decreased collagen density, crosslinking, and thickness) at 15D after tear. No differences were evident at 2D compared to control. Scale bar represents 50 μm. All data are presented as mean ± SD, $p < 0.05$. *, indicates statistical significance compared to control

biopsies in the human supraspinatus [20], which classified acetylcholine receptor (AChR) staining along a range of morphologies (singlet dot, a doublet, a cluster, or a line) and concluded "the trend in innervation status is interpreted as leaving open the possibility that denervation plays a role in RTC injury pathophysiology" [20]. Here, we rigorously examined the NMJ using established methods [54–56] to provide precise, quantifiable measures of morphology. Others have reported no changes in the NMJ using an animal model of RTC tear [19], but that study was conducted in different species (rabbit) and only examined at one time point late after injury (3 months). It is possible that assessing the NMJ at such a late time point accounts for those negative findings, as turnover of AChRs has been reported on a timeline of days [3, 69]. We examined NMJ morphology after tenotomy at a time point when changes at the NMJ occur after injury [55, 63] and found changes during the period when muscle atrophy could not explain the loss in muscle force. We did not examine the nerve axon (i.e., the suprascapular nerve). With retraction of the severed muscles, the suprascapular nerve can be exposed to excessive tension at the suprascapular notch and/or spinoglenoid notch [64]. In animal models, the suprascapular nerve is sometimes cut intentionally, as the outcome from a simultaneous neurotomy-tenotomy better mimics fatty atrophy seen in patients. However, the severity of neurotomy does not allow for study of recovery of muscle contractile function after a tendon tear, and thus was not used in this study. It is possible that neither the nerve nor the NMJ are responsible for the loss in force at 2D as other possible explanations, such as disruption of contractile proteins, are not ruled out.

Fatty infiltration of muscles in patients with RTC tear involves the presence of adipocytes within the muscle (also known as intramuscular adipose tissue). Our findings agree with several studies showing that fatty infiltration after RTC tear is not substantial in the rat [43] compared to the levels seen in humans [5] or rabbits [60] after RTC tear. In addition to the formation of adipocytes in muscles, skeletal muscle fibers have the ability to store lipid in the form of small lipid droplets [9, 58]. While myofibers from patients with RTC tear also have an increase intramyocellular lipid [68], intramyocellular lipid did not increase after RTC tear in our rat model.

The extracellular matrix (ECM) contributes to muscle structure, transduction of mechanical force, remodeling, passive loading, and elasticity [40, 52], but excess accumulation of ECM in muscle (fibrosis) is common in pathological conditions [21, 40]. Fibrosis is evident after RTC tear in some studies [23, 43], but not others [62, 68]. Mechanical properties of tissue are not only affected by the amount of ECM, but also by the organization of ECM components, particularly collagen [2]. Collagen *content*

decrease in muscle mass, paralleling the transient change of NMJ morphology. The NMJ has been implicated as a possible contributing factor to loss of contractile force [19, 20, 47, 59], and the notion of NMJ morphology changing after muscle mechanical strain is not new, but this is one of the very few studies to examine the NMJ after RTC tear. The gross morphology of NMJs has been examined qualitatively in a small sample of

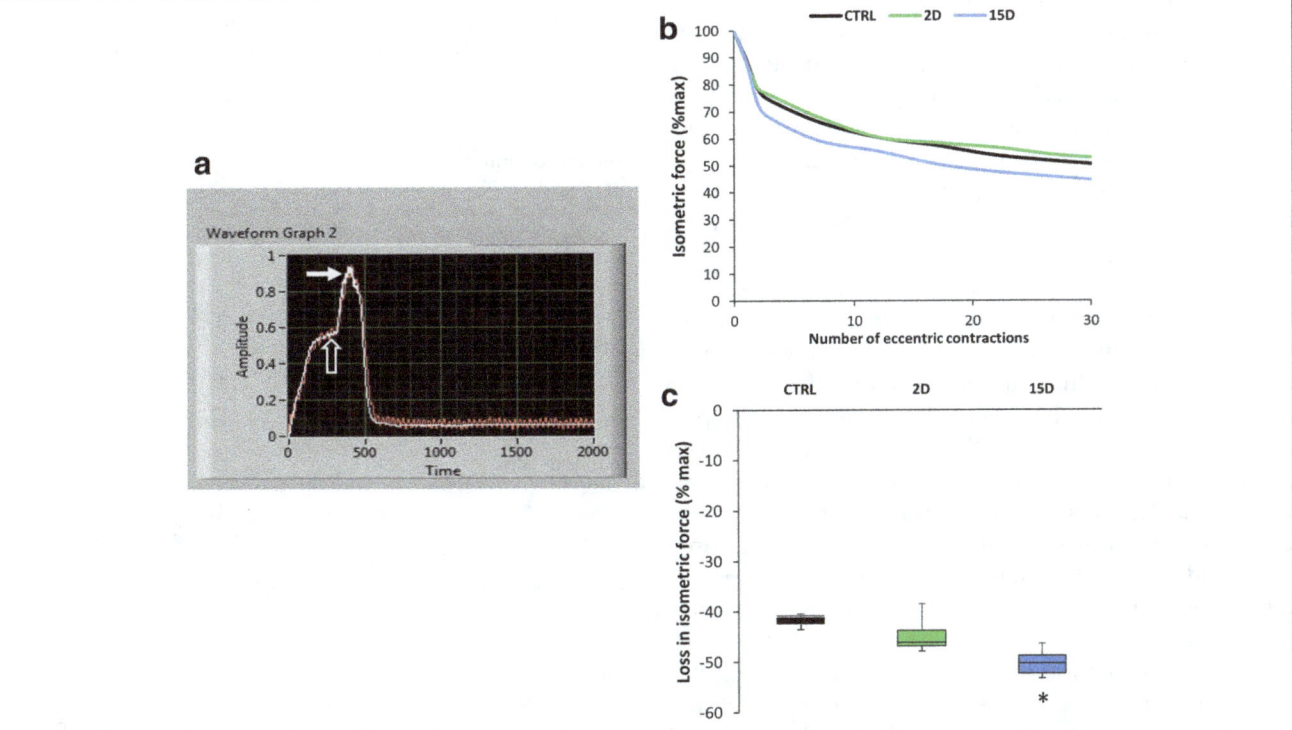

Fig. 6 Tenotomized supraspinatus becomes more susceptible to injury at 15D but not at 2D. The same apparatus used to collect isometric force (Fig. 2) was also used to induce injury. The suprascapular nerve is used to stimulate the supraspinatus maximally while movement of the lever arm resulted in forced linear lengthening of the muscle (15% L_o). **a** Representative screen shot showing force from a single eccentric contraction (closed arrow) superimposed onto a maximal isometric contraction (open arrow; y-axis in volts, which is converted to units of force based on calibration). **b** Representative rep-by-rep isometric force loss for one animal in each group throughout eccentric contraction protocol. **c** The mean loss of force for each group after the injury protocol. Despite an identical injury protocol, there is a greater drop in isometric force after injury at 15D (51.8 ± 2.5%) compared to control. All data are presented as mean ± SD, $p < 0.05$. *, indicates statistical significance compared to control

has been measured after a RTC model in animals, but collagen *organization* has not. Genes involved in collagen turnover (i.e. matrix metalloproteinase and tissue inhibitor metalloproteinase) have an impact on collagen organization, and are upregulated in a rat model of RTC tear [14]. Using the birefringent properties of collagen stained with Picosirious red, we determined that collagen organization was altered 15 days after RTC tear [28, 65]. Decreased crosslinking of collagen is associated with increased collagen turnover, and increased crosslinking could contribute to muscle stiffness, both affecting the mechanical function of the muscle [2]. Although we do not show causality, we found altered collagen organization in the supraspinatus when it was also most susceptible to injury by eccentric contractions.

Eccentric injury commonly induces muscle inflammation and fibrosis, so the repair of a muscle that is apparently healthy, but susceptible to injury, could compound the dysfunction already induced by the RTC tear alone. For instance, one group found that muscle fibers become injured at the time of surgical tendon repair in a rat model of chronic RTC tear [15]. Although, it is currently unknown if susceptibility to injury is preventable,

knowing the timeline of when the muscle is most susceptible to injury could help with decision making for optimal timing for repair, repair tension, and post-operative rehabilitation. It is possible that metabolic changes in the muscle come into play with an injury protocol, however allowing sufficient time between contractions after the protocol should have ruled out muscle fatigue alone as a factor.

A limitation in the rat in this study that prevented us from assessing contractile force at later time points is the spontaneous reattachment to the humerus via a pseudo-tendon. This means our findings are also limited to an acute period after tenotomy. While some investigators make no mention of adhesions or reattachment of the cut rotator cuff tendons in a rat model [24], others report that re-attachment of the supraspinatus tendon occurs spontaneously after tendon transection in rats at time points exceeding 2 weeks [4, 11, 77]. Spontaneous reattachment of the supraspinatus tendon is associated with recovery of muscle mass and collagen content [4, 77]. Efforts to avoid reattachment include removing the distal fragment of tendon [30, 43] or using a membrane [18, 24] to prevent spontaneous reattachment, while other studies make no mention of these deterrents [23, 24, 35–37]. We initially tried using membrane and even a polymer gel (not shown) after tenotomy to prevent spontaneous tendon reattachment. Such methods not only failed to prevent the tendon from scarring down, but also resulted in massive inflammation and an increase of variability in the data. Our experience suggests that removal of the tendon is likely to yield a result that best mimics the human condition of a RTC tear.

Additional limitations include the lack of sham surgery (skin incision and deltoid muscle split, but RTC remains preserved) and the limited window of follow-up mentioned above, making our results more relevant to the acute period after a RTC tear. The birefringent properties of collagen stained with Picosirius red has been previously used to assess collagen organization, but this indirect method is another potential limitation. Finally, the ubiquitin proteasome pathway needs to be more fully studied to determine which ubiquitin ligases are responsible for atrophy during the acute and long-term phases after a RTC tear.

Fiber type composition affects the speed of a muscle contraction, but less so the specific tension (force per unit area). Force depends not only on the size and number of the fibers, but also on muscle architecture. The maximal specific tension of skeletal muscle is considered relatively constant, but we did not assess architectural change or the contractile machinery (actin and myosin content) within fibers. Such variables could also contribute to the findings.

Conclusions

This study describes histological and functional changes in the supraspinatus muscle in a rat model of RTC tear. The most salient findings of this work are the apparent dissociations between atrophy and muscle force soon after a RTC tear, as well as the finding that the supraspinatus becomes more susceptible to contraction-induced injury. Still, knowing when a torn RTC muscle is most susceptible to injury could be useful in surgical and rehabilitation planning, but additional work is needed to elucidate the specific timing and significance of this increased susceptibility to injury in patients.

Abbreviations

15D: 15 days after tenotomy; 2D: 2 days after tenotomy; AChR: Acetylcholine receptor; CTRL: Control; DI: Dispersion index; ECL: Enhanced chemiluminescence agent; ECM: Extracellular matrix; HRP: Horseradish peroxidase; MRI: Magnetic resonance imaging; NA: Number of averages; NMJ: Neuromuscular junction; RARE: Rapid acquisition relaxation-enhanced; RTC: Rotator cuff; T2: Spin-spin relaxation time; TEeff: Effective echo time; TR: Repetition time; α-BTX: α-bungarotoxin

Acknowledgements
Sue Xu, Ph.D. for assistance with MRI.

Funding
This work was supported by the National Institutes of Health by grants to APV (T32AG00026815S1), SRI (AR07592-20), and to RML (R01-AR059179 and R21-AR067872).

Authors' contributions
Developed the concepts or approach: APV, SRI, EES, MNG, RML. Performed experiments or data analysis: APV, SRI; RML. Prepared or edited the manuscript prior to submission: all authors. All authors read and approved the final manuscript.

Competing interests
The authors declare that they have no competing interests.

Author details
[1]Department of Orthopaedics, University of Maryland School of Medicine, AHB, Rm 540, 100 Penn St., Baltimore, MD 21201, USA. [2]Department of Kinesiology, University of Maryland School of Public Health, College Park, USA. [3]Department of Physiology, East Carolina Diabetes and Obesity Institute, Brody School of Medicine, East Carolina University, Greenville, USA.

References
1. Arruda EM, Mundy K, Calve S, Baar K. Denervation does not change the ratio of collagen I and collagen III mRNA in the extracellular matrix of muscle. Am J Physiol Regul Integr Comp Physiol. 2007;292(2):R983–7. doi:10.1152/ajpregu.00483.2006.
2. Avery NC, Bailey AJ. Enzymic and non-enzymic cross-linking mechanisms in relation to turnover of collagen: relevance to aging and exercise. Scand J Med Sci Sports. 2005;15(4):231–40. doi:10.1111/j.1600-0838.2005.00464.x.
3. Avila OL, Drachman DB, Pestronk A. Neurotransmission regulates stability of acetylcholine receptors at the neuromuscular junction. J Neurosci. 1989;9(8):2902–6.
4. Barton ER, Gimbel JA, Williams GR, Soslowsky LJ. Rat supraspinatus muscle atrophy after tendon detachment. J Orthop Res. 2005;23(2):259–65. doi:10.1016/j.orthres.2004.08.018.
5. Beeler S, Ek ET, Gerber C. A comparative analysis of fatty infiltration and muscle atrophy in patients with chronic rotator cuff tears and suprascapular neuropathy. J Shoulder Elb Surg. 2013;22(11):1537–46. doi:10.1016/j.jse.2013.01.028.
6. Bey MJ, Peltz CD, Ciarelli K, et al. In vivo shoulder function after surgical repair of a torn rotator cuff: glenohumeral joint mechanics, shoulder strength, clinical outcomes, and their interaction. Am J Sports Med. 2011;39(10):2117–29. doi:10.1177/0363546511412164.
7. Bodine SC, Baehr LM. Skeletal muscle atrophy and the E3 ubiquitin ligases MuRF1 and MAFbx/atrogin-1. Am J Physiol Endocrinol Metab. 2014;307(6): E469–84. doi:10.1152/ajpendo.00204.2014.
8. Bonaldo P, Sandri M. Cellular and molecular mechanisms of muscle atrophy. Dis Model Mech. 2013;6(1):25–39. doi:10.1242/dmm.010389.
9. Bosma M. Lipid droplet dynamics in skeletal muscle. Exp Cell Res. 2016;340(2):180–6. doi:10.1016/j.yexcr.2015.10.023.
10. Brooks SV, Zerba E, Faulkner JA. Injury to muscle fibres after single stretches of passive and maximally stimulated muscles in mice. J Physiol. 1995;488(Pt 2):459–69. doi:10.1113/jphysiol.1995.sp020980.
11. Buchmann S, Walz L, Sandmann GH, et al. Rotator cuff changes in a full thickness tear rat model: verification of the optimal time interval until reconstruction for comparison to the healing process of chronic lesions in humans. Arch Orthop Trauma Surg. 2011;131(3):429–35. doi:10.1007/s00402-010-1246-5.
12. Camargo PR, Avila MA, Alburquerque-Sendin F, Asso NA, Hashimoto LH, Salvini TF. Eccentric training for shoulder abductors improves pain, function and isokinetic performance in subjects with shoulder impingement syndrome: a case series. Rev Bras Fisioter. 2012;16(1):74–83. doi:10.1590/S1413-35552012000100013.
13. Davies MR, Ravishankar B, Laron D, Kim HT, Liu X, Feeley BT. Rat rotator cuff muscle responds differently from hindlimb muscle to a combined tendon-nerve injury. J Orthop Res. 2015;33(7):1046–53. doi:10.1002/jor.22864.

14. Davis ME, Korn MA, Gumucio JP, et al. Simvastatin reduces fibrosis and protects against muscle weakness after massive rotator cuff tear. J Shoulder Elb Surg. 2015;24(2):280–7. doi:10.1016/j.jse.2014.06.048.

15. Davis ME, Stafford PL, Jergenson MJ, Bedi A, Mendias CL. Muscle fibers are injured at the time of acute and chronic rotator cuff repair. Clin Orthop Relat Res. 2015;473(1):226–32. doi:10.1007/s11999-014-3860-y.

16. de Boer MD, Selby A, Atherton P, et al. The temporal responses of protein synthesis, gene expression and cell signalling in human quadriceps muscle and patellar tendon to disuse. J Physiol. 2007;585(Pt 1):241–51. doi:10.1113/jphysiol.2007.142828.

17. Dwyer T, Razmjou H, Holtby R. Full-thickness rotator cuff tears in patients younger than 55 years: clinical outcome of arthroscopic repair in comparison with older patients. Knee Surg Sports Traumatol Arthrosc. 2015; 23(2):508–13. doi:10.1007/s00167-014-3094-2.

18. Farshad M, Wurgler-Hauri CC, Kohler T, Gerber C, Rothenfluh DA. Effect of age on fatty infiltration of supraspinatus muscle after experimental tendon release in rats. BMC Res Notes. 2011;4:530. doi:10.1186/1756-0500-4-530.

19. Gayton JC, Rubino LJ, Rich MM, Stouffer MH, Wang Q, Boivin GP. Rabbit supraspinatus motor endplates are unaffected by a rotator cuff tear. J Orthop Res. 2013;31(1):99–104. doi:10.1002/jor.22192.

20. Gigliotti D, Leiter JR, Macek B, Davidson MJ, MacDonald PB, Anderson JE. Atrophy, inducible satellite cell activation, and possible denervation of supraspinatus muscle in injured human rotator-cuff muscle. Am J Physiol Cell Physiol. 2015;309(6):C383–91. doi:10.1152/ajpcell.00143.2015.

21. Gillies AR, Lieber RL. Structure and function of the skeletal muscle extracellular matrix. Muscle Nerve. 2011;44(3):318–31. doi:10.1002/mus.22094.

22. Gladstone JN, Bishop JY, Lo IK, Flatow EL. Fatty infiltration and atrophy of the rotator cuff do not improve after rotator cuff repair and correlate with poor functional outcome. Am J Sports Med. 2007;35(5):719–28. doi:10.1177/0363546506297539.

23. Gumucio JP, Davis ME, Bradley JR, et al. Rotator cuff tear reduces muscle fiber specific force production and induces macrophage accumulation and autophagy. J Orthop Res. 2012;30(12):1963–70. doi:10.1002/jor.22168.

24. Gumucio JP, Korn MA, Saripalli AL, et al. Aging-associated exacerbation in fatty degeneration and infiltration after rotator cuff tear. J Shoulder Elb Surg. 2014;23(1):99–108. doi:10.1016/j.jse.2013.04.011.

25. Gwynne-Jones DP, Sims M, Handcock D. Epidemiology and outcomes of acute Achilles tendon rupture with operative or nonoperative treatment using an identical functional bracing protocol. Foot Ankle Int. 2011;32(4): 337–43. doi:10.3113/FAI.2011.0337.

26. Hamer PW, McGeachie JM, Davies MJ, Grounds MD. Evans blue dye as an in vivo marker of myofibre damage: optimising parameters for detecting initial myofibre membrane permeability. J Anat. 2002;200(Pt 1):69–79. doi:10.1046/j.0021- 8782.2001.00008.x.

27. Hinchey JW, Aronowitz JG, Sanchez-Sotelo J, Morrey BF. Re-rupture rate of primarily repaired distal biceps tendon injuries. J Shoulder Elb Surg. 2014; 23(6):850–4. doi:10.1016/j.jse.2014.02.006.

28. Hirshberg A, Sherman S, Buchner A, Dayan D. Collagen fibres in the wall of odontogenic keratocysts: a study with picrosirius red and polarizing microscopy. J Oral Pathol Med. 1999;28(9):410–2. doi:10.1111/j.1600-0714.1999.tb02112.x.

29. Hsu HC, Boardman ND III, Luo ZP, An KN. Tendon-defect and muscle-unloaded models for relating a rotator cuff tear to glenohumeral stability. J Orthop Res. 2000;18(6):952–8. doi:10.1002/jor.1100180615.

30. Ichinose T, Yamamoto A, Kobayashi T, et al. Compensatory hypertrophy of the teres minor muscle after large rotator cuff tear model in adult male rat. J Shoulder Elb Surg. 2016;25(2):316–21. doi:10.1016/j.jse.2015.07.023.

31. Isaac C, Gharaibeh B, Witt M, Wright VJ, Huard J. Biologic approaches to enhance rotator cuff healing after injury. J Shoulder Elb Surg. 2012;21(2): 181–90. doi:10.1016/j.jse.2011.10.004.

32. Jobe FW, Moynes DR. Delineation of diagnostic criteria and a rehabilitation program for rotator cuff injuries. Am J Sports Med. 1982;10(6):336–9. doi:10.1177/036354658201000602.

33. Jonsson P, Wahlstrom P, Ohberg L, Alfredson H. Eccentric training in chronic painful impingement syndrome of the shoulder: results of a pilot study. Knee Surg Sports Traumatol Arthrosc. 2006;14(1):76–81. doi:10.1007/s00167-004-0611-8.

34. Joshi SK, Kim HT, Feeley BT, Liu X. Differential ubiquitin-proteasome and autophagy signaling following rotator cuff tears and suprascapular nerve injury. J Orthop Res. 2014;32(1):138–44. doi:10.1002/jor.22482.

35. Killian ML, Cavinatto L, Shah SA, et al. The effects of chronic unloading and gap formation on tendon-to-bone healing in a rat model of massive rotator

cuff tears. J Orthop Res. 2014;32(3):439–47. doi:10.1002/jor.22519.

36. Killian ML, Cavinatto LM, Ward SR, Havlioglu N, Thomopoulos S, Galatz LM. Chronic degeneration leads to poor healing of repaired massive rotator cuff tears in rats. Am J Sports Med. 2015;43(10):2401–10. doi:10.1177/0363546515596408.

37. Kim HM, Galatz LM, Lim C, Havlioglu N, Thomopoulos S. The effect of tear size and nerve injury on rotator cuff muscle fatty degeneration in a rodent animal model. J Shoulder Elb Surg. 2012;21(7):847–58. doi:10.1016/j.jse.2011.05.004.

38. Kong J, Anderson JE. Dystrophin is required for organizing large acetylcholine receptor aggregates. Brain Res. 1999;839(2):298–304.

39. Laron D, Samagh SP, Liu X, Kim HT, Feeley BT. Muscle degeneration in rotator cuff tears. J Shoulder Elb Surg. 2012;21(2):164–74. doi:10.1016/j.jse.2011.09.027.

40. Lieber RL, Ward SR. Cellular mechanisms of tissue fibrosis. 4. Structural and functional consequences of skeletal muscle fibrosis. Am J Physiol Cell Physiol. 2013;305(3):C241–52. doi:10.1152/ajpcell.00173.2013.

41. Liem D, Buschmann VE, Schmidt C, et al. The prevalence of rotator cuff tears: is the contralateral shoulder at risk? Am J Sports Med. 2014;42(4): 826–30. doi:10.1177/0363546513519324.

42. Liu X, Joshi SK, Samagh SP, et al. Evaluation of Akt/mTOR activity in muscle atrophy after rotator cuff tears in a rat model. J Orthop Res. 2012;30(9): 1440–6. doi:10.1002/jor.21266.

43. Liu X, Manzano G, Kim HT, Feeley BT. A rat model of massive rotator cuff tears. J Orthop Res. 2011;29(4):588–95. doi:10.1002/jor.22096.

44. Lovering RM, McMillan AB, Gullapalli RP. Location of myofiber damage in skeletal muscle after lengthening contractions. Muscle Nerve. 2009;40(4): 589–94. doi:10.1002/mus.21389.

45. Lovering RM, Roche JA, Goodall MH, Clark BB, McMillan A. An in vivo rodent model of contraction-induced injury and non-invasive monitoring of recovery. J Vis Exp. 2011;51:2782. doi:10.3791/2782.

46. Lundgreen K, Lian OB, Engebretsen L, Scott A. Lower muscle regenerative potential in full-thickness supraspinatus tears compared to partial-thickness tears. Acta Orthop. 2013;84(6):565–70. doi:10.3109/17453674.2013.858289.

47. Mallon WJ, Wilson RJ, Basamania CJ. The association of suprascapular neuropathy with massive rotator cuff tears: a preliminary report. J Shoulder Elb Surg. 2006;15(4):395–8. doi:10.1016/j.jse.2005.10.019.

48. McCloy RA, Rogers S, Caldon CE, Lorca T, Castro A, Burgess A. Partial inhibition of Cdk1 in G 2 phase overrides the SAC and decouples mitotic events. Cell Cycle. 2014;13(9):1400–12. doi:10.4161/cc.28401.

49. McMillan A, Shi D, Pratt SJP, Lovering RM. Diffusion tensor MRI to assess damage in healthy and dystrophic skeletal muscle after lengthening contractions. J Biomed Biotechnol. 2011;article ID 970726; doi:10.1155/2011/970726.

50. Oliveira F, Bevilacqua LR, Anaruma CA, Boldrini SC, Liberti EA. Morphological changes in distant muscle fibers following thermal injury in Wistar rats. Acta Cir Bras. 2010;25(6):525–8. doi:10.1590/S0102-86502010000600012.

51. Pandis P, Prinold JA, Bull AM. Shoulder muscle forces during driving: sudden steering can load the rotator cuff beyond its repair limit. Clin Biomech (Bristol, Avon). 2015;30(8):839–46. doi:10.1016/j.clinbiomech.2015.06.004.

52. Patel TJ, Lieber RL. Force transmission in skeletal muscle: from actomyosin to external tendons. Exerc Sport Sci Rev. 1997;25:321–63.

53. Pratt SJ, Lawlor MW, Shah SB, Lovering RM. An in vivo rodent model of contraction-induced injury in the quadriceps muscle. Injury. 2011; doi:10.1016/j.injury.2011.09.015.

54. Pratt SJ, Shah SB, Ward CW, Inacio MP, Stains JP, Lovering RM. Effects of in vivo injury on the neuromuscular junction in healthy and dystrophic muscles. J Physiol. 2013;591(Pt 2):559–70. doi:10.1007/s00018-014-1663-7.

55. Pratt SJ, Shah SB, Ward CW, Kerr JP, Stains JP, Lovering RM. Recovery of altered neuromuscular junction morphology and muscle function in mdx mice after injury. Cell Mol Life Sci. 2014; doi:10.3389/fphys.2015.00252.

56. Pratt SJ, Valencia AP, Le GK SSB, Lovering RM. Pre- and postsynaptic changes in the neuromuscular junction in dystrophic mice. Front Physiol. 2015;6:252. doi:10.1186/1756-0500-6-262.

57. Pratt SJ, Xu S, Mullins RJ, Lovering RM. Temporal changes in magnetic resonance imaging in the mdx mouse. BMC Res Notes. 2013;6(1):262. doi:10.1113/jphysiol.2012.241679.

58. Rivas DA, McDonald DJ, Rice NP, Haran PH, Dolnikowski GG, Fielding RA. Diminished anabolic signaling response to insulin induced by intramuscular lipid accumulation is associated with inflammation in aging but not obesity. Am J Physiol Regul Integr Comp Physiol. 2016;310(7):R561–9. doi:10.1152/ajpregu.00198.2015.

59. Rowshan K, Hadley S, Pham K, Caiozzo V, Lee TQ, Gupta R. Development of fatty atrophy after neurologic and rotator cuff injuries in an animal model of rotator cuff pathology. J Bone Joint Surg Am. 2010;92(13):2270–8. doi:10.2106/JBJS.I.00812.

60. Rubino LJ, Stills HF Jr, Sprott DC, Crosby LA. Fatty infiltration of the torn rotator cuff worsens over time in a rabbit model. Arthroscopy. 2007;23(7): 717–22. doi:10.1016/j.arthro.2007.01.023.

61. Sato EJ, Killian ML, Choi AJ, et al. Architectural and biochemical adaptations in skeletal muscle and bone following rotator cuff injury in a rat model. J Bone Joint Surg Am. 2015;97(7):565–73. doi:10.1002/jor.22646.

62. Sato EJ, Killian ML, Choi AJ, et al. Skeletal muscle fibrosis and stiffness increase after rotator cuff tendon injury and neuromuscular compromise in a rat model. J Orthop Res. 2014;32(9):1111–6. doi:10.2106/JBJS.M.01503.

63. Saxton JM, Clarkson PM, James R, et al. Neuromuscular dysfunction following eccentric exercise. Med Sci Sports Exerc. 1995;27(8):1185–93.

64. Shi LL, Freehill MT, Yannopoulos P, Warner JJ. Suprascapular nerve: is it important in cuff pathology? Adv Orthop. 2012;2012:516985. doi:10.1155/2012/516985.

65. Smith LR, Barton ER. Collagen content does not alter the passive mechanical properties of fibrotic skeletal muscle in mdx mice. Am J Physiol Cell Physiol. 2014;306(10):C889–98. doi:10.1152/ajpcell.00383.2013.

66. Sorichter S, Koller A, Haid C, et al. Light concentric exercise and heavy eccentric muscle loading: effects on CK, MRI and markers of inflammation. Int J Sports Med. 1995;16(5):288–92. doi:10.1055/s-2007-973007.

67. Speer KP, Lohnes J, Garrett WE Jr. Radiographic imaging of muscle strain injury. Am J Sports Med. 1993;21(1):89–95. doi:10.1177/036354659302100116.

68. Steinbacher P, Tauber M, Kogler S, Stoiber W, Resch H, Sanger AM. Effects of rotator cuff ruptures on the cellular and intracellular composition of the human supraspinatus muscle. Tissue Cell. 2010;42(1):37–41. doi:10.1016/j.tice.2009.07.001.

69. Strack S, Petersen Y, Wagner A, et al. A novel labeling approach identifies three stability levels of acetylcholine receptors in the mouse neuromuscular junction in vivo. PLoS One. 2011;6(6):e20524. doi:10.1371/journal.pone.0020524.

70. Takagishi K, Saitoh A, Tonegawa M, Ikeda T, Itoman M. Isolated paralysis of the infraspinatus muscle. J Bone Joint Surg Br. 1994;76(4):584–7.

71. Talaie T, Pratt SJ, Vanegas C, et al. Site-specific targeting of platelet-rich plasma via superparamagnetic nanoparticles. Orthop J Sports Med. 2015; 3(1):2325967114566185. doi:10.1177/2325967114566185.

72. Tetreault P, Levasseur A, Lin JC, De GJ, Nuno N, Hagemeister N. Passive contribution of the rotator cuff to abduction and joint stability. Surg Radiol Anat. 2011;33(9):767–73. doi:10.1007/s00276-011-0807-9.

73. Tokish JM. The mature Athlete's shoulder. Sports Health. 2014;6(1):31–5. doi:10.1177/1941738113514344.

74. Valencia AP, Iyer SR, Pratt SJ, Gilotra MN, Lovering RM. A method to test contractility of the supraspinatus muscle in mouse, rat, and rabbit. J Appl Physiol (1985). 2016;120(3):310–7. doi:10.1152/japplphysiol.00788.2015.

75. van der Linden-van der Zwaag HM, Nelissen RG, Sintenie JB. Results of surgical versus non-surgical treatment of Achilles tendon rupture. Int Orthop. 2004;28(6):370–3. doi:10.1007/s00264-004-0575-9.

76. Vidt ME, Santago AC, Marsh AP, et al. The effects of a rotator cuff tear on activities of daily living in older adults: a kinematic analysis. J Biomech. 2016;49(4):611–7. doi:10.1016/j.jbiomech.2016.01.029.

77. Ward SR, Sarver JJ, Eng CM, et al. Plasticity of muscle architecture after supraspinatus tears. J Orthop Sports Phys Ther. 2010;40(11):729–35. doi:10.2519/jospt.2010.3279.

78. Werner CM, Weishaupt D, Blumenthal S, Curt A, Favre P, Gerber C. Effect of experimental suprascapular nerve block on active glenohumeral translations in vivo. J Orthop Res. 2006;24(3):491–500. doi:10.1002/jor.20011.

79. Xu S, Pratt SJ, Spangenburg EE, Lovering RM. Early metabolic changes measured by 1H MRS in healthy and dystrophic muscle after injury. J Appl Physiol. 2012; doi:10.1152/japplphysiol.00530.2012.

80. Yildiz Y, Aydin T, Sekir U, Kiralp MZ, Hazneci B, Kalyon TA. Shoulder terminal range eccentric antagonist/concentric agonist strength ratios in overhead athletes. Scand J Med Sci Sports. 2006;16(3):174–80. doi:10.1111/j.1600-0838.2005.00471.x.

8

Concomitant glenohumeral pathologies in high-grade acromioclavicular separation (type III – V)

Jochen Markel[†], Tim Schwarting[†], Dominik Malcherczyk, Christian-Dominik Peterlein, Steffen Ruchholtz and Bilal Farouk El-Zayat[*]

Abstract

Background: Acromioclavicular joint (ACJ) dislocations are common injuries of the shoulder associated with physical activity. The diagnosis of concomitant injuries proves complicated due to the prominent clinical symptoms of acute ACJ dislocation. Because of increasing use of minimally invasive surgery techniques concomitant pathologies are diagnosed more often than with previous procedures.

Methods: The aim of this study was to identify the incidence of concomitant intraarticular injuries in patients with high-grade acromioclavicular separation (Rockwood type III – V) as well as to reveal potential risk constellations. The concomitant pathologies were compiled during routine arthroscopically assisted treatment in altogether 163 patients (147 male; 16 female; mean age 36.8 years) with high-grade acromioclavicular separation (Rockwood type III: $n = 60$; Rockwood type IV: n = 6; Rockwood type V: $n = 97$).

Results: Acromioclavicular separation occurred less often in women than men (1:9). In patients under 35, the most common cause for ACJ dislocation was sporting activity (37.4%). Rockwood type V was observed significantly more often than the other types with 57.5% (Rockwood type III = 36.8%, Rockwood type IV 3.7%). Concomitant pathologies were diagnosed in 39.3% of the patients with that number rising to as much as 57.3% in patients above 35 years. Most common associated injuries were rotator cuff injuries (32.3%), chondral defects (30.6%) and SLAP-lesions (22.6%). Of all patients, 8.6% needed additional reconstructive surgery.

Conclusion: Glenohumeral injuries are a much more common epiphenomenon during acromioclavicular separation than previously ascertained. High risk group for accompanying injuries are patients above 35 years with preexisting degenerative disease. The increasing use of minimally invasive techniques allows for an easier diagnosis and simultaneous treatment of the additional pathologies.

Keywords: Acromio-clavicular joint separation, Concomitant injuries, Shoulder arthroscopy

Background

The Acromioclavicular joint (ACJ) is a diarthrodial joint between the distal clavicle and acromion. There is no active motion of the AC joint. Joint movement occurs when the clavicle rotates passively during alteration of scapula placement [1]. Joint stability is achieved with musculoskeletal and ligamentous stabilizers such as the deltoid and trapezoid muscle, capsula, acromioclavicular and coracoclavicular ligaments [2]. During acromioclavicular separation the ligamentous structures rupture first. With higher force the musculoskeletal structures rupture as well [3, 4]. This progression of injury is illustrated in several classification systems of ACJ dislocation (see below).

The occurrence of acromioclavicular joint dislocation highly correlates with physical activity. While injuries of the acromioclavicular joint account for only 3–12% of all shoulder injuries, the incidence rises during sporting activity to up to 40% in contact sports (e.g. Football) [4, 5]. ACJ-dislocation occurs 5 to 10 times more

* Correspondence: elzayat@med.uni-marburg.de
[†]Equal contributors
Center of Orthopaedics and Traumatology, University Hospital Marburg, Baldingerstrasse, 35033 Marburg, Germany

often in men than in women. High risk groups are young and active men [4, 6].

Several classification systems have been described for ACJ separation, starting in 1917 with Cadenat [7]. Today the most commonly used classifications are the Tossy classification of 1963 [8] and the subsequent Rockwood classification of 1984 [9] which adds the aspect of horizontal instability. Both are primarily radiological classifications. The higher the classification, the graver the injury and hence the more likely the stabilizers rupture.

Whereas Rockwood type I and II injuries can almost always be treated conservatively, Rockwood type IV to VI injuries require surgical treatment. Unfortunately there is still discord about the treatment of Rockwood type III injuries in literature. Older studies suggest a similar or even better result of the conservative treatment [10–13]. A consensus of the ISAKOS (International Society of Arthroscopy, Knee Surgery and Orthopedic Sports Medicine) recommends conservative treatment of Rockwood type III injuries and re-evaluation in 3 to 6 weeks [14]. In recent years studies show that early treatment especially in young and active patients improves the clinical outcome [15, 16]. In Germany, there is an increasing tendency to treat Rockwood type III injuries surgically. In a nationwide poll 73% of all queried hospitals stated to prefer surgical treatment to conservative treatment. The most commonly used techniques in Germany are the hook plate with 44% and the arthroscopic TightRope™ with 27% [17]. In comparison of open and minimally invasive techniques no significant difference in outcome has been established [18].

Pauly et al. and Tischer et al. (both 2009) showed that 15.0% to 18.2% of all patients with acromioclavicular separation had suffered concomitant intraarticular injuries (altogether 20 of 117) [19, 20]. Typical concomitant injuries were rotator cuff injuries, SLAP-lesions (Superior Labral tear, Anterior to Posterior) or fractures.

Aim of this study was to reassess this data in a bigger collective and establish the incidence of concomitant lesions in acromioclavicular separation and preeminent risk constellations.

Methods

Between the years 2009 and 2015 163 patients (147 male; 16 female; mean age 36.8 years) suffering from high-grade acromioclavicular separation (Rockwood type III: $n = 60$; Rockwood type IV: n = 6; Rockwood type V: $n = 97$) underwent arthroscopically assisted treatment during which the pathologies were compiled. The obtained data was analyzed descriptively, statistically and the causality of the concomitant pathologies were attributed to three factors (acute, intermediate and degenerative causes). Acute pathology was defined where the trauma was the sole cause for the diagnosed pathology (Intraoperative hemarthrosis and/or reddish blood tinged

pathologies), intermediate pathology had a mixed etiology, and degenerative pathology showed mostly preexisting defects which were only slightly aggravated by the injury. Several subgroup analyses concerning the severity of the AC-separation, sex and age of the patient were conducted.

The data was analyzed with SPSS for Windows, Version 22 (SPSS, Chicago, IL, USA). Probability distribution was determined with the Kolmogorov-Smirnov test. Statistical significance was calculated with the Chi-Square test and in the case of small case numbers, Fisher's exact test was used.

Results

ACJ dislocation was predominantly diagnosed in men (9:1; $p < 0,001$).

Cause of ACJ-dislocation was in 37.4% sporting activity for all patients. Young patients below 35 years suffered an acromioclavicular separation significantly more often during sports (54.5%, $n = 48$) than patients above 35 ($p < 0,001$; see Fig. 1).

3.7% ($n = 6$) of all patients suffered a Rockwood type IV injury, 36.8% ($n = 60$) Rockwood type III while Rockwood type V injuries were observed significantly more often than the other grades ($p = 0,015$) with 57.5% ($n = 97$; see Fig. 2).

Concomitant pathologies were found in 39.3% ($n = 64$) of the patients with that number rising to as much as 57.3% ($n = 43$) and significantly higher (p < 0,001) in the age group above 35 years (see Fig. 3).

An average of 1.9 injuries per patient with a total of 124 accompanying pathologies occurred. In the following the absolute total of pathologies will be counted, not considering the fact that in many patients several concomitant injuries at once could be found. Typical constellations were chondral defects on the humerus as well as the glenoid and several rotator cuff injuries at once. Of these 64 patients, 21.9% ($n = 14$) needed additional reconstructive surgery (e.G. *rotator* cuff and SLAP repair).

The incidence of rotator cuff injuries accounted for 32.3% ($n = 40$) of all concomitant injuries.

Chondral defects were diagnosed in 30.6% ($n = 38$) and SLAP-lesions in 22.6% ($n = 28$) of all injuries (see Fig. 4). Accompanying pathologies were attributed to preexisting degeneration in 70.0% ($n = 42$) of the cases.

Subgroup analysis showed no difference concerning etiology, kind and frequency of concomitant injuries during AC-separation between the sexes and between the different Rockwood types.

Specific concomitant pathologies in the subgroup of patients above 35 years were SLAP-lesions ($p < 0,001$), lesions of the M. subscapularis ($p < 0,001$), injuries of the long biceps tendon ($p = 0,002$) and glenoidal chondral defects (p = 0,029). All pathologies in the age group

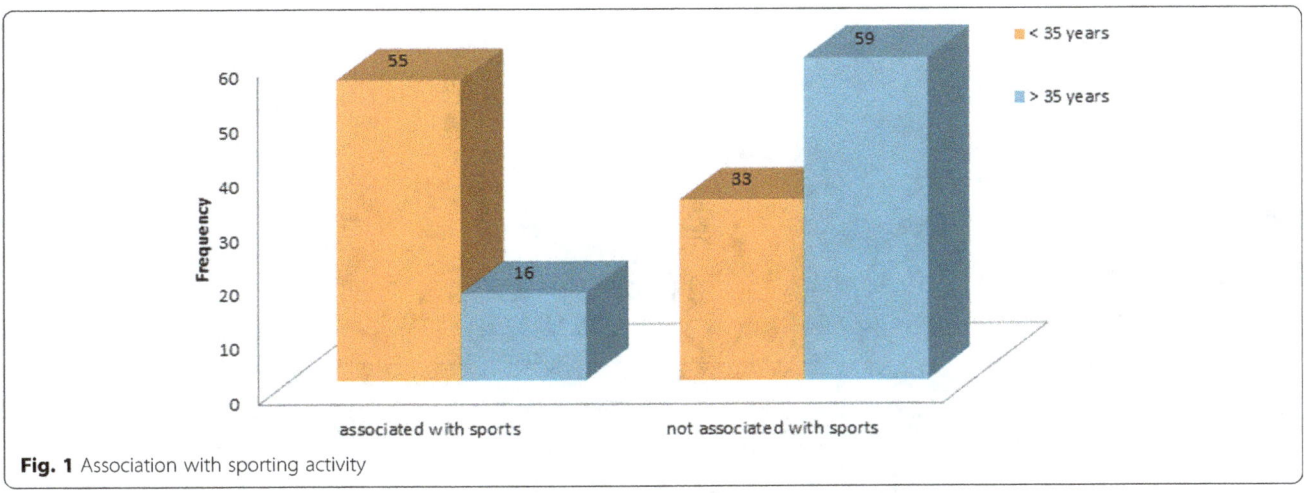

Fig. 1 Association with sporting activity

above 35 years were significantly more likely to have been degenerative ($p < 0,001$).

Discussion

To date there are only two publications discussing concomitant injuries in ACJ separations, with small collectives. In the present study a collective of 163 patients with ACJ separations is presented.

As in recent literature [4, 6], men in the present collective were much more likely than women to having suffered acromioclavicular separation ($p < 0,001$).

Etiology of ACJ-dislocation was sporting activity in 37.4% for both sexes and all age groups. In the younger age group acromioclavicular separation occurred significantly more often ($p < 0,001$) during sporting activity (54.5%). This is also consistent with current data [4, 5]. In the older age group ACJ separation did not necessarily occur during sporting activity and no predominant trauma mechanism could be found. With higher age the rate of preexisting degenerative defects is higher as well. Therefore a rising incidence of ACJ separation even during minor trauma is plausible.

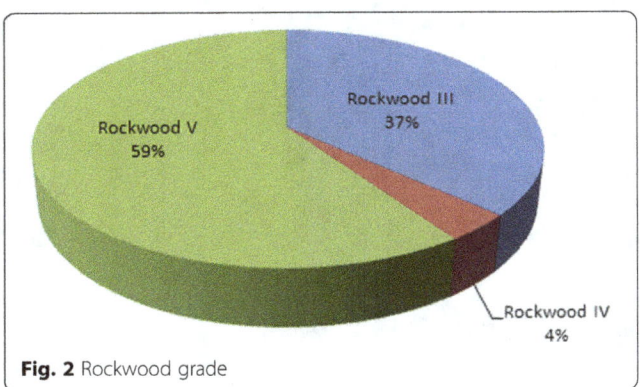

Fig. 2 Rockwood grade

In our study group Rockwood type V injuries were most common with 57.5%. Recent studies have shown mostly Rockwood type III injuries as the most common type of acromioclavicular separation [10]. Since only surgically treated patients were included into the study group the real total of Rockwood type III patients will most likely be higher. There is no definite conclusion about accompanying injuries in all Rockwood III patients (regardless if conservatively or surgically treated). Additional studies concerning concomitant pathologies in conservatively treated Rockwood III cases should be performed (e.g. MRI studies).

Most interestingly there was no difference of frequency or etiology of concomitant pathologies between the different Rockwood types. The pathomechanism of the ACJ separation would suggest that with rising force during impact it is more likely for intraarticular lesions to occur. In our study group this was not the case.

To date there are only two studies which compiled the frequency of intraarticular lesions associated with ACJ separation. These studies by Tischer et al. (2009) [20] and Pauly et al. (2009) [19] show a combined 17.1% ($n = 20/117$) of concomitant injuries. In this study group, concomitant pathologies were found in 39.3% ($n = 64$) of all patients with that number rising to as much as 57.3% ($n = 43$) and thus significantly higher ($p < 0,001$) in patients above 35 years. A contributing factor may be that in the studies mentioned above only the most relevant accompanying injuries were collected (e.g. no chondral defects). If omitting chondral defects for comparison, the rate of accompanying pathologies would still be 29.4% in the present study collective. Biggest discrepancy was found in prevalence of rotator cuff lesions which were diagnosed more often in this collective, whereas

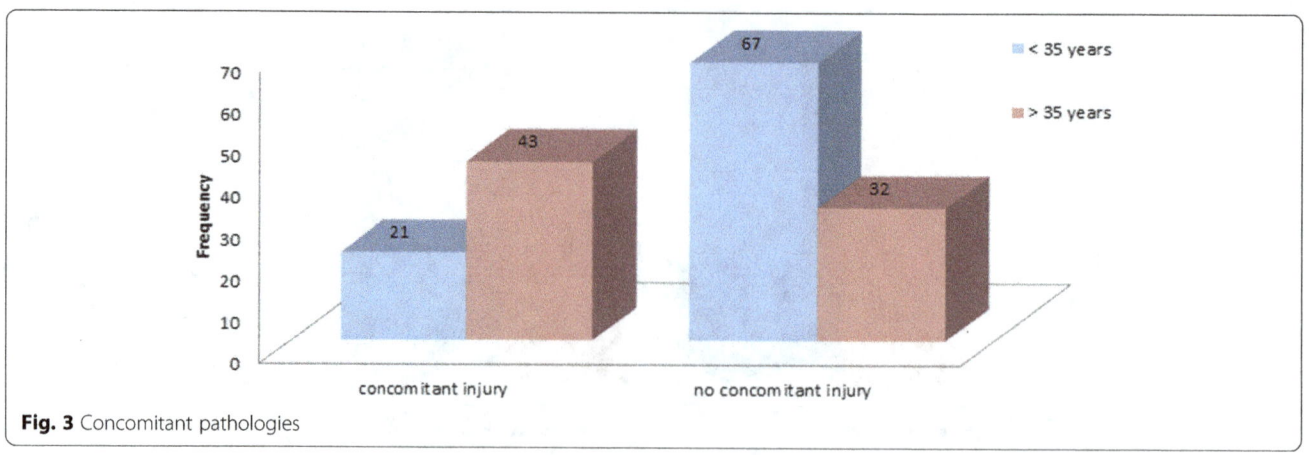

Fig. 3 Concomitant pathologies

SLAP-lesions occurred in comparable frequency. Possibly, the slightly higher mean age in this group is a contributing factor to the higher rate of rotator cuff lesions.

8.6% of all patients needed reconstructive surgery (e.G. *rotator* ruff- and/or SLAP-repair) in addition to the treatment of the ACJ dislocation. If surgery had not been performed arthroscopically, it is likely that at least in some cases diagnosis and treatment would have been delayed/not performed.

Accompanying pathologies were sorted into the above mentioned three groups. Most commonly preexisting degeneration was found in the age group above 35 years (70.0%). As expected, no dominant etiology of the pathology was detected in patients below 35 years.

The subgroups for sex and the different Rockwood types showed no difference concerning etiology, kind and frequency of concomitant pathologies.

Conclusion

The present study shows that the incidence of concomitant injuries in acromioclavicular separation has been underestimated. In almost 40% of all patients with ACJ-dislocation a concomitant injury could be diagnosed during the preceding diagnostic arthroscopy. In the age group above 35 years the incidence of an accompanying injury rises to 57.3%. Most commonly diagnosed pathologies were rotator cuff injuries, SLAP-lesions and chondral defects. 70% of all concomitant injuries could be attributed to a mostly degenerative etiology. Preeminent risk group to having suffered an accompanying injury are patients above 35 with degenerative defects. 21.9% of all patients with concomitant pathology needed additional reconstructive surgery.

In patients with ACJ separation diagnostic shoulder arthroscopy should be integrated as standard procedure for detection and treatment of concomitant pathologies.

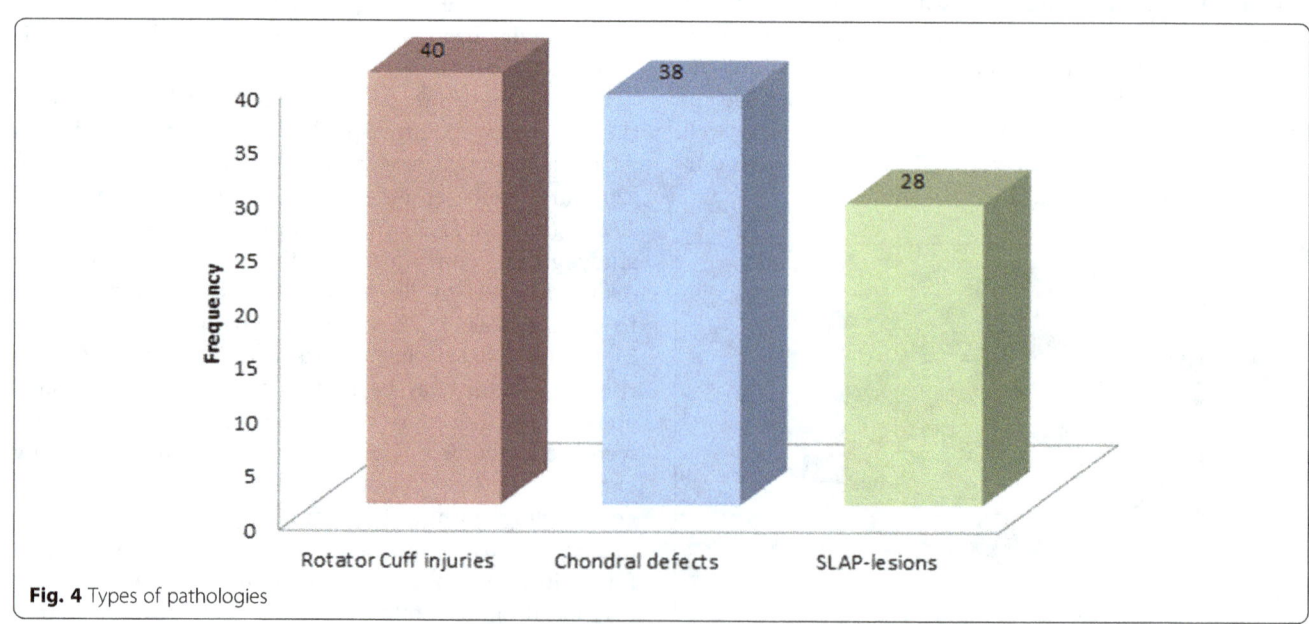

Fig. 4 Types of pathologies

Abbreviations

AC: Acromioclavicular; ACJ: Acromioclavicular Joint; ISAKOS: International Society of Arthroscopy, Knee Surgery and Orthopedic Sports Medicine; M: Musculus, muscle; MRI: Magnetic Resonance Imaging; SLAP: Superior Labral tear, Anterior to Posterior

Acknowledgements

Not Applicable.

Funding

There was no external funding or sponsoring in this study. All costs were funded through the Center of Orthopaedics and Trauma Surgery, University Hospital Marburg, Germany.

Authors' contributions

All authors read and approved the final manuscript. BFE and JM participated in the study design, carried out the study, interpreted the results, and drafted the manuscript. SR, TS, CDP and DM helped with data collection, the draft of the manuscript and critical revision as well as interpretation of the results. JM, CDP and TS set up the protocol, carried out the study and participated in interpretation of the results, performed the statistical data analysis as well as supported in the draft of the manuscript. All authors read and approved the final manuscript.

Competing interests

The authors declare that they have no competing interests' in relation to this study.

References

1. Flatow EL. The biomechanics of the acromioclavicular, sternoclavicular, and scapulothoracic joints. Instructional course lectures 42, S. 1993:237–45.
2. Wellmann M, Smith T. Epidemiologie, Anatomie, Biomechanik und Bildgebung von Akromioklavikulargelenkverletzungen. Unfallchirurg. 2012; 115(10):867–71.
3. Bontempo NA, Mazzocca AD. Biomechanics and treatment of acromioclavicular and sternoclavicular joint injuries. Br J Sports Med. 2010; 44(5):361–9.
4. Enad JG, Gaines RJ, White SM, Kurtz CA. Arthroscopic superior labrum anterior-posterior repair in military patients. Journal of shoulder and elbow surgery/American Shoulder and Elbow Surgeons. 2007;16(3):300–5.
5. Willimon SC, Gaskill TR, Millett PJ. Acromioclavicular joint injuries: anatomy, diagnosis, and treatment. Phys Sportsmed. 2011;39(1):116–22.
6. Pallis M, Cameron KL, Svoboda SJ, Owens BD. Epidemiology of acromioclavicular joint injury in young athletes. Am J Sports Med. 2012; 40(9):2072–7.
7. Cadenat FM. The treatment of dislocations and fractures of the outer end of the clavicle. In: Int Clin 1, S; 1917. p. 145–69.
8. Tossy JD, Mead NC, Sigmond HM. Acromioclavicular separations: useful and practical classification for treatment. Clinical orthopaedics and related research 28, S. 1963:111–9.
9. Rockwood CA. The shoulder. 3rd ed. Philadelphia: Saunders; 2004.
10. Press J, Zuckerman JD, Gallagher M, Cuomo F. Treatment of grade III acromioclavicular separations. Operative versus nonoperative management. Bulletin (Hospital for Joint Diseases (New York, NY)) 56 (2), S. 1997:77–83.
11. Schlegel TF, Burks RT, Marcus RL, Dunn HK. A prospective evaluation of untreated acute grade III acromioclavicular separations. The American journal of sports medicine 29 (6), S. 2001:699–703.
12. Spencer EE Jr. (2007): Treatment of grade III acromioclavicular joint injuries: a systematic review. Clin Orthop Relat Res 455:38–44..
13. Wojtys EM, Nelson G. Conservative treatment of grade III acromioclavicular dislocations. In: Clinical orthopaedics and related research (268), S; 1991. p. 112–9.
14. Beitzel, Knut; Mazzocca, Augustus D.; Bak, Klaus; Itoi, Eiji; Kibler, William B.; Mirzayan, Raffy et al. (2014): ISAKOS upper extremity committee consensus statement on the need for diversification of the Rockwood classification for acromioclavicular joint injuries. In: Arthroscopy : the journal of arthroscopic & related surgery : official publication of the Arthroscopy Association of North America and the international arthroscopy association 30 (2), S. 271–278.
15. Gstettner C, Tauber M, Hitzl W, Resch H. Rockwood type III acromioclavicular dislocation: surgical versus conservative treatment. In: Journal of shoulder and elbow surgery/American shoulder and elbow surgeons 17 (2), S; 2008. p. 220–5.
16. Leidel BA, Braunstein V, Kirchhoff C, Pilotto S, Mutschler W, Biberthaler P. Consistency of long-term outcome of acute Rockwood grade III acromioclavicular joint separations after K-wire transfixation. J Trauma. 2009; 66(6):1666–71.
17. Balke M, Schneider MM, Akoto R, Bäthis H, Bouillon B, Banerjee M. Die akute Schultereckgelenkverletzung. Unfallchirurg 118 (10), S. 2015:851–7.
18. Kraus N, Minkus M, Scheibel M. Schultereckgelenksprengungen. In: Trauma Berufskrankh 16 (4), S; 2014. p. 251–7.
19. Pauly S, Gerhardt C, Haas NP, Scheibel M. Prevalence of concomitant intraarticular lesions in patients treated operatively for high-grade acromioclavicular joint separations. Knee surgery, sports traumatology, arthroscopy : official journal of the ESSKA. 2009;17(5):513–7.
20. Tischer T, Salzmann GM, El-Azab H, Vogt S, Imhoff AB. Incidence of associated injuries with acute acromioclavicular joint dislocations types III through V. Am J Sports Med. 2009;37(1):136–9.

9

Compression-rate-dependent nonlinear mechanics of normal and impaired porcine knee joints

Marcel Leonardo Rodriguez and LePing Li[*] ⓘ

Abstract

Background: The knee joint performs mechanical functions with various loading and unloading processes. Past studies have focused on the kinematics and elastic response of the joint with less understanding of the rate-dependent load response associated with viscoelastic and poromechanical behaviors.

Methods: Forty-five fresh porcine knee joints were used in the present study to determine the loading-rate-dependent force-compression relationship, creep and relaxation of normal, dehydrated and meniscectomized joints.

Results: The mechanical tests of all normal intact joints showed similar strong compression-rate-dependent behavior: for a given compression-magnitude up to 1.2 mm, the reaction force varied 6 times over compression rates. While the static response was essentially linear, the nonlinear behavior was boosted with the increased compression rate to approach the asymptote or limit at approximately 2 mm/s. On the other hand, the joint stiffness varied approximately 3 times over different joints, when accounting for the maturity and breed of the animals. Both a loss of joint hydration and a total meniscectomy greatly compromised the load support in the joint, resulting in a reduction of load support as much as 60% from the corresponding intact joint. However, the former only weakened the transient load support, but the latter also greatly weakened the equilibrium load support. A total meniscectomy did not diminish the compression-rate-dependence of the joint though.

Conclusions: These findings are consistent with the fluid-pressurization loading mechanism, which may have a significant implication in the joint mechanical function and cartilage mechanobiology.

Keywords: Articular cartilage, Compression-rate dependence, Knee joint mechanics, Mechanical test, Meniscus, Poromechanics

Background

The knowledge of joint mechanics is essential for understanding the mechanism of joint injury and disease. Applications of this knowledge also include joint reconstruction and replacement. Articular cartilage is essential for the normal mechanical function of a diarthrodial joint. The load response of articular cartilage is highly compression-rate dependent. For a given magnitude of compressive strain, the reaction force is substantially greater if the strain is applied at a higher rate until the force approaches its asymptote. This rate-dependent response is well observed from the mechanical tests of

cartilage disks and elaborated in modeling [1–3]. The rate-dependence is also found in tensile tests of articular cartilage [4, 5]. However, these tests have been performed using small tissue explants. The rate-dependence has not been sufficiently investigated at the joint level to account for the complex structure of the joint and provide physiologically relevant data.

A series of experimental techniques have been used to study the mechanics of the knee joint. Hand-held probes are used during knee arthroscopy to evaluate cartilage properties [6–8]. Non-invasive methods, such as electro-arthrography [9] and T2 relaxation maps of magnetic resonance imaging [10], are also used to determine the integrity of the tissue structure. These measurements

* Correspondence: Leping.Li@ucalgary.ca
Department of Mechanical and Manufacturing Engineering, University of Calgary, 2500 University Drive, N.W, Calgary, AB T2N 1N4, Canada

target at cartilage properties rather than the mechanical response of the joint.

The mechanical testing using entire knee joint specimens is still the most direct and convenient measurement to gain the mechanical response of the joint [11–13]. Static assessment of cadaveric knee joints shows the role of the Medial Collateral Ligament (MCL) to primarily restrain valgus loading and stabilize external rotation [14–16]. Impact tests have been used to study the influence of braces on the MCL elongation for dynamic conditions, the multiple failure modes of the Posterior Cruciate Ligament (PCL) on a high-speed crash, and the increased anteromedial strain in the Anterior Cruciate Ligament (ACL) under combined impulsive knee compression, flexion and valgus moments [17–19].

The mechanical function of menisci has also been widely studied using joint testing [20–22]. A meniscectomized knee joint under compression shows a reduced contact area and increased peak pressure as compared with the intact joint, while any meniscal transplantation with only one horn secured gives intermediate values for both peak pressure and contact area [21–23]. Naturally, the contact area increases with force applied to the joint [24]. Cadaveric knee joint measurements showed that a significant fraction of the load is transmitted through the menisci [25]. In addition, a tibial flexion osteotomy increases cartilage pressure and causes an anterior shift in tibial resting position [26, 27].

Animal joints are widely used in the mechanical tests due to great availability, low cost and low biological risk as compared to the use of cadaveric joints. In addition, large animal stifle joints have a biological similarity to human knee joints [28, 29]. Porcine stifle joints are a popular choice for testing as the porcine knee has a similar size and anatomy to human's [30, 31].

The mechanical response of the knee joint has been mostly studied for elastic or traumatic behavior [32–34]. Few studies have considered both transient and long-term mechanical behaviors [35]. The effect of loading rates on the joint response has only been addressed in the injury models of the joint. For example, two compression rates, 1 and 500 mm/s, were tested in a murine model of post-traumatic osteoarthritis [36]. Different injuries were seen when a compression of 1.7 mm was applied, respectively, at the two rates.

The investigation of rate-dependent mechanical behavior is essential for the understanding of the knee joint mechanics and the consequence of surgical procedures because the joint experiences a variety of loadings applied at different rates. The objective of the present study was to quantify experimentally the compressive loading-rate-dependent mechanical behavior of the knee joint and the subsequent creep and relaxation of the joint associated with the poromechanical behavior of the

tissues in the joint. Only compressive loadings were considered in the study to highlight the influence of fluid pressurization in articular cartilages and menisci.

Methods

Porcine stifle joints were used as they have anatomy similarities to human's and are available in a large quantity required in the present study. Fresh porcine joints with sealed joint capsules were purchased within 24 h of the slaughter of the animals (Irricana Meat Market, Red Deer Lake Meat Processing and Ryan's Meats, Alberta, Canada). The ankle joint was partially retained to keep the tibia and fibula together. The joints were kept in sealed bags with Phosphate Buffered Saline (PBS) and stored in a fridge at 4 °C before testing in 1–3 days.

Compression tests of the joints were performed on an 858 Mini Bionix® II material testing system (MTS, Minnesota, USA). Two custom-made hollow steel cylinders, each welded at one end to a square flat plate, were used to fix the joint to the MTS (Fig. 1), as described below. All muscles were removed from the distal tibia and

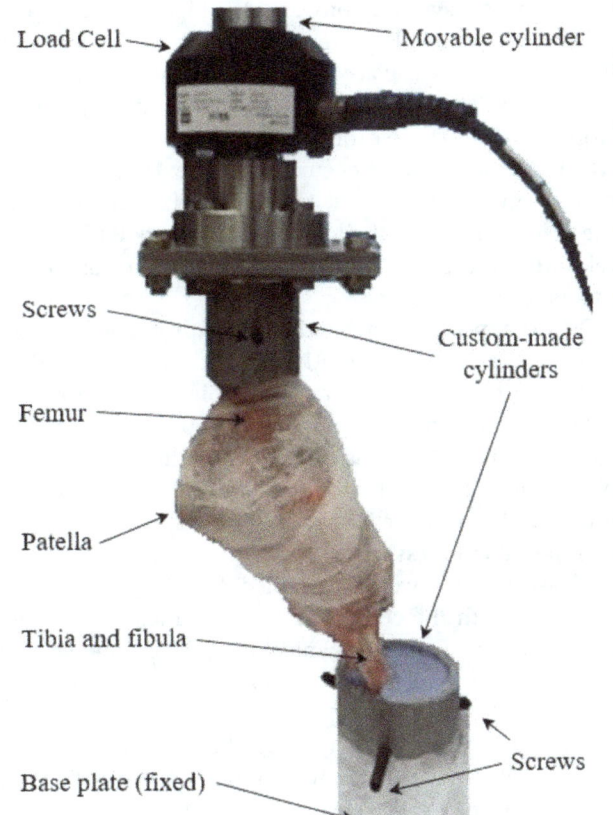

Fig. 1 Experimental setup for the porcine knee joint test on MTS. The joint was initially fixed at its natural angle to custom-made adapters with screws and dental cement. The lower cylinder was fixed to the base of the MTS, while the upper one was able to move in the vertical direction only. A force was applied by the movable cylinder of the MTS

proximal femur so the ends of the specimen could be fixed in the hollow cylinders using dental cement (Fastray™ LC, Bosworth, IL, USA). Three alloy steel set screws were tightened to the bone surface before cementing, to prevent sliding between cement and cylinder or bone. The femur was fixed to the cylinder first in a fume hood, and the cement was let set for 10 min before the cylinder holding it was attached to a force transducer (MTS® 661.19F-02) using an adaptor. After the force transducer was installed in the movable cylinder of the MTS, the custom-made cylinder for the ankle joint was positioned appropriately on the MTS base to maintain the natural angle of the joint while the pig stands, which was approximately 40° [31]. The ankle joint was then fixed to the cylinder with screws and cement and finally let set for 15 min. This fixing procedure minimized malalignment and prestresses in the joint. Since the cementing of the ankle joint had to be done on the MTS, a fan was used to expel the cement fume to the fume hood using a long hose. PBS-soaked gauzes were used to cover the joint in order to keep it hydrated during the preparation and test (Fig. 1).

Station Manager®, a software developed by the MTS, was used to control the vertical motion of the load cell. Both force and displacement control modes are available. For safety reasons, the testing machine was set to stop if a compressive or tensile force reached 800 N, which did not actually occur during any tests. The sampling frequencies were set to 10–100 Hz, depending on the loading rate, for the loading phase, and 1 Hz for the relaxation/creep phase to record at least dozens of data points for each phase.

Before applying a targeted loading protocol, the joint was subjected to preconditioning with a cyclic loading, to ensure that the structure of the joint was at a repeatable reference state [37, 38]. After applying a compressive force of 20 N to ensure contact within the joint, the preconditioning was performed at 0.25 Hz with an amplitude of 400 μm for 30 cycles. The response tended to be repeatable in less than 10 cycles.

Measurements were performed for different loading protocols with intact, dehydrated, and meniscectomized joints. Six groups of mechanical tests were done with 45 joints in total (Table 1) as described below.

(1) A pilot study ($n = 13$) was conducted to determine the appropriate magnitude of ramp compression within the elastic range and compression rates necessary to approximate the full range of rate-dependent response. Eleven joints were tested with an 800-μm ramp compression at six rates respectively, 10, 50, 100, 500, 1000 and 2000 μm/s, from the lowest to highest rate, followed by a 20-min relaxation period. Two additional joints were loaded with a higher ramp compression of 1200 μm at up to 5000 μm/s (Table 1). The joint remained unloaded for at least 20 min between tests on the same joint to allow tissue recovery from synovial fluid loss and deformation. The loading protocol was repeated for 2–3 times with the same specimen among some of these joints (7/13).

(2) A ramp compression of 1200 μm with four compression rates, 10, 100, 1000 and 2000 μm/s, was chosen for most further tests after the pilot study. The relaxation phase was extended to 35 min for the increased compression of 1200 μm. The relaxation phase was skipped in some tests in order to complete multiple compression rates for the same specimen during the same day (Table 1).

(3) Different loading sequences were tested with the same joint specimens, when various compression rates were applied, respectively, from the lowest to highest rate, from the highest to lowest rate and randomly starting from a middle rate ($n = 5$).

(4) The static response was simulated with the equilibrium response of relaxation tests, because a zero compression rate cannot be possibly performed. A joint was slowly compressed (~10 μm/s) to 300, 600, 900 and 1200 μm, respectively, and each of the four compressions was followed by a relaxation of 30–45 min to static equilibrium ($n = 7$, Table 1).

(5) The force-displacement relationship was examined with repeated tests on the same intact and dehydrated joints ($n = 3$). First, the fully hydrated intact joint was tested. Second, the joint capsule was carefully opened to drain the synovial fluid partially: dry kitchen paper towels were inserted above and below the menisci by lifting the femur slightly, followed by a small joint compression to squeeze out some fluid from the tissues. Finally, the towels were removed, and the same loading protocol was repeated on the joint after the fluid loss.

(6) Tests were repeated on the same joints before and after meniscus removal ($n = 12$, Table 1). A ramp compression of either 1200 or 800 μm was applied in the displacement-control tests with or without the relaxation phase ($n = 8$). A force of 500 N was applied in 20 s and kept constant for 30–60 min in the creep loading protocol with additional specimens ($n = 4$). After the test of each intact joint, small incisions were made to reach and cut the meniscal attachments and remove the menisci from the joint, while the specimen remained on the MTS. The joint was then tested with the same loading protocol. The locations of the incisions were chosen to keep the synovial fluid in the joint capsule.

Table 1 Summary of six groups of mechanical tests performed for specific purposes

Tests	Intact				Dehydration	Meniscectomy		
Purpose of Tests	(1) Pilot study	(2) Rate dependence	(3) Altered test sequence	(4) Static response	(5) Fluid pressure support	(6) Load support of menisci		
Applied peak force/displacement	800 µm	1200 µm	1200 µm	1200 µm	1200 µm	1200 µm	800 µm	500 N
Rates in loading phase	10, 50, 100, 500, 1000, 2000 µm/s	10, 100, 1000, 2000, 5000 µm/s	10, 100, 1000, 2000 µm/s	< 10 µm/s	10, 100, 1000, 2000 µm/s	10, 100, 1000 µm/s	10, 100, 1000 µm/s	25 N/s
Minutes for relaxation/creep phase	20	35 (3 joints); 0 (2 joints)	0 (no relaxation)	30–45	0	30–60	30–60 (3 joints); 0 (3 joints)	30–60
Joint angle	~40°	~40°	~40°	~40°	~40°	~40°	30°	30°
Number of joints	11	5	5	7	3	2	6	4

The total number of joints was 45. The tests of dehydrated and meniscectomized joints were performed after the mechanical tests of the corresponding intact joints

All tests were performed when the joints were held at their natural angles (~40°) with a 10-kN force transducer until the shared load cell failed ($n = 35$; Table 1). Although the failure of the load cell was unlikely related to the loading tests in this study, we reduced the joint angle to 30° to reduce the horizontal reaction and bending moment in the system, which were potential risks for the force transducer. We further reduced the maximum ramp compression from 1200 back to 800 μm in the sixth group of tests (Table 1). A new force transducer of 15-kN was used thereafter ($n = 10$). The resolution is 1% in force for this type of transducers according to the manufacturer.

The joints were carefully opened and visually inspected for tissue damage and degeneration after the mechanical tests. Only two joints from all tests were found to be abnormal: one had a small cut in the joint capsule resulting in a synovial fluid loss, another had a frozen joint capsule because the lab refrigerator was accidentally set to an unusually low temperature. The one with a damaged joint capsule showed a much smaller reaction force than other joints. The one with a frozen joint capsule showed a much weaker rate-dependence in the load response. Therefore, the measurements from these two joints were excluded from Table 1.

Finally, all statistical analyses were performed with Minitab 17.1.0 (Minitab Inc., PA, USA). The General Linear Model in the software includes a two-way ANOVA (analysis of variance) that was used, for example, to determine the significance of our results on the compression-magnitude, compression-rate and the combined effect of the two variables.

Results

The force-displacement data for various rates were reproducible when the same loading protocol was repeated on the same joints ($n = 7$ which includes all joints in Group 1 that were subjected to repeated tests). For example, the relative error was 4.0% at 800 μm, and increased to 7.4% at 400 μm compression when averaged over all compression-rates for all repeated tests. No significant difference was found between repeated tests as shown in a two-way ANOVA ($p = 0.93$). The deviations produced by different loading sequences were also insignificant (two-way ANOVA $p = 0.88$; $n = 5$, Group 3). The relative error was 2.2% and 6.3%, respectively, at 1200 μm and 600 μm compression. These findings validated the testing system including the fixing procedure. They also indicated that the loadings were within the elastic limit of the joints and that the waiting periods between tests on the same joints were sufficient for the tissue recovery from the previous loading.

The average force-compression relationship is shown for five compression rates (Fig. 2a). For the clarity of the

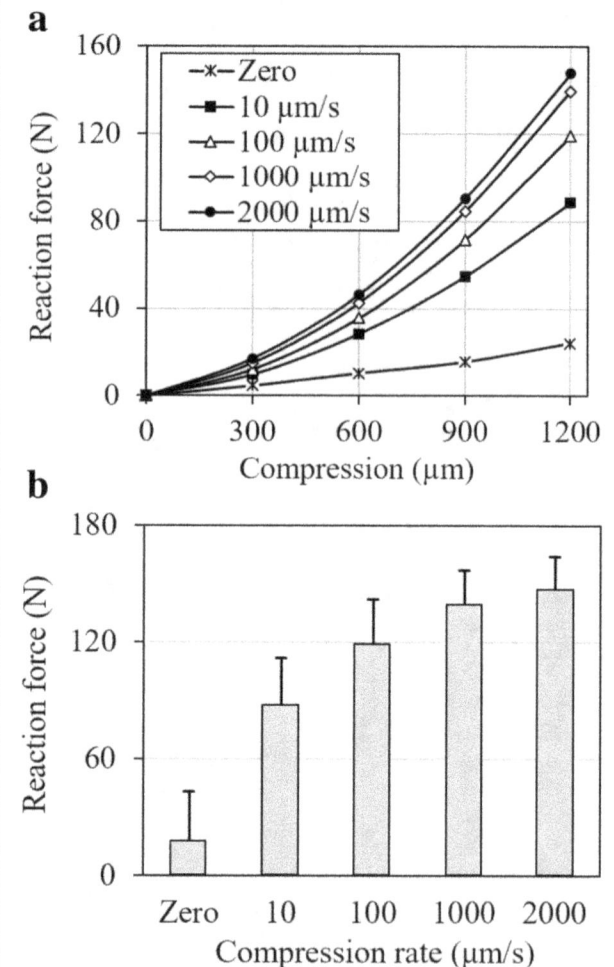

Fig. 2 Average reaction force in the joint as a function of (**a**) compression magnitude and (**b**) compression rate ($n = 6$). The data for the zero compression rate were taken from the equilibrium responses of the relaxation tests of six joints when each joint was compressed, respectively, by 300, 600, 900 and 1200 μm. **b** shows the reaction for the 1200-μm compression: the average forces were 24, 88, 119, 139 and 148 N, when the equal compression of 1200 μm was applied, respectively, at a compression rate of 0, 10, 100, 1000 and 2000 μm/s (specimens were obtained from the same source)

figure, the deviations are shown separately for 1200-μm compression only (Fig. 2b), which also shows the force as a function of compression rate. A two-way ANOVA showed a significant dependence of the reaction force on the compression-magnitude, compression-rate and the interaction between the two factors ($p < 0.001$ for all).

The reaction force was reduced by approximately 60% for all four compression-rates even when the synovial fluid was only partially removed (Fig. 3). An ANOVA analysis showed a significant dependence of the reaction force on the joint hydration ($p < 0.001$). Moreover, after the fluid loss from the tissues, the toe region of the force-displacement curve became more obvious and the

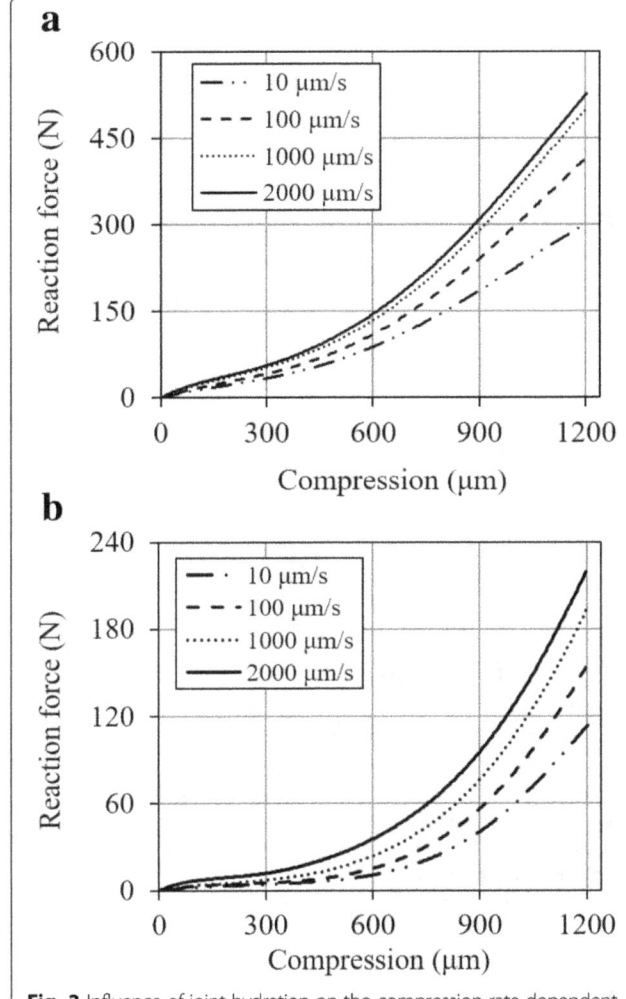

Fig. 3 Influence of joint hydration on the compression-rate-dependent response of a knee joint: **a** intact joint capsule; **b** drained joint capsule. Note that the vertical axis of (**b**) is scaled to 40% of that of (**a**)

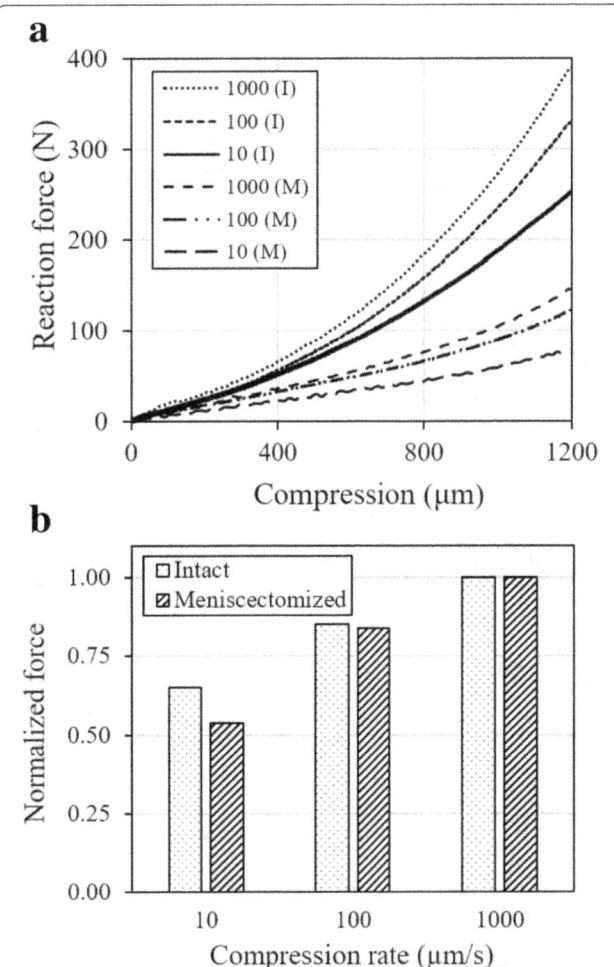

Fig. 4 Influence of meniscectomy on the load support of the joint. The joint was first tested with intact joint capsule (I) and then after meniscectomy (M). **a** Typical reaction force as a function of compression for three compression rates, 10, 100 and 1000 μm/s respectively; **b** Normalized reaction force at 1200-μm compression: the force was normalized by the maximum obtained, respectively, from the intact and meniscectomized joint

force continued to increase substantially from 1000 to 2000 mm/s (Fig. 3b).

The reaction force for any compression rate was significantly reduced after meniscectomy ($p < 0.001$). At the compression of 1200 μm, the force was reduced by over 60% with meniscectomy (Fig. 4a). On the other hand, a larger percent variation in the rate-dependence was observed after meniscectomy (Fig. 4b). The long-term response was also altered by meniscectomy (Fig. 5). After the initial ramp compression, reaction force decayed rapidly within the first five minutes relaxation (Fig. 5a). The knee compression at equilibrium was increased by almost 40% with meniscectomy when a 500-N force was applied (Fig. 5b).

The reaction forces varied approximately 3 folds among different groups of joints (Fig. 6), which was most likely related to the age and breed of the animals that were not made available for this study. For this reason, only the joints obtained from the same source were used to

evaluate the mean and deviation values (Fig. 2). Interestingly, the percent variations for different intact joints were similar as a function of either compression-magnitude or compression-rate (Fig. 7).

Discussion

Forty-five porcine stifle joints were tested to determine the compression-rate-dependent force-compression relationship, creep or relaxation behavior of the normal, dehydrated, and meniscectomized knee joints. The joints were loaded with a flexion angle but only the vertical motion of the femur was possible. The testing system and loading protocols were reasonably examined with repeatable results.

The force-compression relationship of normal joints was predominantly determined by the compression rate

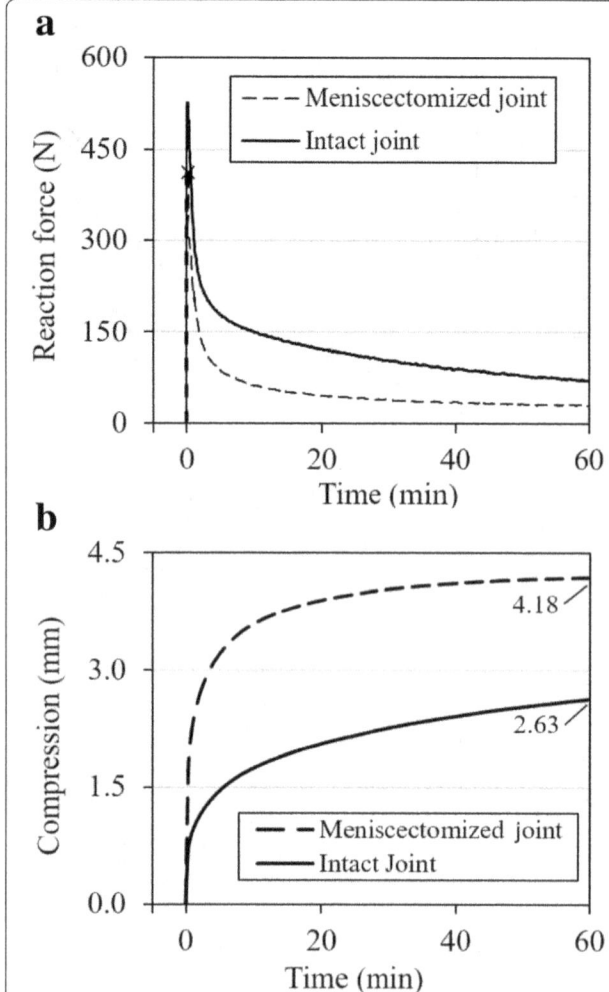

Fig. 5 Typical transient responses of a knee joint before and after meniscectomy. **a** Relaxation test: the joints were compressed by 800 μm at a rate of 100 μm/s prior to relaxation. The peak forces were 419.8 ± 129.1 and 187.4 ± 112.3 N (n = 6), respectively, before and after meniscal removal of the same joints (× marks the peak force for the meniscectomized joint). **b** Creep test: the joints were loaded to 500 N in 20 s prior to creep. The maximum knee compressions were 3.24 ± 0.70 and 4.56 ± 0.98 mm (n = 4), respectively, before and after the meniscal removal

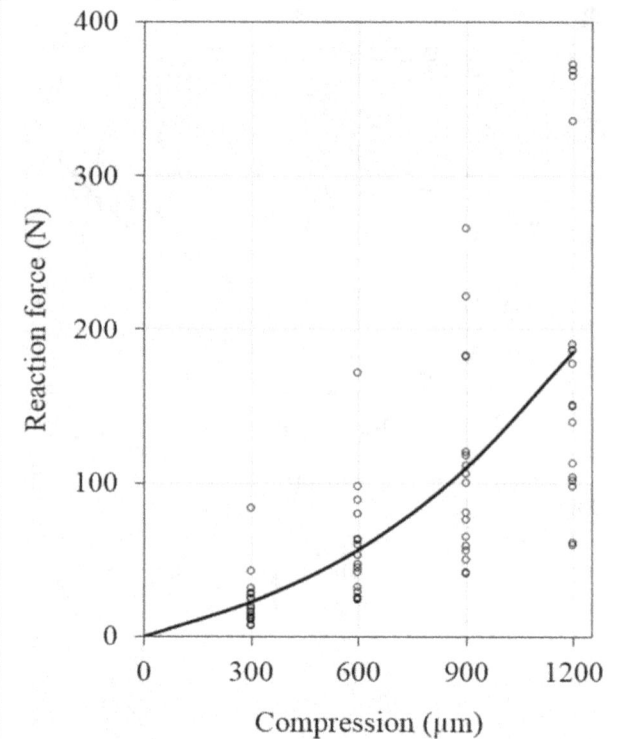

Fig. 6 Force-compression data variation potentially caused by different ages and breeds of the pigs. The curve shows the average over the 17 intact joints, including 2, 5, 5, 3 and 2, respectively, from test Groups 1, 2, 3, 5 and 6 (Table 1). Data were taken from all joints (regardless of the sources) tested at the natural angle (~40°) with a compression of 1200 μm applied at 1000 μm/s

(Figs. 2, 3a, 4 and 7). For a given magnitude of knee compression, the force increased with the compression rate rapidly until after 100 μm/s; it then increased slowly towards its asymptote (Fig. 2b); little increase was seen after 2000 μm/s, as indicated in the pilot study with a compression rate of 5000 μm/s (Table 1). In other words, a full-range of compression-rate-dependence has been approximated in the present study. On the other hand, the nonlinear behavior was also rate-dependent: the load response was almost linear at a nearly static compression; it became strongly nonlinear at a fast compression.

A comparison of these results with that from the literature is only partially available. Compression test data from cartilage discs showed over 10 times variation in stress over strain-rate for a given strain-magnitude of 10% [1]. Similarly, the dynamic modulus of cartilage tested in unconfined compression at 10 Hz cyclic loading was 24 times equilibrium modulus [39]. The present study indicated a weaker compression-rate dependence at the joint level than at the tissue level, likely due to non-uniform tissue compression and meniscus load support in the joint, as compared to uniform compression in the simple tissue test. Interestingly, the present study showed a variation of stress as a function of strain-rate that agrees with a model prediction. The model predicted a faster increase in the stress when the strain-rate gradually increases until around the vicinity of 5%/s then a slower increase towards to the asymptote [40]. The present study showed a similar trend (Fig. 2, 100 μm/s likely corresponds to ~5%/s average strain-rate in the joint), where the reaction force was only increased by 24% (119 to 148 N) when the compression-rate increased from 100 to 2000 μm/s (Fig. 2b). This result also compares well with the result from unconfined compression tests where

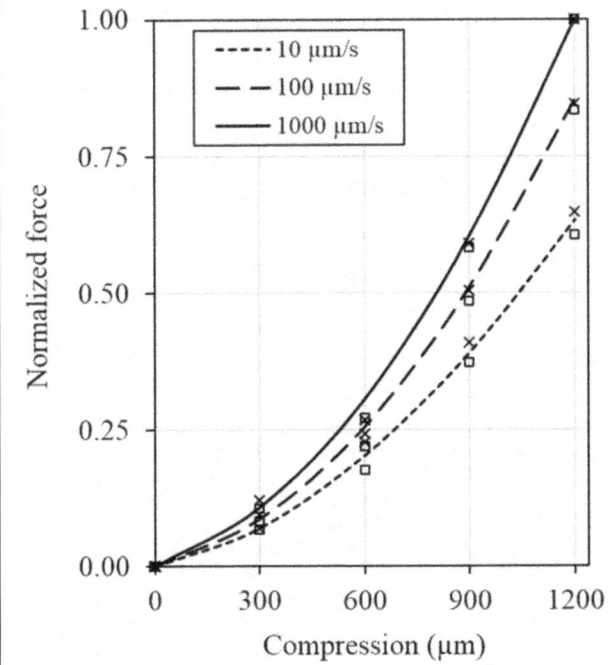

Fig. 7 Normalized reaction force at three compression rates for the normal intact joints. The lines show the average results taken from Fig. 2a, while the symbols show the results for individual joints (□: Figs. 3a; ×: 4a). The value shown was normalized by the reaction force at 1200-μm compression applied at 1000 μm/s in each case

the average dynamic modulus was only increased by 34% (48.2 to 64.8 MPa) when the frequency increased from 0.1 to 40 Hz [41]. Note that the present study only concerned with elastic deformation, as the variation of stress with strain-rate may be reversed at the strain level that causes the interruption of the collagen network [42].

The tissue hydration played a key role in the load support of the knee joint as indicated by the reaction force for a given joint compression. Fluid loss in the tissues not only reduced the load support of the joint, but also altered its nonlinear mechanical behavior including a more obvious toe region and a delayed asymptote for the compression rate (Fig. 3b vs 3a). This observation may be explained by fluid pressurization in the issues: some partially saturated region became fully saturated and pressurized with tissue compression. Therefore, the force increased faster with further compression. The fluid-pressure load support in the tissue and joint was explored previously [43, 44]. Therefore, only three joints were used in the present study (Table 1) to demonstrate the phenomenon and the compromised load support was not quantitatively correlated to the amount of fluid loss in the joint. On the other hand, it is understood from the literature that a partial fluid loss does not affect the equilibrium response of the joint because tissue hydration has little influence on the response at low

compression rates [45, 46] when the load is mainly supported by the tissue matrix [47, 48]. Thus, the dehydration tests were only performed for the loading phase without creep or relaxation phases.

The load support of the joint was compromised consistently over all compression rates after a total meniscectomy. For the compression of 1200 μm, the total meniscectomy reduced approximately 60% of the load support as compared to that of the same intact joint at the same compression rate (Fig. 4a). The reduction was slightly greater at lower compression rates (68% and 62% reductions at 10 and 1000 μm/s respectively). The menisci were known to improve the congruency in the knee and thus provide a better load support in the joint [49–52]. Our result compares well with the previous data from partially degenerate human and healthy pig knees that showed menisci bearing 45–75% of the joint load [53]. Interestingly, the patterns of rate-dependence for normal and meniscectomized joints were similar (Fig. 4b). The slightly larger variation in the meniscectomized joint was probably caused by a greater contact area change during loading as compared to the normal joint. Furthermore, a meniscectomy also altered the rate of creep and relaxation and greatly reduced the load support of the knee at equilibrium (Fig. 5) while the fluid loss does not affect the equilibrium response. This observation was supported by modeling results that showed changes in fluid pressurization after both total and partial meniscectomy [54, 55].

The mechanical responses of all normal joints were found to have similar patterns of compression-rate dependence (Fig. 7), although the stiffness of the joint in compression varied over 3 times among the joints (Fig. 6). This implied that the rate-dependent response was governed by the same mechanisms regardless of differences in the age or size of the joints tested in the study. The load response was mainly determined by cartilages and menisci in the present test conditions. It has been understood from constitutive modeling that the interplay between fibril-reinforcement and fluid pressurization governs the mechanical behavior of articular cartilage in unconfined compression [3, 56]. The necessity of implementing this fluid pressurization mechanism in cartilages and menisci was also demonstrated with a human knee joint model [57]. The mechanism was partially validated in the present study when the fluid loss in cartilages and menisci greatly reduced the load support of the joint (Fig. 3).

There were a few limitations with the present study. First, the age and breed of the animals were not available, because all the pigs were butchered for meat. Second, only one flexion angle was tested for each joint due to the constraint of the adapters; the corresponding loading condition is similar to that of a standing animal.

Third, the system could only record the vertical reaction force and thus the knee response to the transverse loading and bending was not investigated. Finally, the horizontal force and bending moment in the joint required the use of large load cells (10-kN and 15-kN), although the vertical force was well below 1 kN. As a result, we were not able to obtain good data for a very slow compression at 1 μm/s (the data for static compression were taken from the equilibrium response of relaxation tests). However, these limitations do not compromise the qualitative results of the present study.

Conclusions

The force-compression relationship of the fresh porcine joint is highly compression-rate-dependent, which is demonstrated in the present study to be greatly influenced by the fluid pressurization in the cartilaginous tissues. This phenomenon has been previously observed in the mechanical testing with cartilage explants that are immersed in PBS. The present results have been obtained using the whole joints with sealed joint capsules and thus the cartilaginous tissues are intact, saturated with only synovial fluid and subjected to realistic contact and loading conditions. Accordingly, a weaker rate-dependence has been observed in the joint than explant tests, while the trend of variation on the strain-rate is similar.

This study has also confirmed the role of menisci in the creep and relaxation behavior of the joint, in addition to the previous finding in the load share in the joint.

Although no animal models will ultimately match human joints, we expect similar mechanical behaviors for the human knee joints, as predicted by our computer simulations of the human joint. Since our daily life involves loading and unloading in the joint at different rates, the results presented here may help understand the injury, repair and mechanobiology of the knee joint.

Abbreviations

ACL: Anterior cruciate ligament; ANOVA: Analysis of variance; MCL: Medial collateral ligament; MTS: Material testing system; PBS: Phosphate buffered saline; PCL: Posterior cruciate ligament

Acknowledgments

We appreciate Dr. Walter Herzog's great support with his lab facility and technical assistance from Tim Leonard and Andrew Sawatsky.

Funding

The Natural Sciences and Engineering Research Council of Canada.

Authors' contributions

MLR performed the study under the supervision of LPL. MLR collected all data, while LPL played a key role in the study design and manuscript writing. Both authors wrote, revised and approved the manuscript.

Competing interests

LePing Li is a member of the editorial board of this journal.

References

1. Oloyede A, Flachsmann R, Broom N. The dramatic influence of loading velocity on the compressive response of articular cartilage. Connect Tissue Res. 1992;27(4):211–24.
2. Langelier E, Buschmann MD. Increasing strain and strain rate strengthen transient stiffness but weaken the response to subsequent compression for articular cartilage in unconfined compression. J Biomech. 2003;36(6):853–9.
3. Li LP, Shirazi-Adl A, Buschmann MD. Investigation of mechanical behavior of articular cartilage by fibril reinforced poroelastic models. Biorheology. 2003;40(1):227–33.
4. Verteramo A, Seedhom B. Zonal and directional variations in tensile properties of bovine articular cartilage with special reference to strain rate variation. Biorheology. 2004;41(3):203–13.
5. Ahsanizadeh S, Li LP. Strain-rate-dependent non-linear tensile properties of the superficial zone of articular cartilage. Connect Tissue Res. 2015;56(6):469–76.
6. Lyyra T, Jurvelin J, Pitkänen P, Väätäinen U, Kiviranta I. Indentation instrument for the measurement of cartilage stiffness under arthroscopic control. Med Eng Phys. 1995;17(5):395–9.
7. Kiviranta P, Lammentausta E, Töyräs J, Kiviranta I, Jurvelin J. Indentation diagnostics of cartilage degeneration. Osteoarthr Cartil. 2008;16(7):796–804.
8. Dudda M, Hauser J, Muhr G, Esenwein S. Low-intensity pulsed ultrasound as a useful adjuvant during distraction osteogenesis: a prospective, randomized controlled trial. J Trauma. 2011;71(5):1376–80.
9. Préville AM, Lavigne P, Buschmann MD, Hardin J, Han Q, Djerroud L, Savard P. Electroarthrography: a novel method to assess articular cartilage and diagnose osteoarthritis by non-invasive measurement of load-induced electrical potentials at the surface of the knee. Osteoarthr Cartil. 2013;21(11):1731–7.
10. Kwack K, Min B, Cho J, Kim J, Yoon S, Kim S. T2 relaxation time mapping of proximal tibiofibular cartilage by 3-tesla magnetic resonance imaging. Acta Radiol. 2009;50(9):1049–56.
11. Desio SM, Burks RT, Bachus KN. Soft tissue restraints to lateral patellar translation in the human knee. Am J Sports Med. 1998;26(1):59–65.
12. Lee S, Aadalen K, Malaviya P, Lorenz E, Hayden J, Farr J, Cole B. Tibiofemoral contact mechanics after serial medial meniscectomies in the human cadaveric knee. Am J Sports Med. 2006;34(8):1334–44.
13. Papaioannou G, Nianios G, Mitrogiannis C, Fyhrie D, Tashman S, Yang KH. Patient-specific knee joint finite element model validation with high-accuracy kinematics from biplane dynamic roentgen stereogrammetric analysis. J Biomech. 2008;41(12):2633–8.
14. Paulos L, France E, Rosenberg T, Jayaraman G, Abbott P, Jaen J. The biomechanics of lateral knee bracing. Part I: response of the valgus restraints to loading. Am J Sports Med. 1987;15(5):419–29.
15. Griffith C, LaPrade R, Johansen S, Armitage B, Wijdicks C, Engebretsen L. Medial knee injury: part 1, static function of the individual components of the main medial knee structures. Am J Sports Med. 2009;37(9):1762–70.
16. Thaunat M, Pioger C, Chatellard R, Conteduca J, Khaleel A, Sonnery-Cottet B. The arcuate ligament revisited: role of the posterolateral structures in providing static stability in the knee joint. Knee Surg Sports Traumatol Arthrosc. 2014;22(9):2121–7.
17. Erickson A, Yasuda K, Beynnon B, Johnson R, Pope M. An in vitro dynamic evaluation of prophylactic knee braces during lateral impact loading. Am J Sports Med. 1993;21(1):26–35.
18. Balasubramanian S, Beillas P, Belwadi A, Hardy WN, Yang KH, King AI, Masuda M. Below knee impact responses using cadaveric specimens. Stapp Car Crash Journal. 2004;48:71–88.
19. Withrow TJ, Huston LJ, Wojtys EM, Ashton-Miller JA. The effect of an impulsive knee valgus moment on in vitro relative ACL strain during a simulated jump landing. Clin Biomech. 2006;21(9):977–83.
20. Bylski-Austrow D, Ciarelli M, Kayner D, Matthews L, Goldstein S. Displacements of the menisci under joint load: an in vitro study in human knees. J Biomech. 1994;27(4):421–31.
21. Krause W, Pope M, Johnson R, Wilder D. Mechanical changes in the knee after meniscectomy. Journal of Bone and Joint Surgery Am. 1976;58(5):599–604.
22. Kurosawa H, Fukubayashi T, Nakajima H. Load-bearing mode of the knee joint: physical behavior of the knee joint with or without menisci. Clin Orthop Relat Res. 1980;149:283–90.
23. Chen M, Branch T, Hutton WI. It important to secure the horns during lateral meniscal transplantation? A cadaveric study. Arthroscopy : the journal of Arthroscopic & Related. Surgery. 1996;12(2):174–81.
24. Haut RC. Contact pressures in the patellofemoral joint during impact loading on the human flexed knee. J Orthop Res. 1989;7(2):272–80.

25. Ahmed AM, Burke DL. In-vitro measurement of static pressure distribution in synovial joints-part I: Tibial surface of the knee. J Biomech Eng. 1983;105(3):216–25.

26. Agneskirchner J, Hurschler C, Stukenborg-Colsman C, Imhoff A, Lobenhoffer P. Effect of high tibial flexion osteotomy on cartilage pressure and joint kinematics: a biomechanical study in human cadaveric knees. Arch Orthop Trauma Surg. 2004;124(9):575–84.

27. Giffin J, Vogrin T, Zantop T, Woo S, Harner C. Effects of increasing tibial slope on the biomechanics of the knee. Am J Sports Med. 2004;32(2):376–82.

28. Gregory MH, Capito N, Kuroki K, Stoker AM, Cook JL, Sherman SL. A review of translational animal models for knee osteoarthritis. Arthritis. 2012;2012:764621. https://doi.org/10.1155/2012 /764621.

29. Brill R, Wohlgemuth W, Hempfling H, Bohndorf K, Becker U, Welsch U, Roemer F. Dynamic impact force and association with structural damage to the knee joint: an ex-vivo study. Ann Anat. 2014;196(6):456–63.

30. Seo J, Li G, Shetty G, Kim J, Bae J, Jo M, Nha K. Effect of repair of radial tears at the root of the posterior horn of the medial meniscus with the pullout suture technique: a biomechanical study using porcine knees. Arthroscopy : the journal of Arthroscopic & Related. Surgery. 2009;25(11):1281–7.

31. Proffen BL, McElfresh M, Fleming BC, Murray MMA. Comparative anatomical study of the human knee and six animal species. Knee. 2012;19(4):493–9.

32. Eckstein F, Lemberger B, Gratzke C, Hudelmaier M, Glaser C, Englmeier KH, Reiser M. In Vivo cartilage deformation after different types of activity and its dependence on physical training status. Ann Rheum Dis. 2005;64(2):291–5.

33. Hosseini A, Van de Velde S, Kozanek M, Gill T, Grodzinsky A, Rubash H, Li G. In-vivo time-dependent articular cartilage contact behavior of the tibiofemoral joint. Osteoarthr Cartil. 2010;18(7):909–16.

34. Hosseini A, Van De Velde S, Gill TJ, Li G. Tibiofemoral cartilage contact biomechanics in patients after reconstruction of a ruptured anterior cruciate ligament. J Orthop Res. 2012;30(11):1781–8.

35. Halonen K, Mononen M, Jurvelin J, Töyräs J, Salo J, Korhonen R. Deformation of articular cartilage during static loading of a knee joint - experimental and finite element analysis. J Biomech. 2014;47(10):2467–74.

36. Lockwood K, Chu B, Anderson M, Haudenschild D, Christiansen B. Comparison of loading rate-dependent injury modes in a murine model of post-traumatic osteoarthritis. J Orthop Res. 2014;32(1):79–88.

37. Cheng S, Clarke E, Bilston L. The effects of preconditioning strain on measured tissue properties. J Biomech. 2009;42(9):1360–2.

38. Yoo L, Kim H, Gupta V, Demer J. Quasilinear viscoelastic behavior of bovine extraocular muscle tissue. Invest Ophthalmol Vis Sci. 2009;50(8):3721–8.

39. Park S, Ateshian GA. Dynamic response of immature bovine articular cartilage in tension and compression, and nonlinear viscoelastic modeling of the tensile response. J Biomech Eng. 2006;128(4):623–30.

40. Li LP, Herzog W. Strain-rate dependence of cartilage stiffness in unconfined compression: the role of fibril reinforcement versus tissue volume change in fluid pressurization. J Biomech. 2004;37(3):375–82.

41. Park S, Hung CT, Ateshian GA. Mechanical response of bovine articular cartilage under dynamic unconfined compression loading at physiological stress levels. Osteoarthr Cartil. 2004;12:65–73.

42. Kaplan JT, Neu CP, Drissi H, Emery NC, Pierce DM. Cyclic loading of human articular cartilage: the transition from compaction to fatigue. J Mech Behav Biomed Mater. 2017;65:734–42.

43. Li LP, Korhonen RK, Iivarinen J, Jurvelin JS, Herzog W. Fluid pressure driven fibril reinforcement in creep and relaxation tests of articular cartilage. Med Eng Phys. 2008;30(2):182–9.

44. Gu KB, Li LP. A human knee joint model considering fluid pressure and fiber orientation in cartilages and menisci. Med Eng Phys. 2011;33(4):497–503.

45. Race A, Broom ND, Robertson P. Effect of loading rate and hydration on the mechanical properties of the disc. Spine. 2000;25(6):662–9.

46. Párraga Quiroga JM, Wilson W, Ito K, van Donkelaar CC. Relative contribution of articular cartilage's constitutive components to load support depending on strain rate. Biomech Model Mechanobiol. 2017;16(1):151–8.

47. Mow VC, Kuei SC, Lai WM, Armstrong CG. Biphasic creep and stress relaxation of articular cartilage in compression: theory and experiments. J Biomech Eng. 1980;102(1):73–84.

48. Oloyede A, Broom N. Stress-sharing between the fluid and solid components of articular cartilage under varying rates of compression. Connect Tissue Res. 1993;30(2):127–41.

49. Fithian DC, Kelly MA, Mow VC. Material properties and structure-function relationships in the menisci. Clin Orthop Relat Res. 1990;252:19–31.

50. McDermott ID, Masouros SD, Amis AA. Biomechanics of the menisci of the knee. Curr Orthop. 2008;22(3):193–201.

51. Andrews S, Shrive N, Ronsky J. The shocking truth about meniscus. J Biomech. 2011;44:2737–40.

52. Walker PS, Erkman MJ. The role of the menisci in force transmission across the knee. Clin Orthop Relat Res. 1975;109:184–92.

53. Shrive NG, O'Connor JJ, Goodfellow JW. Load-bearing in the knee joint. Clin Orthop Relat Res. 1978;131:279–87.

54. Kazemi M, Li LP, Savard P, Buschmann MD. Creep behavior of the intact and meniscectomy knee joints. J Mech Behav Biomed Mater. 2011;4(7):1351–8.

55. Kazemi M, Li LP, Buschmann MD, Savard P. Partial meniscectomy changes fluid pressurization in articular cartilage in human knees. J Biomech Eng. 2012;134(2):021001.

56. Li LP, Buschmann MD, Shirazi-Adl A. The asymmetry of transient response in compression versus release for cartilage in unconfined compression. ASME. J Biomech Eng. 2001;123(5):519–22.

57. Li LP, Gu KB. Reconsideration of the use of elastic models to predict the instantaneous load response of the knee joint. Proc Inst Mech Eng H J Eng Med. 2011;225(9):888–96.

10

Knee arthrodesis versus above-the-knee amputation after septic failure of revision total knee arthroplasty: comparison of functional outcome and complication rates

Sven Hungerer[1,2]* , Martin Kiechle[1], Christian von Rüden[1,2], Matthias Militz[1], Knut Beitzel[3] and Mario Morgenstern[1,2,4]

Abstract

Background: After septic failure of total knee arthroplasty (TKA) and multiple revision operations resulting in impaired function, bone and/or soft-tissue damage a reconstruction with a revision arthroplasty might be impossible. Salvage procedures to regain mobility and quality of life are an above-the-knee amputation or knee arthrodesis. The decision process for the patient and surgeon is difficult and data comparing arthrodesis versus amputation in terms of function and quality of life are scarce. The purpose of this study was to analyse and compare the specific complications, functional outcome and quality of life of above-the-knee amputation (AKA) and modular knee-arthrodesis (MKA) after septic failure of total knee arthroplasty.

Methods: Eighty-one patients treated with MKA and 32 patients treated with AKA after septic failure of TKA between 2003 and 2012 were included in this cohort study. Demographic data, comorbidities, pathogens and complications such as re-infection, implant-failure or revision surgeries were recorded in 55MKA and 20AKA patients. Functional outcome with use of the Lower-Extremity-Functional-Score (LEFS) and the patients reported general health status (SF-12-questionnaire) was recorded after a mean interval of 55 months.

Results: A major complication occurred in more than one-third of the cases after MKA and AKA, whereas recurrence of infection was with 22% after MKA and 35% after AKA the most common complication. Patients with AKA and MKA showed a comparable functional outcome with a mean LEFS score of 37 and 28 respectively ($p = 0.181$). Correspondingly, a comparable physical quality of life with a mean physical SF-12 of 36 for AKA patients and a mean score of 30 for MKA patients was observed ($p = 0.080$). Notably, ten AKA patients that could be fitted with a microprocessor-controlled-knee-joint demonstrated with a mean LEFS of 56 a significantly better functional outcome than other amputee patients ($p < 0.01$) or MKA patients ($p < 0.01$).

Conclusion: Naturally, the decision process for the treatment of desolate situations of septic failures following revision knee arthroplasty is depending on various factors. Nevertheless, the amputation should be considered as an option in patients with a good physical and mental condition.

Keywords: Prosthetic joint infection, Revision total knee arthroplasty, Knee-arthrodesis, Above-the-knee amputation

* Correspondence: sven.hungerer@bgu-murnau.de
[1]BG Unfallklinik Murnau, Prof. Küntscher Str. 8, Murnau 82418, Germany
[2]Institute of Biomechanics, Paracelsus Medical University Salzburg and BG Unfallklinik Murnau, Prof. Küntscher Str. 8, Murnau 82418, Germany
Full list of author information is available at the end of the article

Background

Prosthetic joint infections (PJI) following total knee arthroplasty (TKA) pose a devastating complication, since eradication of infection and restoration of functionality present a significant challenge to both patients and surgeons [1, 2]. Despite tremendous efforts and targeted therapy, infection reoccurs in up to 14 to 28% after revision TKA and causes severe morbidity as well as substantial treatment costs [3, 4]. If infection cannot be eradicated or if multiple revision TKAs led to loss of soft-tissue, extreme bone defects or instability as well as deficiency of the extensor apparatus successful reconstruction or control of infection using revision TKA may no longer be possible [5, 6]. In these cases knee-arthrodesis or above-the-knee amputation (AKA) are beside resection arthroplasty often the only treatment options [2, 5]. Wu et al. performed a systematic review on treatment options in persistent infection after failed revision TKA and concluded that arthrodesis should strongly be considered in this case to control infection and to maximize function [7]. In contrast, Rohner et al. recently reported an infection persistence of 50%, substantially impaired quality of life and pain after knee-arthrodesis. They concluded that bone fusion following septic failure of revision TKA should be regarded with scepticism [2]. On the other hand, poor functional outcome and high complication rates of more than 30% are also described for AKA after TKA [8–10]. There are scant data on directly comparing functionality and complication rates of AKA and knee-arthrodesis performed after septic failure of TKA. Solely, one retrospective study compared the functional outcome of bone fusion and AKA after PJI in small numbers [11]. There is no study comparing AKA with access to modern orthotics and modular knee arthrodesis (MKA) in this situation. Knee-arthrodesis with modular endoprosthesis provides advantages over bone fusion including immediate fixation and weight bearing as well as modularity, which allows the reconstruction of segmental deficits [12].

Therefore the central aims of our study was to analyse the clinical course, complications, functionality and quality of life of AKA and MKA after septic failure of TKA. We hypothesize that neither AKA nor MKA after septic failure of TKA is superior in terms of functional outcome and complication rates and that the treatment decision process should be judged individually according to the patients` overall condition and the local bone and soft-tissue status.

Methods

All patients treated in our department over a ten-years time period (2003–2012) with MKA or AKA after septic failure of revision TKA were included in this retrospective cohort study. Additional inclusion criteria were:

minimum follow-up interval of 12-month, a sufficient patient data set and complete radiographic imaging studies. A PJI was diagnosed according to the American Academy of Orthopaedic Surgeons clinical practice guideline [13].

Demographic data was collected and the overall medical condition of the patient was evaluated using the Charlson comorbidity index (CCI) [14]. The initial infecting pathogens detected in the underlying PJI were documented. Patients were seen in regular visits (minimum visits after surgery: 6 weeks, 6 months, 1 year) and underwent physical and radiographic examination.

In patients with KA the following items were documented: implant positioning and leg length discrepancy. Distance arthrodesis was performed with a modular system (Peter Brehm GmbH, Weisendorf, Germany). Major complications after arthrodesis such as re-infection, implant-failure /–loosening or fracture were documented and surgical revisions like implant exchange, debridement or amputation were quoted. A recurrence or persistent infection was defined when local and/ or systemic signs of infection or one of the mentioned diagnosis criteria for PJI were present [13]. Loosening was defined as migration of the implant and the presence of a radiolucent liner larger than 2 mm [2]. Survival of the implant or arthrodesis was deemed to be the absence of above-mentioned complications or surgical revisions.

In patients with AKA the following was documented: level of amputation, fitted with a functional prosthesis and type of prosthesis (mechanic and microprocessor-controlled-knee-joint). Major complications after amputation such as stump healing disorder, recurrence of infection and revision amputation were recorded.

In 58 patients functional outcome was assessed with use of the Lower Extremity Functional Scale (LEFS) [15] and the SF-12 [16]. According to previous validation studies the SF-12 is comparable to the SF-36 for assessing patients` physical (Physical Component Summary; PCS) and emotional quality of life (Mental Component summary; MCS) [17]. The LEFS describes the functionality of the lower extremity (maximum score of 80 equates to the best functional outcome) [15]. Patients, in which amputation was performed after MKA, were excluded from analysis of functional outcome.

Statistical analysis

Statistical analysis was performed using SPSS® Statistics for Windows 19.0 (IBM Corp., Armonk, New York, U.S.A.). Results in this study are presented as mean values with standard deviation. Significance for categorical data was calculated using the Pearson's chi-squared test. Analysis of variance was used to detect differences between the groups. Numeric data were tested for normal distribution with the Kolmogorov Smirnov Test. Assuming parametric data, statistical differences were tested using the paired T-test for independent variables. A result was considered to be statistically significant with p-value <0.05. Implant survival was calculated by Kaplan-Meier survival plot. The functional outcome, assessed with the LEFS was defined the primary aim. The complication rate, as well as the patients` physical (PCS) and emotional quality of life (MCS) were defined secondary aims.

Results

Overview – Patient cohorts

In the time period between 2003 and 2012 we treated 127 patients with knee-arthrodesis and 157 patients with AKA due to various indications. Patients undergoing knee-arthrodesis or AKA due to other indication than PJI were excluded from this study. In total in 32 patients AKA and in 81 MKA was performed after septic failure of revision TKA and therefore patients were included in the current study. In six patients knee-arthrodesis after PJI was performed by bone fusion using an external fixator, plates or an intramedullary nail and they were excluded from this investigation (Fig. 1).

Modular knee arthrodesis – Clinical course and complications

Demographic data and infection characteristics of MKA patients are summarized in Table 1. After MKA, three patients (4%) died postoperatively and death was related to the underlying infection or a serious postoperative

complication. Six patients reportedly died in the first year after arthrodesis. In total, 17 patients with MKA were lost to follow-up examination, leaving 55 patients for analysis.

During the follow-up period loosening occurred after eight (15%) arthrodeses. A peri-implant fracture was seen in four patients (7%) and a technical implant failure in one patient (2%). Re-infection was observed in 12 cases (22%). An amputation had to be performed due to persisting or recurrent infection in six patients (11%) (Table 2). In nine patients at least one re-arthrodesis had to be performed due to periprosthetic fracture, implant loosening or re-infection. This was leading to a total number of 93 arthrodeses in 81 patients. An overall survival rate for all 93 modular arthrodeses was after one year 86%, after five years 71% and after ten years 61% (Table 1).

Above-the-knee amputations –clinical course and complications

Demographic data and infection characteristics of amputee patients are summarized in Table 3. After AKA four patients (13%) died postoperatively and death was related to the underlying disease or a serious postoperative complication. Two patients reportedly died in the first year after in AKA. In total, five patients (16%) with AKA were lost to follow-up examination, leaving 20 patients for analysis (Table 3). At follow-up 80% of the patients were fitted with a functional prosthesis ($n = 16$), six of them with a mechanic knee joint (30%) and ten with a

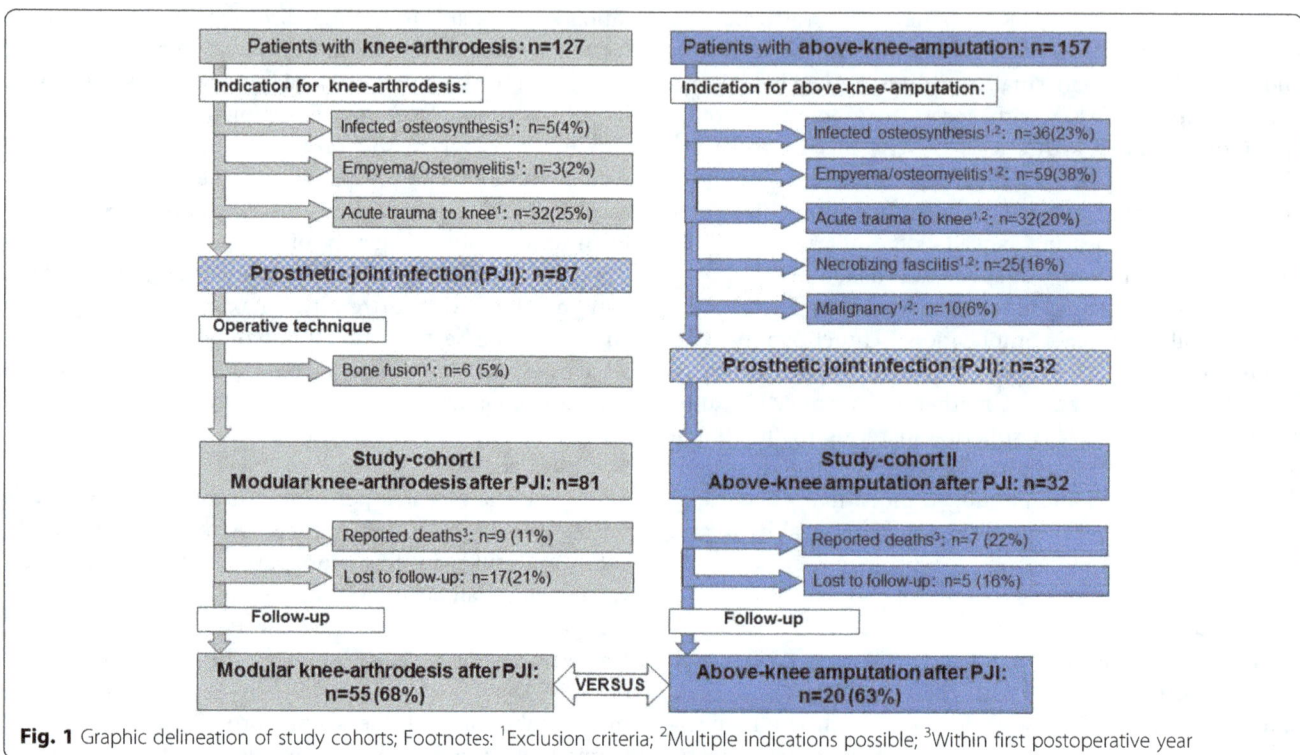

Fig. 1 Graphic delineation of study cohorts; Footnotes: [1]Exclusion criteria; [2]Multiple indications possible; [3]Within first postoperative year

Table 1 Modular knee-arthrodesis (MKA) after prosthetic joint infection (PJI): demographic and clinical data, implant survival rate

Characteristic	MKA after PJI
Number of patients, n	81
Demographic data	
Mean age (in years), mean (sd; Min - Max)	68.6 (11.2; 29–85)
Male sex, n (%)	43 (53.1)
Charlson Comorbidity Index, mean (sd)	4.8 (2.0)
Death within 1st year, n (%)	9 (11.1)
Lost to follow-up, n (%)	17 (21.0)
Patients with min. Follow-up, n (%)	55 (67.9)
Disease causing pathogens[a]	
S. aureus, n (%)	25 (30.9)
S. epidermidis, n (%)	31 (38.3)
Others[2], n (%)	25 (30.9)
Leg length discrepancy after MKA in cm, mean (sd)	1.8 (1.4)
Survival rate (SR) for MKA after PJI	
One – year SR	85.6%
Five – years SR	71.1%
Ten – years SR	60.9%

[a]Disease causing pathogen isolated in PJI leading MKA

microprocessor-controlled-knee-joint (50%). After initial AKA a revision surgery with irrigation and debridement was required due to non-healing stumps or recurrent infections in seven patients (35%). Re-amputation had to be performed in four cases (20%) (Table 2).

Comparison of complications and functional outcome of MKA and AKA

Patients with AKA showed a tendency towards a higher postoperative death rate with 13% when compared with patients with MKA (4%) ($p = 0.081$). Major complications, which required surgical revision, were seen in both cohorts equally, in 36% after MKA ($n = 20$) and in 35% after AKA ($n = 7$) ($p = 0.91$). Recurrence of in infection was the most common complication and occurred within follow-up interval in 22% after MKA ($n = 12$) and in 35% after AKA ($n = 7$) ($p = 0.25$). Due to this, amputation had to be performed in six cases after MKA (11%) and re-amputation was necessary in four (20%) after AKA ($p = 0.31$).

The functional outcome and quality of life, which were assessed in average 53 months after MKA and 62 months after AKA showed now significant differences between both procedures. Patients after amputation reached an average LEFS of 37 points and a mean PCS of 36, whereas after arthrodesis a mean LEFS of 28 points ($p = 0.181$) and a PCS of 30 ($p = 0.080$) could be observed. In both cohorts a comparable mental quality of life could be observed with a mean MCS for AKA and MKA of 47 and 46, respectively ($p = 0.755$) (Table 2). In total ten AKA patients could be fitted

Table 2 Modular knee-arthrodesis (MKA) versus Above-the-knee amputation (AKA) after prosthetic joint infection (PJI): clinical course, complications, functional outcome and quality of life

Characteristic	MKA after PJI	p-value	AKA after PJI
Patients with min. Follow-up (12 month), n (%)	55 (67.9)		20 (62.5)
Follow-up interval in month			
• Mean (sd)	53 (26)		62 (40)
• Min-Max	12–119		12–112
Complications			
Patients with major complication, n (%)	20 (36.4)	0.91	7 (35.0)
Recurrence of infection, n (%)	12 (21.8)	0.25	7 (35.0)
(Re-) Amputation, n (%)	6 (10.9)	0.31	4 (20.0)
MKA Loosening, n (%)	8 (14.5)	n/a	–
MKA Implant failure, n (%)	1 (1.8)	n/a	–
Peri-implant fracture, n (%)	4 (7.3)	n/a	–
Patients with functional follow up, n (%)	48 (59.3%)		10 (31.3%)
Functional follow-up examination			
LEFS[a], mean (sd)	28 (13.7)	0.181	37 (26.4)
Physical SF-12, mean (PCS) (sd)	30 (9.1)	0.080	36 (14.5)
Mental SF-12, mean (MCS) (sd)	46 (11.2)	0.755	47 (12.0)

[a]LEFS = Lower Extremity Functional Scale. A maximum score of 80 equates to the best functional outcome

Table 3 Above-the-knee amputation (AKA) after prosthetic joint infection (PJI): demographic and clinical data, level of AKA and orthotics

Characteristic	AKA after PJI
Number of patients, n	32
Demographic data	
Mean age (in years), mean (sd; Min – Max)	63.4 (14.4; 29–85)
Male sex, n (%)	17 (53.1)
Charlson Comorbidity Index, mean (sd)	5.5 (2.1)
Death within 1st year, n (%)	7 (21.8)
Lost to follow-up, n (%)	5 (15.6)
Patients with min. Follow-up, n (%)	20 (62.5)
Disease causing pathogens[a]	
S. aureus, n (%)	11 (34.4)
S. epidermidis, n (%)	9 (28.1)
Others, n (%)	12 (37.5)
Level of AKA	
Proximal, n (%)	5 (15.6)
Midshaft, n (%)	11 (34.4)
Distal, n (%)	16 (50.0)
Fitted with functional prosthesis[b], n (%)	16 (80.0)
Mechanic knee joint, n (%)	6 (30.0)
Microprocessor knee joint, n (%)	10 (50.0)

[a]Disease causing pathogen isolated in PJI leading to AKA
[b]Out of 20 patients, which were available for FUP

with a modern microprocessor-controlled-knee-joint. This sub-group showed a significantly better functional outcome with a mean LEFS of 56, compared to patients with a mechanic knee joint (mean LEFS: 20, $p < 0.01$) or those who received an arthrodesis ($p < 0.01$). Four patients that couldn't be fitted with prosthesis had with a mean LEFS of 14 a significantly compromised outcome when compared with MKA patients ($p < 0.01$).

In amputee patients age at surgical amputation was associated with a significantly lower functional outcome and quality of life at final follow-up examination ($p < 0.01$). Patients aged less than 60 years could all be fitted with prosthesis and reached a mean LEFS of 56, patients aged 60 to 69 years showed a mean LEFS of 36 and those who were aged between 70 and 79 years had a mean LEFS of just 14. All patients aged older than 80 years at amputation were lost to follow-up. In contrast, in patients receiving arthrodesis age did not significantly influence the functional outcome, since the age groups of below 60 years, 60 to 69 years, 70 to 79 years and more than 80 years showed a comparable LEFS value of 28, 30, 28 and 27 respectively.

Discussion

If infection after septic failure of TKA cannot be controlled or multiple revisions led to extensive bone or soft-tissue damage, salvage of a failed TKA remains difficult and the only alternatives to regain mobility and quality of life for the patient are AKA or KA [7, 10, 18–20]. Previous research does not provide a proper answer, if knee-arthrodesis or AKA with proper orthotic care is superior in terms of functional outcome, quality of life and postoperative complications. Therefore we compared these parameters in patients with AKA and knee-arthrodesis after PJI and revealed that as well AKA as knee-arthrodesis patients suffered an equally high rate of major complications of around 35%. Correspondingly, patients with AKA and knee-arthrodesis after septic failure of revision TKA showed a comparably compromised functional outcome and physical quality of life, whereas AKA patients that were fitted with a microprocessor-controlled-knee-joint reached a significantly better functional outcome, compared to all other amputee patients or those who received arthrodesis. Therefore, patients with a proper physical and mental state that will be able to mobilize with proper orthotics may benefit from an AKA. In amputee patients increasing age was associated with a lower functional outcome and decreasing number of patients fitted with prosthesis. In contrast, in arthrodesis patients age did not influence the functional outcome.

In literature a comparable complication rate of 31–32% after AKA [10, 21] and 30–50% after knee-arthrodesis is reported [2, 11]. Recurrence of infection was the most common complication in our study populations, which surprisingly occurred with 35% more frequently after AKA, than after MKA (22%). It is astonishing that reinfection is less common after MKA, despite a huge implant is present. Infection in MKA led in 15% to implant loosening and in 50% of these cases no re-arthrodesis was possible and amputation had to be performed. The implant survival rate of MKA was after one year 86%, after five years 71% and after ten years 61%. These results are considerably higher than literature data, which showed survivorship of MKA of 50% and 25% at five and ten years, respectively [12].

Death, which was related to the underlying disease or a serious postoperative complication, occurred in 4% after MKA and in 13% after AKA. This and the higher re-infection rate may be explained that patients with AKA had a more compromised overall health status and that the underlying infection was more often caused by a more virulent pathogen, such as *S. aureus*. It is widely accepted that in uncontrolled and occasionally life-threatening infections amputation is the preferred treatment option.

In literature on knee-arthrodesis after PJI, contrary results about functional outcome and quality of life as well as high complication rates are reported [2, 7, 11, 18, 22]. It has to be noted that in several above-cited studies knee-arthrodesis was performed with bone fusion using external fixator or intramedullary nail. A specific problem of multiple revision TKAs is an increasing bone defect and therefore a direct bony fusion would result in a leg length discrepancy of more than 5 cm. Such a leg length discrepancy, is known as a major factor to reduce the functional outcome and quality of life [5, 7]. In our cohort we performed arthrodesis with modular endoprostheses. This technique provides above-mentioned advantages over bone fusion and allows the reconstruction of segmental deficits and consequently adaption of a leg length discrepancy [12, 23].

Conway et al. concluded in a literature review on knee-arthrodesis, that a patient with successful knee-arthrodesis may be able to walk effectively, particularly in comparison to AKA [18]. Further studies reported a very poor functional outcome after amputation above septic failure of TKA [8–10]. But, the listed studies and the studies cited by Conway et al. analysed amputations which were mainly performed in the 1970's until the 1990's. Functional results of this era are meanwhile obsolete and can't be compared with nowadays. Meanwhile considerable engineering process with development of microprocessor-controlled knee-joints improved functional outcome and quality of life after AKA [24]. Our AKA cohort was fitted in 80% with prosthesis and mainly with a microprocessor-controlled -knee-joint, which may explain the deviating functional results compared to previous studies. In contrast, in the study of Sierra et al., who reported a poor functional outcome for AKA, just 36% of the patients were fitted with prosthesis [10]. Chen et al. stated a worse functional outcome for AKA when comparing with knee-arthrodesis after PJI. But in their AKA cohort also just 30% were fitted with prosthesis and no details are provided on the type of prosthesis.

The good functional outcome of our AKA population may also be explained by the fact that they showed a lower mean age with 63 years when compared to the MKA cohort (69 years). The age at amputation is significantly influencing the later functional outcome, as proven by our results.

The major limitation of the current study is that the patients are not prospectively randomized to one cohort. However, a randomization is ethically not acceptable. The decision process is depended on a multitude of factors such as soft tissue and bony situation, infection parameters, overall medical condition and the patients` preference. Nevertheless, the knowledge of the prognosis and what the individual patient has to expect from a MKA or an AKA in terms of quality of life or complication rates are important aspects in this decision process. Both cohorts were not matched in terms of age and gender, because AKA and MKA are rare procedures and matched cohorts with a representative sample-size are

only feasible in a multi-center study. Further limitation is a lack of the pre-operative documentation of functional status and quality of life and ta functional outcome score. However, a pre-operative functional status has a limited value, because at this stage most of the patients are bedridden due to the underlying PJI. Furthermore the aim of the study was to compare the functional outcome between the two surgical procedures and not within one cohort. Another limitations are the inhomogeneous follow-up intervals and the high lost to follow-up rate of 32% after MKA and 37% after AKA. The inhomogeneous follow-up intervals are a consequence of the retrospective study design. The high drop out rate is explained by the advanced age of a part of patients at inclusion and is consequently accounting for a limited number of patients available for follow-up examination. At follow-up, the mean LEFS was 37 for AKA patients and 28 for MKA patients, but statistical analysis could not show any significant difference. The missing significance may be explained by the limited power of the study. Nevertheless, the current data provide basic information for a proper sample size calculation for a multicentre study. A multicentre study is needed for more reliable outcome data and the indications for AKA or MKA after septic failure of revision arthroplasty are rare and drop out rates in this cohort are high.

Conclusion

Patients treated with AKA and MKA after septic failure of revision TKA showed a comparable functional outcome, quality of life and postoperative complication rate. Younger amputee patients, that could be fitted with microprocessor-controlled-knee-joint presented a significantly better functional outcome than MKA patients. If AKA patients could not be fitted with a prosthesis functional outcome was devastating. In unsalvageable situations of septic failure after TKA the treatment decision process is depending on the patients' expectations, overall medical condition, physical strength, severity of infection and soft-tissue envelope. Taking these factors into account each case has to be evaluated carefully to determine which treatment option might lead to the best achievable outcome. For the daily clinical routine these data should be considered in the decision-making amputation vs. modular arthrodesis: Younger patients in a proper physical and mental state may benefit from an AKA with proper orthotics, whereas in physically compromised older patients arthrodesis seems to be the superior treatment.

Abbreviations
AKA: Above the knee amputation; CCI: Charlson comorbidity index; LEFS: Lower Extremity Functional Scale; MCS: Mental component summary; MKA: Modular knee prosthesis; PCS: Physical component summary; PJI: Prosthetic joint infection; TKA: Total knee arthroplasty

Acknowledgements
Not applicable.

Funding
This study was not funded.

Authors' contributions
MM₁, MK, CVR, KB and SH searched literature, drafted the manuscript, participated in conception, design and coordination. MM₂, MK and SH contributed to acquisition of data, analysis and interpretation of data. SH supervised the whole study. All authors read and approved the final manuscript.

Competing interests
The authors declare that they have no competing interests.

Author details
[1]BG Unfallklinik Murnau, Prof. Küntscher Str. 8, Murnau 82418, Germany. [2]Institute of Biomechanics, Paracelsus Medical University Salzburg and BG Unfallklinik Murnau, Prof. Küntscher Str. 8, Murnau 82418, Germany. [3]Department of Orthopedic Sports Medicine, Technische Universität München, Isamningerstr. 22, 81675 Munich, Germany. [4]Department of Orthopaedic Surgery and Traumatology, University Hospital Basel, Spitalstr. 21, 4031 Basel, Switzerland.

References
1. Matar WY, Jafari SM, Restrepo C, Austin M, Purtill JJ, Parvizi J. Preventing infection in total joint arthroplasty. The Journal of bone and joint surgery American volume. 2010;92(Suppl 2):36–46.
2. Rohner E, Windisch C, Nuetzmann K, Rau M, Arnhold M, Matziolis G. Unsatisfactory outcome of arthrodesis performed after septic failure of revision total knee arthroplasty. The Journal of bone and joint surgery American volume. 2015;97(4):298–301.
3. Mittal Y, Fehring TK, Hanssen A, Marculescu C, Odum SM, Osmon D. Two-stage reimplantation for periprosthetic knee infection involving resistant organisms. The Journal of bone and joint surgery American volume. 2007; 89(6):1227–31.
4. Mortazavi SM, Vegari D, Ho A, Zmistowski B, Parvizi J. Two-stage exchange arthroplasty for infected total knee arthroplasty: predictors of failure. Clin Orthop Relat Res. 2011;469(11):3049–54.
5. Jones RE, Russell RD, Huo MH. Alternatives to revision total knee arthroplasty. The Journal of bone and joint surgery British volume. 2012;94(11 Suppl A):137–40.
6. Gottfriedsen TB, Schroder HM, Odgaard A. Knee arthrodesis after failure of knee Arthroplasty: a Nationwide register-based study. The Journal of bone and joint surgery American volume. 2016;98(16):1370–7.
7. CH W, Gray CF, Lee GC. Arthrodesis should be strongly considered after failed two-stage reimplantation TKA. Clin Orthop Relat Res. 2014;472(11): 3295–304.
8. Isiklar ZU, Landon GC, Tullos HS. Amputation after failed total knee arthroplasty. Clin Orthop Relat Res. 1994;299:173–8.
9. Pring DJ, Marks L, Angel JC. Mobility after amputation for failed knee replacement. The Journal of bone and joint surgery British volume. 1988; 70(5):770–1.
10. Sierra RJ, Trousdale RT, Pagnano MW. Above-the-knee amputation after a total knee replacement: prevalence, etiology, and functional outcome. J Bone Joint Surg Am. 2003;85-A(6):1000–4.
11. Chen AF, Kinback NC, Heyl AE, McClain EJ, Klatt BA. Better function for fusions versus above-the-knee amputations for recurrent periprosthetic knee infection. Clin Orthop Relat Res. 2012;470(10):2737–45.
12. Angelini A, Henderson E, Trovarelli G, Ruggieri P. Is there a role for knee arthrodesis with modular endoprostheses for tumor and revision of failed endoprostheses? Clin Orthop Relat Res. 2013;471(10):3326–35.
13. Della Valle C, Parvizi J, Bauer TW, DiCesare PE, Evans RP, Segreti J, Spangehl M, Watters WC, 3rd, Keith M, Turkelson CM et al: American Academy of Orthopaedic surgeons clinical practice guideline on: the diagnosis of periprosthetic joint infections of the hip and knee. The Journal of bone and joint surgery American volume 2011, 93(14):1355–1357.
14. Charlson ME, Pompei P, Ales KL, MacKenzie CR. A new method of classifying prognostic comorbidity in longitudinal studies: development and validation. J Chronic Dis. 1987;40(5):373–83.
15. Binkley JM, Stratford PW, Lott SA, Riddle DL. The lower extremity functional scale (LEFS): scale development, measurement properties, and clinical application. North American Orthopaedic rehabilitation research network. Phys Ther. 1999;79(4):371–83.
16. Ware J Jr, Kosinski M, Keller SD. A 12-item short-form health survey: construction of scales and preliminary tests of reliability and validity. Med Care. 1996;34(3):220–33.
17. Jenkinson C, Layte R, Jenkinson D, Lawrence K, Petersen S, Paice C, Stradling J. A shorter form health survey: can the SF-12 replicate results from the SF-36 in longitudinal studies? J Public Health Med. 1997;19(2):179–86.
18. Conway JD, Mont MA, Bezwada HP. Arthrodesis of the knee. J Bone Joint Surg Am. 2004;86-A(4):835–48.
19. Rao N, Crossett LS, Sinha RK, Le Frock JL. Long-term suppression of infection in total joint arthroplasty. Clin Orthop Relat Res. 2003;414:55–60.
20. Thornhill TS, Dalziel RW, Sledge CB. Alternatives to arthrodesis for the failed total knee arthroplasty. Clin Orthop Relat Res. 1982;170:131–40.
21. Fedorka CJ, Chen AF, McGarry WM, Parvizi J, Klatt BA. Functional ability after above-the-knee amputation for infected total knee arthroplasty. Clin Orthop Relat Res. 2011;469(4):1024–32.
22. Bargiotas K, Wohlrab D, Sewecke JJ, Lavinge G, Demeo PJ, Sotereanos NG. Arthrodesis of the knee with a long intramedullary nail following the failure of a total knee arthroplasty as the result of infection. The Journal of bone and joint surgery American volume. 2006;88(3):553–8.
23. Somayaji HS, Tsaggerides P, Ware HE, Dowd GS. Knee arthrodesis–a review. Knee. 2008;15(4):247–54.
24. Bellmann M, Schmalz T, Blumentritt S. Comparative biomechanical analysis of current microprocessor-controlled prosthetic knee joints. Arch Phys Med Rehabil. 2010;91(4):644–52.

11

Posterior shoulder dislocation with associated reverse Hill-Sachs lesion: treatment options and functional outcome after a 5-year follow up

Markus Guehring[1], Simon Lambert[2], Ulrich Stoeckle[1] and Patrick Ziegler[1]* (iD)

Abstract

Background: The current study describes several surgical techniques for the treatment of the reverse Hill - Sachs lesion after posterior shoulder dislocation; we also aimed to present long term results followed for a minimum of five years.

Methods: This study is a prospective case series of 17 patients who were treated in our clinic between 2008 and 2011. Patients with a defect size smaller than 25% of the articular surface were treated conservatively. An endoprosthesis of the glenohumeral joint was implanted in patients with a defect size bigger than 40%. All remaining patients were treated by a variety of operative techniques, depending on the quality of the bone and size of the defect.

Results: Twelve of seventeen patients had a defect size of the humeral articular surface between 25% and 40% with a mean age of 39 years. Depending on the defect size these patients were treated with retrograde chondral elevation, antegrade cylindrical graft or a graft of the iliac bone crest with an open approach. All the procedures showed fair results, e.g. the open approach with a graft of the iliac bone crest (2010: Dash 3.89, Constant 90.33, Rowe 86. 67; 2015: Dash 2.22, Constant 92.00, Rowe 93.33).

Conclusion: The open approach is not a disadvantage for the functional outcome. The treatment algorithm should involve the superficial size of the defect as well as the depth of the defect and the time interval between the dislocation and the surgical treatment.

Trial registration: 223/2012BO2, 02 August 2010.

Keywords: Posterior shoulder dislocation, Defect size, Osteosynthesis, Outcome

Background

Posterior shoulder dislocation is a rare injury, comprising 2% to 5% of all shoulder dislocations [1, 2] and up to 10% in patients with shoulder instability (mostly polar type II and III according to the Stanmore instability classification). The spectrum of posterior dislocation ranges from acute traumatic dislocation to chronic irreducible dislocations, and in combination with a proximal humeral fracture [3]. An extreme muscle contraction (seizures or electric shock), a direct or indirect trauma that occurs with flexion, adduction and internal rotation of the affected arm, is pathognomonic for the posterior shoulder dislocation [4–6].

Cooper first described the typical clinical signs of the posterior shoulder dislocation: dorsal protrusion of the humeral head in accordance with a flattened front shoulder and prominent coracoid, significantly limited or even repealed external rotation, or fixed internal rotation and restricted abduction under 90 degrees [7]. However, in contrast to the anterior shoulder dislocation, there may be very little obvious deformity of the shoulder girdle. Accordingly, the posterior shoulder dislocation is not detected in the primary examination in 60% to 79% of the

* Correspondence: patrick.ziegler333@googlemail.com
[1]Department for Traumatology and Reconstructive Surgery, BG Trauma Center Tübingen, University of Tübingen, Schnarrenbergstr 95, 72076 Tuebingen, Germany
Full list of author information is available at the end of the article

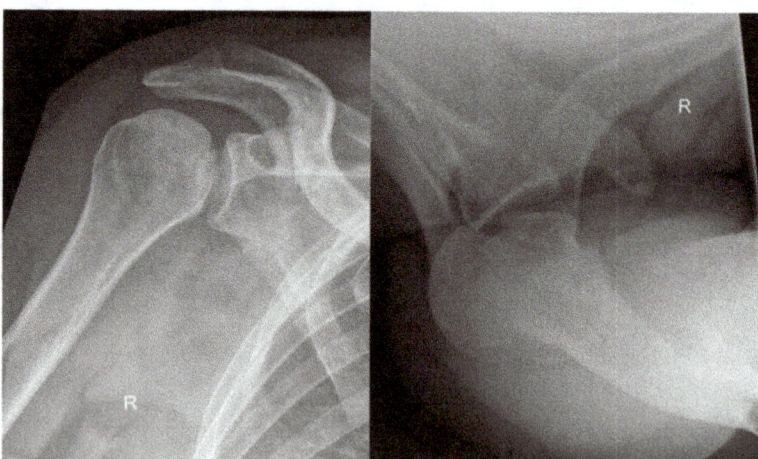

Fig. 1 Axial and ap view of posterior shoulder dislocation

cases [1, 2, 8]. Periods of over 10 years between disloca-tion and diagnosis are described in the literature [4].

A radiological examination in two views is obligatory (anteroposterior (a-p) and axial; Fig. 1). If pain precludes an axial x-ray because of limited abduction, a 'scapular-Y' view is recommended, even if there is marked pain. In the a.-p. view the posterior dislocation classically appears as a 'light-bulb' but this is not diagnostic and dislocation is thus sometimes difficult to detect [9]. Moreover, a careful clinical examination (lack of external rotation in a patient with a history of a shoulder injury) is mandatory. Computed tomography (CT) is essential for evaluating the injury and for preoperative planning regarding bone defects in the humeral head (Fig. 2). A magnetic resonance imaging scan (MRI), with contrast, is useful to diagnose lesions of the labrum and rotator cuff [1, 2, 4], particularly of the incarcerated tendon of the long head of biceps in irreducible dislocations [4]. Compared to anterior shoulder dislocations with defects in the anterior labrum and capsule (that is, soft tissue

lesions), posterior dislocation typically causes bone le-sions (the anterior humeral head impression fracture„ otherwise known as the "reverse Hill-Sachs lesion", McLaughlin lesion, or "l'encoche de Malgaigne") [5]. Other injuries such as lesions of the posterior labrum, or fractures the posterior glenoid rim are described [10–12]. Treatment depends on the size of the bone defect, the duration of the dislocated condition, and the functional demand of the patient [13].

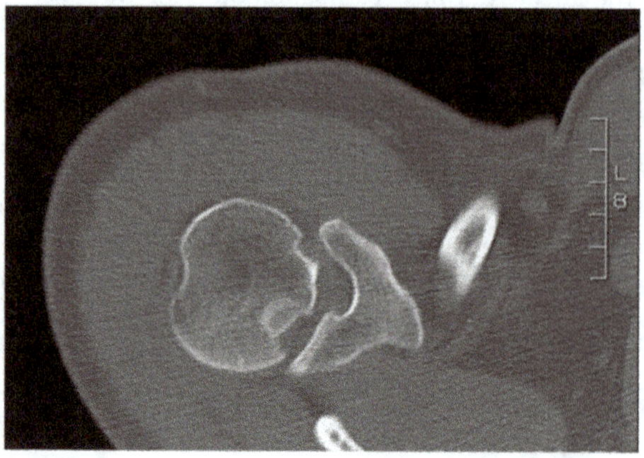

Conservative treatment is possible with a stable situ-ation after closed reduction and no significant bone defect. Subsequently, the affected shoulder should be immobi-lized in internal rotation or neutral position over a short period of time [6, 14]. Depending on the size, the reverse Hill-Sachs lesion is a risk factor for re-dislocation and therefore a surgical treatment is normally recommended [15]. For the treatment of the bone defect in the region of

Fig. 2 CT scan after posterior shoulder dislocation

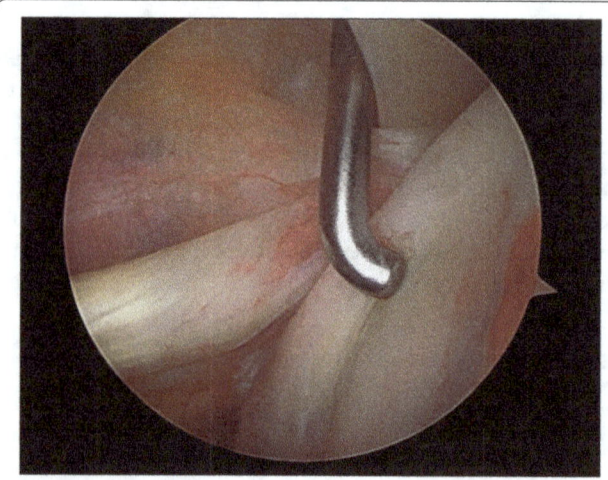

Fig. 3 Diagnostic arthroscopy after posterior shoulder dislocation to detect cartilage defects

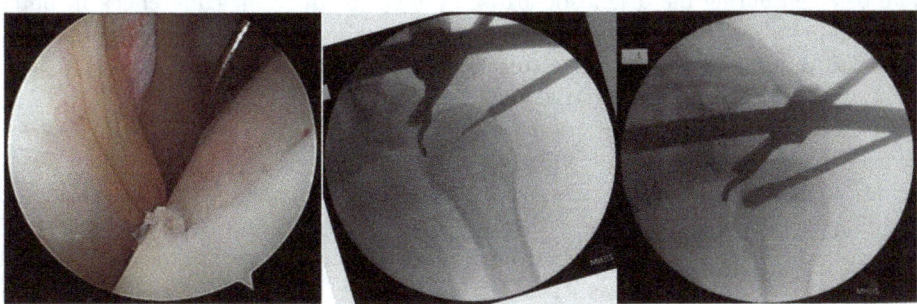

Fig. 4 Arthroscopic retrograde elevation with target device from cruciate ligament surgery

the humeral head, a variety of surgical procedures are described in the literature: filling the defect by tendon transposition of the subscapularis muscle [5], medial transposition of the lesser tuberosity [16] or allograft [17]; rotational osteotomy [18]; and hemi- or total arthroplasty [19, 20] are options.

The choice of the surgical technique depends on the size of the bone defect. With a stable shoulder joint and a defect of less than 25% of the articular surface, conservative treatment normally shows a satisfactory outcome. Reconstruction of the anatomical joint surface is recommended for defects between 25% and 40% of the articular surface. Lesions with greater defects than 40% of the articular surface should be treated with shoulder prosthesis [16, 19]. The literature of posterior dislocations of the shoulder largely comprises case reports or small series, while studies with a significant number of patients are rare. The aims of the present study are: to evaluate the anatomical reconstruction of the articular surface in a homogeneous patient population; and to evaluate the long-term functional outcomes in the cohort.

Methods

Between January 2008 and December 2011, 17 patients were treated with a posterior shoulder dislocation. The diagnosis was confirmed by using two orthogonal x-rays of the shoulder joint (anteroposterior (AP) and axial views). Closed reduction of the dislocation was attempted immediately under analgesia and sedation. A CT scan, to evaluate the size of the reverse Hill-Sachs lesion, was undertaken if closed reduction was not possible using the method of Cicak et al [21]. Five patients were excluded from this study. Four patients with defects of less than 25% of the articular surface in whom the joint was stable after open reduction were treated conservatively. One patient with a defect greater than 40% of the articular surface had a total shoulder arthroplasty. The remaining twelve patients had a reverse Hill-Sachs compression fracture involving 25–40% of the articular surface of the humeral head following a traumatic posterior shoulder dislocation.

All patients were male with a mean age of 39 years (range 17–55). The postoperative results were evaluated after a mean of one and five years following intervention using the Constant score [22], the Rowe score [23] and the DASH (disability of the arm, shoulder and hand) score [24]. The subjective perception of pain was evaluated by a VAS (visual analogue scale). No patient had multidirectional instability, prior shoulder surgery, or a neuromuscular disorder.

Diagnostic arthroscopy of the affected shoulder was attempted in all cases. The depth of the bone defect and the cartilage of the humeral articular surface were noted, together with associated injuries of the labrum and the rotator cuff. If no deep lesions of the

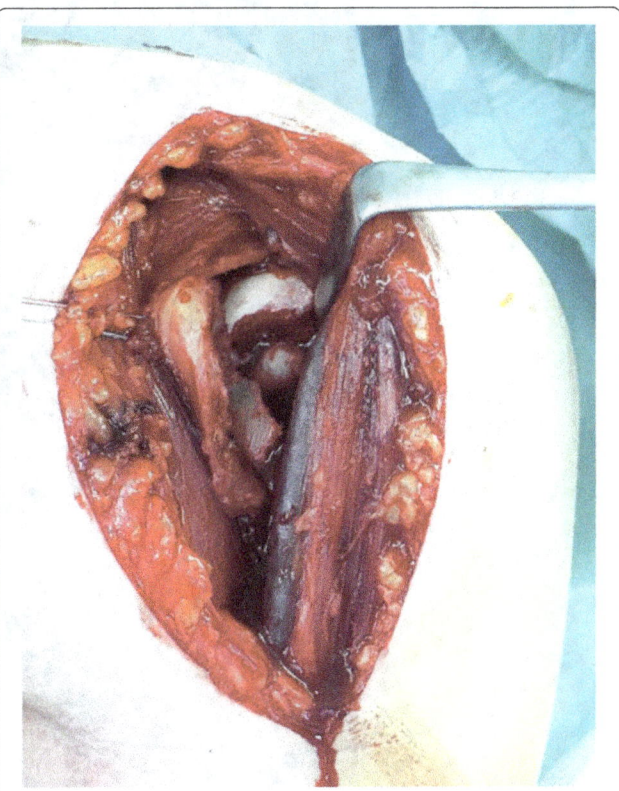

Fig. 5 Open approach for the treatment with an iliac bone crest graft

cartilage surface were detected during the diagnostic arthroscopy (ICRS classification grade 0–2, Fig. 3) and the time between the shoulder dislocation and the operative treatment was less than 14 days, we elected to restore the joint surface by retrograde elevation with arthroscopic assistance using a target device from the knee ligament surgery (Fig. 4). Larger cartilage lesions (ICRS classification grade 3 + 4) were treated during open debridement [25] using a deltopectoral approach in all cases (Fig. 5). If the interval between the accident and operative treatment was less than 14 days the joint surface was reconstructed with antegrade cortico-cancellous cylindrical grafts. If the interval was more than 14 days the defect was reconstructed using an autologous iliac crest fixed by small fragment screws (Fig. 6). The therapeutic algorithm is shown in Fig. 7.

Statistical analysis

Statistical analysis was performed in SPSS (version 22.0, SPSS Inc., Chicago, US). The t-test was used to calculate differences between the one and five year evaluations of pain and function. Differences in outcome between the surgical techniques were calculated using the Kruskal-Wallis variance method.

Results

The cause of the posterior shoulder dislocation was a high energy trauma in 75% (8 cases). The average length of in-hospital stay was 7.6 (4-24) days (Table 1).

In five cases with an ICRS score of 0–2 (42%), arthroscopically-assisted elevation of the articular surface was performed. Four patients had ICRS grade 3 or higher cartilage lesions, and were treated by antegrade cortico-cancellous cylindrical grafts. Three patients had polytrauma and had definitive treatment of the shoulder more than 14 days after injury using iliac crest cortico-cancellous graft. There were no postoperative infections, bleeding or nerve injuries, and no complication after harvesting the iliac bone graft. There were no re-dislocations over the period of review.

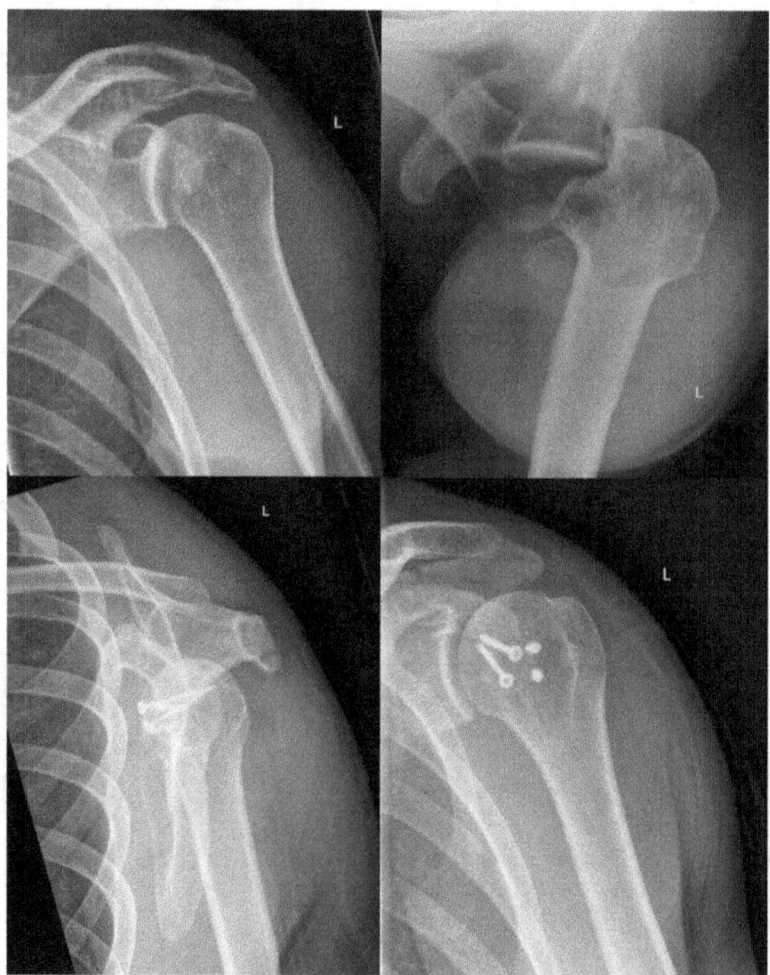

Fig. 6 Before and after reconstruction with an autologous graft of the iliac crest with small fragment screws

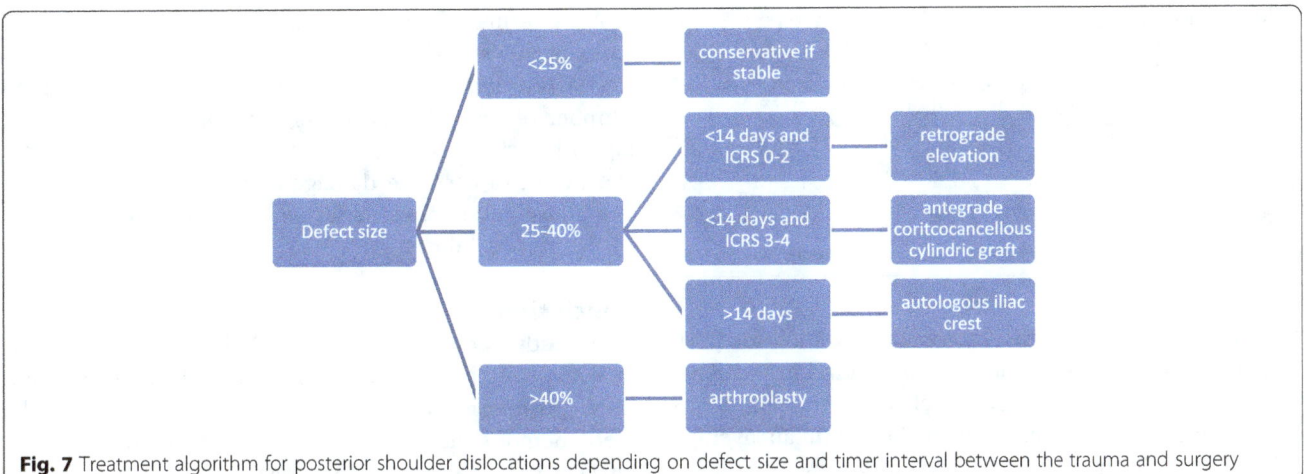

Fig. 7 Treatment algorithm for posterior shoulder dislocations depending on defect size and timer interval between the trauma and surgery

A complete minimum follow up of five years was achieved in all patients. There was an improvement in outcomes at five years compared with the one year results: 5.28 points in the DASH score, 7.58 points in the Constant score, 8 points in the ROWE score and 0.86 points on the VAS on average (Table 2). Patients who were treated with a corticocancellous graft of the iliac crest had the best results after one and five years within the small group of patients (year one: Dash 3.89, Constant 90.33, Rowe 86.67; year five: Dash 2.22, Constant 92.00, Rowe 93.33). This could be demonstrated in all evaluated scores as well as in the VAS (year one, 0.67; year five, 0.5) (Tables 3 and 4).

Discussion

Optimal treatment of the reverse Hill-Sachs lesion after posterior shoulder dislocation remains controversial. Due to the rare entity of this injury pattern, high numbers of cases in clinical trials are difficult to generate [17, 26]. The cause of traumatic, non-epileptic posterior dislocation is usually a direct force applied to the adducted and extended arm in internal rotation [3] while the mechanism in epilepsy is considered to be a high muscular force generating internal rotation in an adducted arm [27, 28]. Posterior dislocation of the humeral head may cause a posterior-directed shearing of the labrum or the bony glenoid rim [29, 30] but is primarily characterized by the osteochondral impression fracture of the ventromedial articular surface of the humeral head, the so-called reverse Hill-Sachs lesion [5, 31]. Concomitant neurovascular injuries or lesions of the rotator cuff occur much rarely after posterior dislocation [30, 32]. We observed two lesions of the labrum requiring operative treatment in addition to the reverse Hill-Sachs lesion in this study. These were detected during the diagnostic arthroscopy and accordingly fixed by suture anchors. We did not detect any rotator cuff injuries.

The treatment of posterior instability with a reverse Hill-Sachs lesion considers the arc of stability relative to the arc of rotation of the humeral head with respect to the glenoid surface. The treatment therefore largely depends on the size of the humeral head defect [33]. The surgical strategies are either: the optimization of the surface arc of rotation by restoration of the sphericity of the humeral head (and thereby optimizing the arc of stability), or the restriction of motion of the humeral head relative to the glenoid so that the arc of stability becomes equivalent to the more limited arc of rotation. Various techniques have been described to reconstruct

Table 1 Epidemiological data of the patients included in the study

Criteria	Specification	Total	
Total number of patients	Reverse Hill-Sachs lesion[n]	12	
Age	total [y (range)]	39 (17–55)	
Gender	male [n]	12	100%
	female [n]	0	0%
Treatment	Arthroscopic reduction and retrograde elevation [n]	5	42%
	Open reduction antegrade cylindric graft [n]	4	33%
	Iliac bone crest	3	25%
Cause of injury	High energy trauma [n]	9	75%
	Low energy trauma [n]	2	17%
	Eplilepsy [n]	1	8%

Table 2 Functional outcome and the VAS after one and five years showed better results in the five year follow up in all evaluated scores

Score	2010	2015
DASH	10.49 ± 2.57	5.21 ± 1.37
Constant	81.92 ± 3.10	89.50 ± 2.72
ROWE	72.92 ± 5.56	87.92 ± 3.61
VAS	1.67 ± 0.36	0.81 ± 0.19

Table 3 Functional outcome and the VAS showed the best results for patients treated with an iliac bone crest graft in 2015

Score 2015	Retrograde elevation (n = 5)	Antegrade cylindric graft (n = 4)	Iliac bone crest (n = 3)	p
DASH	7.33 ± 2.64	4.79 ± 2.02	2.22 ± 1.21	.39
Constant	89.80 ± 4.66	87.25 ± 5.59	92.00 ± 4.61	.84
ROWE	85.00 ± 7.25	87.50 ± 6.29	93.33 ± 3.33	.89
VAS	0.94 ± 0.30	0.88 ± 0.43	0.50 ± 0.29	.67

the joint surface defect by osteochondral allograft [34]. Miniaci and Gish performed osteochondral transplantation using fresh-frozen, size-matched allograft in 18 patients with a defect greater than 25% with an average follow-up of 50 months. The allografts were fixed with Kirschner wires [35]. Outcomes were reasonable with an average Constant score of 78.5 points. Several complications such as osteoarthritis, secondary sintering, subluxation and wire migration were noted. In another series, Diklic et al. recorded an average Constant score of 86.8 points with a follow-up period of 54 months after reconstruction using femoral allograft and fixation with cannulated screws [36]. Gerber and Lambert showed an average Constant score of 82 points in a group of 4 patients after reconstruction of the articular surface by femoral allograft [17]. Krackhart et al. recommended fixing the subscapularis tendon with suture anchors into the defect [37]. This leads to restriction of internal rotation [38].

Only patients with a defect size between 25 and 40% of the joint surface after posterior shoulder dislocation were included in our study. The patients were reviewed at a mean of one year and five years after surgery. Irrespective of the operative technique used in the present study, we observed a fair outcome with a mean Constant score of 81.92 and 89.50 points respectively. Over time, all of the scores showed an improvement, with low pain scores, related to exercise, at both time points. The best outcome for patients at both time-points was observed after using an autologous iliac crest cortico-cancellous bone graft. This could result from a lower secondary sintering rate of cortico-cancellous bone graft compared to retrograde elevation of the articular surface or antegrade cylindrical osteochondral grafting. These findings have

to be interpreted carefully due to the small number of cases of this study.

The limiting factor of this study remains the small number of cases. Nevertheless, we believe the treatment algorithm shown in Fig. 7 is very useful, since it includes the extent of cartilage damage and the interval between the injury and surgical treatment, in addition to the size of the humeral defect.

Conclusion

This study shows the results and techniques of reconstructive treatment options for reverse Hill-Sachs lesion after posterior shoulder dislocation. The best results were demonstrated in the reconstruction of the joint surface by autologous iliac crest grafts. The open approach does not appear to be a disadvantage for the functional outcome despite the invasiveness. In our opinion, the treatment algorithm of the reverse Hill - Sachs lesion should involve the superficial size of the defect, as well as the depth of the defect and the time interval between the dislocation and the surgical treatment.

Abbreviations

CT: Computed tomography; DASH: Disability of the arm, shoulder and hand; ICRS: International Cartilage Repair Society; MRI: Magnetic resonance imaging; SD: Standard Deviation; VAS: Visual analogue scale

Acknowledgements

Not applicable

Funding

There is no funding source.

Authors' contributions

MG has initiated the study, has made the data collection and interpretation. PZ has made the statistics, written the manuscript and has analyzed most of the data. SL and US have helped with analyzing the data and supervised the development of the study. All authors read and approved the final manuscript.

Competing interests

The authors declare that they have no competing interests.

Author details

[1]Department for Traumatology and Reconstructive Surgery, BG Trauma Center Tübingen, University of Tübingen, Schnarrenbergstr 95, 72076 Tuebingen, Germany. [2]Shoulder and Elbow Service, Royal National Orthopaedic Hospital, Stanmore HA7 4LP, UK.

Table 4 Functional outcome and the VAS showed the best results for patients treated with an iliac bone crest graft in 2010

Score 2010	Retrograde elevation (n = 5)	Antegrade cylindric graft (n = 4)	Iliac bone crest (n = 3)	p
DASH	12.17 ± 4.21	13.33 ± 5.28	3.89 ± 0.56	.18
Constant	79.00 ± 3.70	79.25 ± 7.33	90.33 ± 2.33	.31
ROWE	76.00 ± 8.57	58.75 ± 8.00	86.67 ± 8.33	.11
VAS	1.80 ± 0.37	2.25 ± 0.85	0.67 ± 0.33	.21

References

1. Kowalsky MS, Levine WN. Traumatic posterior glenohumeral dislocation: classification, pathoanatomy, diagnosis, and treatment. Orthop Clin North Am. 2008;39(4):519–33.
2. Hatzis N, Kaar TK, Wirth MA, Rockwood CA Jr. The often overlooked posterior dislocation of the shoulder. Tex Med. 2001;97(11):62–7.

Posterior shoulder dislocation with associated reverse Hill-Sachs lesion: treatment options and functional...

83

3. Robinson CM, Aderinto J. Posterior shoulder dislocations and fracture-dislocations. J Bone Joint Surg Am. 2005;87(3):639–50.

4. Hawkins RJ, Neer CS, 2nd, Pianta RM, Mendoza FX. Locked posterior dislocation of the shoulder. J Bone Joint Surg Am 1987;69(1):9–18.

5. Mc LH. Posterior dislocation of the shoulder. J Bone Joint Surg Am. 1952; 24(3):584–90.

6. Itoi E, Hatakeyama Y, Kido T, Sato T, Minagawa H, Wakabayashi I, Kobayashi M. A new method of immobilization after traumatic anterior dislocation of the shoulder: a preliminary study. J Shoulder Elb Surg. 2003;12(5):413–5.

7. Cooper A. On the dislocations of the os humeri upon the dorsum scapulae, and upon fractures near the shoulder joint. Guy's Hosp Rep. 1839;4:265–84.

8. Rowe CR, Zarins B. Chronic unreduced dislocations of the shoulder. J Bone Joint Surg Am. 1982;64(4):494–505.

9. Pfister U, Rohner H, Weller S. Diagnosis and therapy of traumatic posterior shoulder dislocations. Unfallchirurgie. 1985;11(1):12–6.

10. Irlenbusch L, Pyschik M, Hein W, Brehme K. Possibilities for the operative treatment of traumatic posterior shoulder dislocation. Unfallchirurg. 2008; 111(6):464–8.

11. O'Connor SJ, Jacknow AS. Posterior dislocation of the shoulder. AMA Arch Surg. 1956;72(3):479–91.

12. Wilson JC, Mc KF. Traumatic posterior dislocation of the humerus. J Bone Joint Surg Am. 1949;160(72):31A–1.

13. Schliemann B, Muder D, Gessmann J, Schildhauer TA, Seybold D. Locked posterior shoulder dislocation: treatment options and clinical outcomes. Arch Orthop Trauma Surg. 2011;131(8):1127–34.

14. Seybold D, Gekle C, Fehmer T, Pennekamp W, Muhr G, Kalicke T. Immobilization in external rotation after primary shoulder dislocation. Chirurg. 2006;77(9):821–6.

15. Bock P, Kluger R, Hintermann B. Anatomical reconstruction for reverse hill-Sachs lesions after posterior locked shoulder dislocation fracture: a case series of six patients. Arch Orthop Trauma Surg. 2007;127(7):543–8.

16. Hawkins RJ, fractures ARLD p h. Selecting treatment, avoiding pitfalls. Orthop Clin North Am. 1987;18(3):421–31.

17. Gerber C, Lambert SM. Allograft reconstruction of segmental defects of the humeral head for the treatment of chronic locked posterior dislocation of the shoulder. J Bone Joint Surg Am. 1996;78(3):376–82.

18. Surin V, Blader S, Markhede G, Sundholm K. Rotational osteotomy of the humerus for posterior instability of the shoulder. J Bone Joint Surg Am. 1990;72(2):181–6.

19. Checchia SL, Santos PD, Miyazaki AN. Surgical treatment of acute and chronic posterior fracture-dislocation of the shoulder. J Shoulder Elb Surg. 1998;7(1):53–65.

20. Sperling JW, Pring M, Antuna SA, Cofield RH. Shoulder arthroplasty for locked posterior dislocation of the shoulder. J Shoulder Elb Surg. 2004;13(5): 522–7.

21. Cicak N. Posterior dislocation of the shoulder. J Bone Joint Surg Br. 2004; 86(3):324–32.

22. Constant CR, Gerber C, Emery RJ, Sojbjerg JO, Gohlke F, Boileau P. A review of the constant score: modifications and guidelines for its use. J Shoulder Elb Surg. 2008;17(2):355–61.

23. Jensen KU, Bongaerts G, Bruhn R, Schneider S. Not all Rowe scores are the same! Which Rowe score do you use? J Shoulder Elb Surg. 2009;18(4):511–4.

24. Germann G, Wind G, Harth A. The DASH(disability of arm-shoulder-hand) questionnaire–a new instrument for evaluating upper extremity treatment outcome. Handchir Mikrochir Plast Chir. 1999;31(3):149–52.

25. Brittberg M, Winalski CS. Evaluation of cartilage injuries and repair. J Bone Joint Surg Am. 2003;85-A(Suppl 2):58–69.

26. Martinez AA, Calvo A, Domingo J, Cuenca J, Herrera A, Malillos M. Allograft reconstruction of segmental defects of the humeral head associated with posterior dislocations of the shoulder. Injury. 2008;39(3):319–22.

27. DeToledo JC, Seizures LMR, decubitus I. Aspiration, and shoulder dislocation: time to change the guidelines? Neurology. 2001;56(3):290–1.

28. DeToledo JC, Lowe MR, Ramsay RE. Restraining patients and shoulder dislocations during seizures. J Shoulder Elb Surg. 1999;8(4):300–2.

29. Ovesen J, dislocation SJOP s. Muscle and capsular lesions in cadaver experiments. Acta Orthop Scand. 1986;57(6):535–6.

30. Roberts A, Wickstrom J. Prognosis of posterior dislocation of the shoulder. Acta Orthop Scand. 1971;42(4):328–37.

31. Edelson G, Kelly I, Vigder F, Reis ND. A three-dimensional classification for fractures of the proximal humerus. J Bone Joint Surg Br. 2004;86(3):413–25.

32. Mestdagh H, Maynou C, Delobelle JM, Urvoy P, Butin E. Traumatic posterior dislocation of the shoulder in adults. Apropos of 25 cases. Ann Chir. 1994; 48(4):355–63.

33. Moroder P, Plachel F, Tauber M, Habermeyer P, Imhoff A, Liem D, Lill H, Resch H, Gerhardt C, Scheibel M. Risk of engagement of bipolar bone defects in posterior shoulder instability. Am J Sports Med. 2017;45(12): 2835–9. 363546517714456

34. Kropf EJ, Tjoumakaris FP, Sekiya JK. Arthroscopic shoulder stabilization: is there ever a need to open? Arthroscopy. 2007;23(7):779–84.

35. Miniaci A, Gish G. Management of Anterior Glenohumeral Instability Associated with Large Hill–Sachs Defects. Tech Shoulder Elbow Surg. 2004;5:170–5.

36. Diklic ID, Ganic ZD, Blagojevic ZD, Nho SJ, Romeo AA. Treatment of locked chronic posterior dislocation of the shoulder by reconstruction of the defect in the humeral head with an allograft. J Bone Joint Surg Br. 2010;92(1):71–6.

37. Krackhardt T, Schewe B, Albrecht D, Weise K. Arthroscopic fixation of the subscapularis tendon in the reverse Hill-Sachs lesion for traumatic unidirectional posterior dislocation of the shoulder. Arthroscopy. 2006;22(2):227. e1- e6

38. Verma NN, Sellards RA, Romeo AA. Arthroscopic reduction and repair of a locked posterior shoulder dislocation. Arthroscopy. 2006;22(11):1252. e1–5

12

Determinants of patient satisfaction following reconstructive shoulder surgery

Sascha J. Baettig[†], Karl Wieser[*†] and Christian Gerber

Abstract

Background: Obtaining patient satisfaction is a key goal of surgical treatment. It was the purpose of this study to identify pre-, peri- and postoperative factors determining patient satisfaction after shoulder surgery, quantify their relative importance and thereby allow the surgeon to focus on parameters, which will influence patient satisfaction.

Methods: We retrospectively reviewed 505 patients, who underwent either rotator cuff repair ($n = 216$) or total shoulder arthroplasty ($n = 289$). We examined 21 patient-specific and socio-demographic parameters as well as 31 values of the Constant-Score with regard to their impact on patient satisfaction.

Results: In the univariable analysis higher patient satisfaction was correlated with higher age, private health insurance, light physical work, retirement, primary surgery, non-smoking, absence of chronic alcohol abuse, absence of peri- or postoperative complications, operation performed by the medical director as well as various Constant Score sub-values ($p < 0.05$). In the multivariable analysis absence of peri- or postoperative complications ($p = 0.008$), little postoperative pain ($p = 0.0001$), a large range of postoperative active abduction ($p = 0.05$) and a high postoperative subjective shoulder value ($p = 0.0001$) were identified as independent prognostic factors for high satisfaction.

Conclusion: After reconstructive shoulder surgery particular attention should be paid to prevention of complications, excellent perioperative pain control and restoration of abduction during rehabilitation. This study is first step towards a preoperative prediction model of a subjectively successful surgery as well as a tool to exclude irrelevant parameters in clinical routine.

Keywords: Patient satisfaction, Determinants, Shoulder surgery, Rotator cuff repair, Shoulder arthroplasty, Reconstructive shoulder surgery, Satisfaction, Factors

Background

Subjective outcome parameters such as self-assessment of function, quality of life or patient satisfaction have become fundamental tools for outcome assessment of orthopaedic interventions [1]. Patient satisfaction is a reliable indicator of health care quality, enabling the comparison between different health care providers [2]. Patient reported outcomes may guide patients to choose their health care provider and could substantially influence competition in health care markets [3] [4]. Objective treatment success is essential, but not the only condition, which generates patient satisfaction [5, 6].

Many factors such as age [7–10], gender [7], marital status [11], occupation [8, 9, 11, 12], workers' compensation status [7–9, 13–17], presence of revision surgery after a previously failed operation [7], preoperative expectations [11], postoperative pain [8, 11, 12, 18, 19] and postoperative range of motion (i.e. internal rotation [8, 12], anteversion/elevation [10, 12, 18, 19] had already been identified to influence patient satisfaction after shoulder surgery. However, the majority of the above mentioned studies had substantial limitations in scope and or validity. But there exist a few other studies with excellent quality, which examine determinants of patient satisfaction after surgery in other articulations for example the knee [20, 21].

Patient satisfaction plays a pivotal and not thoroughly studied role in assessing surgical outcome. The identification of positive and negative predicting factors could

* Correspondence: karl.wieser@balgrist.ch
†Equal contributors
Orthopaedic Department, Balgrist University Hospital, University of Zurich, Forchstrasse 340, 8008 Zurich, Switzerland

lead to preoperative prediction models for determining the probability of an (un-)desired surgical outcome. It appears particularly important also to know parameters, which do not affect patients' postoperative satisfaction because it may help surgeon and therapist to avoid wasting energy in efforts not leading to improvement of patient satisfaction.

The purpose of this study was to systematically analyse as many allegedly relevant determinants in one evaluation and study their true influence on patient satisfaction following operative treatment of rotator cuff tears or osteoarthritis in a multivariable regression model.

Methods

Setting and patient selection

We retrospectively reviewed the shoulder database to identify patients, who had been treated in our institution, either with open or arthroscopic rotator cuff repair or implantation of a total or reverse shoulder arthroplasty between January 1999 and December 2011. In this time period we performed approximately 2500 surgeries, after randomization we selected 600 patients for the evaluation in this study. Patients with prospectively recorded, complete pre- and postoperative Constant Scores (CS), subjective shoulder value (SSV) and a documented postoperative patient satisfaction were included in this study. Out of the 600 selected patients, 505 patients met the mentioned criteria. For a patient with multiple monitoring consultations, we selected the data closest to 24 months after the index surgery for final analysis. Postoperative scores or patients' satisfaction obtained earlier than 12 or later than 60 months after index surgery were excluded. This study was approved by the Swiss Ethics Committees on research involving humans (KEK-ZH-2014-0377).

Independent factors potentially influencing patient satisfaction extracted from patients' charts comprised: (1) Age, (2) BMI, (3) gender, (4) marital status, (5) health insurance status, (6) occupation, (7 and 8) affected/dominant side, (9) opposite shoulder affected, (10) nature of injury (labour vs. leisure trauma vs. non-traumatic orthopaedic disease), (11) chronic nicotine abuse (> 10 pack-years), (12) chronic alcohol abuse (male: > 30 g; female: > 20 g/day [22]), (13) clinical position of the responsible surgeon, (14) length of follow-up, (15) number of non shoulder-specific previous operations, (16) Diabetes mellitus, (17) revision or primary surgery, (18) psychopharmacological drug use, (19) immunosuppressive medication, (20) peri- and/or postoperative complications (surgical site infection, iatrogenic neurological lesion, hematoma evacuation, extended intensive care unit stay), (21) chronic comorbidities (symptomatic cardio-vascular disease, COPD, asthma, autoimmune disease, neurologic (Parkinson disease, multiple sclerosis,

dementia), infectious disease (HIV, hepatitis A/B), endocrinological diseases, chronic cervical or lumbosacral pain syndrome, gastrointestinal diseases, gout and chronic renal insufficiency). The decisive date for gathering the information for parameters (4, 5, 6, 11, 12, 18, 19, 21) was the time of surgery. In addition, all values of the pre- and postoperative Constant Scores, the amount of improvement (delta) of those values as well as the pre- and postoperative SSV were analysed regarding their implication on patient satisfaction.

Outcome measure

We identified 505 patients, who underwent either rotator cuff repair ($n = 216$) or shoulder arthroplasty (total or reverse) ($n = 289$) and met the above mentioned inclusion criteria for this investigation. The study comprised 271 men and 234 women. The age of the 505 patients ranged from 17 to 90 years old (mean: 61.4 years, SD: 12.3 years). The surgery had involved 71% dominant shoulders. The mean time period between surgery and the measurement of the patients' satisfaction was 23.6 months (range: 12–60 months) (Table 1). Our primary target variable was patient satisfaction, which was documented at the postoperative consultation closest to 24 months after index surgery. The patients graded their satisfaction as: not satisfied, rather dissatisfied, rather satisfied and very satisfied (Table 2).

Statistical methods

Statistical analysis was performed under the supervision of an experienced biomedical statistician using IBM SPSS Statistics, Version 21.0, Armonk, NY. The level of

Table 1 Patients'Characteristics

Variable	Data
Number of patients analysed in total	505
Mean age of the patient collective	61.4 years (range 17–90 years)
Mean time period between surgery and satisfaction measurement	23.6 months
Gender	Male = 271, Female = 234
Family Status	Married = 328, Single = 169
Number of patients retired	194 (38.4%)
Number of patients with a traumatic origin of injury	340 (67.3%)
Mean BMI of the patient collective	26.9 (range 15.7–48.0)
Number of patients smoking	89 (17.6%)
Affected side	Right = 339, Left = 166
Number of patients with the dominant shoulder involved	358 (70.9%)
Mean preoperative Constant Score	40.4 (range 2.0–100.0) points
Mean postoperative Constant Score	59.6 (range 3.0–100.0) points

Table 2 Patients' satisfaction

Patients' satisfaction	Rotator cuff reconstruction	Arthroplasty
Highly satisfied patients	60 (27,8%)	122 (42.2%)
Rather satisfied patients	50 (23.1%)	80 (27.7%)
Rather dissatisfied patients	52 (24.1%)	57 (19.7%)
Dissatisfied patients	54 (25%)	30 (10.4%)
	216 (100%)	289 (100%)

significance was set at ($p < 0.05$). Due to the numerous statistical comparisons we calculated an additional Bonferroni-corrected level of significance ($p = 0.00095$). To increase the significance and validity of the evaluation particularly with regard to the multivariable regression model we divided the patients in a satisfied (including rather satisfied and very satisfied, $n = 312$) and dissatisfied (including rather satisfied and not satisfied, $n = 193$) group. Pearson Chi squared test was performed for categorical determinants in the univariable analysis. The effect of the numeric values was analysed with the non-parametric test of Mann and Whitney. Univariable significant variables were integrated in a logistic regression dependent on likelihood-quotients (calculated backwards), to identify independent prognostic factors of patients' satisfaction. For the delta of score sub-values a multivariable analysis was not accurate due to its dependency on pre- and postoperative values.

Results
Univariable analysis
The univariable analysis revealed that, higher age ($p = 0.0001$), private health insurance (p = 0.0001), primary surgery (p = 0.0001), non-smoking ($p = 0.001$), absence of intra- or postoperative complications (p = 0.001) and the absence of chronic alcoholism ($p = 0.039$) were associated with high patient satisfaction. Retired patients or patients with light physical work were significantly more satisfied than manual workers and especially significantly more than patients, who were job seeking or had ongoing workers compensation claims ($p = 0.0001$). Furthermore, patients treated by the medical director showed a higher satisfaction than patients treated by a senior surgeon or senior consultant ($p = 0.045$). Pursuant to our results there was no significant correlation between patients satisfaction and BMI ($p = 0.886$), gender ($p = 0.238$), marital status ($p = 0.442$), affected side ($p = 0.502$), dominance ($p = 0.521$), opposite shoulder affected ($p = 0.363$), nature of the injury ($p = 0.139$), more than 2 previous non shoulder-specific operations ($p = 0.548$), chronic comorbidity ($p = 0.382$), diabetes mellitus ($p = 0.171$), regular consumption of psychotropic drugs ($p = 0.741$) and immunosuppressive medication ($p = 0.177$). Compared to the "Bonferroni-corrected" level of significance ($p = 0.00095$) following determinants forfeit their

significance: non-smoking, the absence of chronic alcoholism, the absence of intra- and postoperative complications and the status of the responsible surgeon (Tables 3 and 4).

The analysis of the *pre*operative (Constant) score identified the following factors to be associated with higher patient satisfaction: higher activities of daily living ($p = 0.0001$), higher preoperative subjective shoulder value (p = 0.0001) and a higher range of external rotation ($p = 0.008$). All constituent parts of the *post*operative Constant Score (including postoperative subjective shoulder value) had an influence on higher patient satisfaction except the range of the internal ($p = 0.118$) and external rotation ($p = 0.982$). Lastly, a higher improvement (delta) of the Constant Score had a positive influence on patient satisfaction. Compared to the "Bonferroni-corrected" level of significance ($p = 0.00095$) the preoperative age-adjusted Constant Score, the preoperative range of external rotation and the improvement of internal rotation loose their significance. (Table 4).

Multivariable analysis
Multivariable analysis retained as independent determinants: absence of intra- or postoperative complications ($p = 0.008$), low postoperative pain ($p = 0.0001$), high postoperative subjective shoulder value (p = 0.0001) and a large range of postoperative abduction ($p = 0.05$). Primary surgery ($p = 0.062$) and a high range of preoperative external rotation ($p = 0.064$) showed a trend to higher satisfaction but missed the level of significance (Tables 3 and 4).

Discussion
Subjective outcome research has become much more relevant over the last decades [11]. A key capacity of patient satisfaction is the opportunity to critically assess medical outcome or treatment methods. It offers new tools to compare procedures and health care providers or enables the validation of health care quality of an existing environment [8]. The purpose of this study was to investigate how patient satisfaction after a rotator cuff repair or an implantation of a shoulder arthroplasty is composed and to establish a list with all determinants of ultimate patient satisfaction an orthopaedic surgeon should consider. We confirmed our hypothesis and identified various determinants and score values, which are associated with patient satisfaction.

Despite a rather large study population of 505 patients we are aware of potential limitations of this study. First this is a retrospective study of data, which were prospectively collected in a standardized fashion. Patients who wish or consent to undergo surgery may be more positive than those who have elected not to be operated on and who are not included in this study. Further, we

Table 3 Results

Univariable analysis				Multivariable
Determinant	Number of pat.	Satisfied patt. *	*p*-value	*p*-value
Type of operation			0.0001**	0.0001
Rotator cuff	216	51%		
Totalarthroplasty	289	73%		
Gender			0.238	n.s.
Male	271	59%		
Female	234	65%		
Marital status			0.442	n.s.
Single	169	64%		
Married	328	60%		
Health insurance			0.0001**	n.s.
Statutory	226	53%		
Private	266	69%		
Occupation			0.0001**	n.s.
Light physical work	195	64%		
Heavy physical work	90	47%		
Retired	194	69%		
Job-seeking/IV-Ins.	22	36%		
Affected side			0.502	n.s.
Right	339	61%		
Left	166	64%		
Dominance			0.521	n.s.
Dominant	358	61%		
Adominant	147	64%		
Opposite shoulder affected			0.363	n.s.
No	428	63%		
Yes	77	57%		
Nature of the injury			0.139	n.s.
Trauma during leisure time	294	59%		
Trauma during labour time	46	61%		
Non-traumatic orthopaedic disease	165	68%		
Revision surgery			0.0001**	0.062***
Yes	225	49%		
No	280	72%		
Non shoulder-specific previous operations			0.548	n.s.
Less than 2	306	61%		
More than 2	197	63%		
Smoking			0.001	n.s.
No	416	65%		
Yes	89	46%		
Alcohol abuse			0.039	n.s.
No	468	63%		
Yes	37	46%		

Table 3 Results *(Continued)*

Univariable analysis				Multivariable
Responsible surgeon			0.045	n.s.
Senior surgeon	70	61%		
Senior consultant	137	53%		
Medical director	298	66%		
Chronic Comorbidity			0.382	n.s.
No	371	61%		
Yes	134	65%		
Diabetes mellitus			0.171	n.s.
No	475	63%		
Yes	30	50%		
Psychotropic drugs			0.741	n.s.
No	417	62%		
Yes	88	60%		
Immunosuppressive medication			0.177	n.s.
No	478	61%		
Yes	27	74%		
Complications (intra-,postOP)			0.001	0.008
No	459	64%		
Yes	46	39%		

*Contains only very satisfied and satisfied patients
**Significant compared to "Bonferroni-corrected" p-value ($p = 0.00095$)
***Without significance

selected patients with complete data sets: this may contain a bias as patients not reporting back may have other perceptions of satisfaction. However, overall satisfaction of our population is compared to other studies rather reduced [18] and as well to other orthopaedic interventions [23]. This fact is probably related with the selection criteria because dissatisfied Patient had more frequent consultations and more complete data. Further, we are aware of other potential influencing factors like orthopaedic disease, type of surgery, which we excluded on purpose from the analysis as we really focused on other independent factors influencing the patients satisfaction.

Despite these limitations we were able to identify factors, which showed neither in the multi- nor univariable analysis any influence on patients satisfaction:

Gender does not play a relevant role in the determination of patient satisfaction. This fact is agreed upon in the orthopaedic literature for rotator cuff repairs [9, 11, 12, 24], implantations of hemi- and total arthroplasties [8] or shoulder stabilisations [19, 25]. In addition, our findings are in accordance with the results of the study of Tashjian et al. [11], which shows that *marital status* is not a relevant determinant of patient satisfaction after rotator cuff repair. Furthermore, we found in our

evaluation that the *affected side*, the *dominance*, the case of *both shoulders affected* or the *nature of the injury* does not play a decisive role for the patients' postoperative satisfaction. This result corresponds with the result of Kim et al. [9] concerning the determinant dominance of the affected shoulder.

It has been postulated in literature that psychosocial factors, especially preoperative psychological distress, such as depression, is associated with poor clinical outcome [26–28]. We have tried to incorporate various psychiatric diagnoses in a single variable and investigated the effect of psychotropic drugs on patient postoperative satisfaction. A correlation between those variables could, however, not be confirmed in our evaluation. In addition, we scrutinized the potential effect of different *chronic comorbidities*. In accordance with the results of Tashjian et al. [11] and Jacobs et al. [18] we were unable to find a correlation. Pursuant to our knowledge, this is the first study, which has analysed specific determinants like the presence of *immunosuppressive medication* or *non-orthopaedic previous surgeries*. However, none of these determinants showed an influence on the resulting satisfaction.

Despite all other sub-values of the postoperative Constant score, neither *postoperative internal- nor*

Table 4 Result Scores

Determinant	Average value	Higher satisfaction with:	p-value	Multivariable Analysis
Age	61.4	higher	0.0001[**]	n.s.
Length of follow-up	23.6		0.226	
BMI	26.9		0.886	n.s.
Preoperative Constant Score				
Pain (0–15 pts.)	6.2	higher [*]	0.45	n.s.
Activities of daily living (0–10 pts.)	4	higher	0.0001[**]	n.s.
Reach of the hand (0–10 pts.)	6.2		0.857	n.s.
Anteversion (0–10 pts.)	5.5		0.901	n.s.
Abduction (0–10 pts.)	4.9		0.857	n.s.
External rotation (in degrees)	30.4	higher	0.008	n.s.
Internal rotation (in degrees)	29.7		0.423	n.s.
Force (0–25 pts.)	3.7		0.628	n.s.
Total CS (0–100 pts.)	40.4		0.331	n.s.
Total CS, age-adjusted (%)	50		0.05	n.s.
Preoperative subjective shoulder value (%)	36.3	higher	0.0001[**]	n.s.
Postoperative Scores				
Pain (0–15 pts.)	10.5	higher [*]	0.0001[**]	0.0001
Activities of daily living (0–10 pts.)	6.9	higher	0.0001[**]	n.s.
Reach of the hand (0–10 pts.)	8.2	higher	0.0001[**]	n.s.
Anteversion (0–10 pts.)	7.1	higher	0.0001[**]	n.s.
Abduction (0–10 pts.)	6.8	higher	0.0001[**]	0.05
External rotation (in degrees)	35		0.118	n.s.
Internal rotation (in degrees)	22.6		0.982	n.s.
Force (0–25 pts.)	6.8	higher	0.0001[**]	n.s.
Total CS (0–100 pts.)	59.6	higher	0.0001[**]	n.s.
Total CS, age-adjusted (%)	74.2	higher	0.0001[**]	n.s.
Postoperative subjective shoulder value (%)	63.3	higher	0.0001[**]	0.0001
Changes Constant Score				
Pain	4.3		0.0001[**]	***
Activities of daily living	2.9		0.0001[**]	***
Reach of the hand	2		0.0001[**]	***
Anteversion	1.1		0.0001[**]	***
Abduction	1.9		0.0001[**]	***
External rotation	4.6		0.0001[**]	***
Internal rotation	−7.1		0.049	***
Force	3.1		0.0001[**]	***
Total Constant Score (Pts.)	19.2		0.0001[**]	***

[*]A high pain score means low effective pain in the measurement of the Constant Score
[**]Significant compared to "Bonferroni-corrected" p-value ($p = 0.00095$)
[***]Multivariable analysis is not possible

external rotation showed a correlation with higher patient satisfaction. Although previous reports did show a positive correlation between internal rotation and patients satisfaction [8, 12], postoperative external rotation was also found to be of little importance regarding patients satisfaction [12, 18, 19]. A possible explanation for the unexpectedly missing correlation between patients' satisfaction and internal and external rotation might be the fact, that it is not the maximum amount of rotation but the absence of a necessary minimal achievement, which indisputably will influence patient satisfaction.

Furthermore this investigation revealed factors, which seem to have some influence on patients satisfaction (significant influence in univariable analysis) but might be confounded and influenced by other factors (no significant influence in multivariable analysis):

Age as a determinant is being discussed very controversially in the orthopaedic literature. Our results indicate a higher satisfaction of older patients, which is in accordance to the results of Chen et al. [8] and Kim et al. [9] for shoulder arthroplasties and rotator cuff repairs. Watson et al. [7] proposes that younger patients have higher demands and expectations of their shoulder and are therefore more easily dissatisfied with imperfect healing. There is, however also a number of publications, which deny a correlation between increasing age and higher patient satisfaction [12, 14, 19, 24, 25].

In our study, patients with a *private health care insurance* reached a significantly higher patient satisfaction than patients with a statutory health insurance. Furthermore, *patients receiving treatment by the chief of the department* seem to reach a higher satisfaction level than patients treated by (senior) consultants.

Our finding that *employed and retired patients* tend to be more satisfied than *unemployed and disabled patients* are in accordance with the results of the studies by Kim et al. [9] and Tashjian et al. [11]. Furthermore our data confirms the often reported correlation between *workers' compensation claims* and a lower patient satisfaction [7–9, 13–17, 29, 30]. Also *postoperative anteversion/elevation* is an established determinant of the patient satisfaction in the orthopaedic literature [10, 12, 18, 19]. The results of our evaluation further support this correlation.

Also chronic alcohol abuse or a history of smoking (more than 10 pack-years) was associated with a low patient satisfaction. The later finding is contrary to the findings of Tashjian et al. [11]. A possible explanation for our result is the known impaired healing potential and the diminished collagen production of a chronic smoker [31–33].

Finally we were able to identify factors, which turned out to independently influence patients' satisfaction (significant correlation in uni- and multivariable analysis):

As expected, remaining *pain* was identified to negatively influence patient satisfaction. This is in consensus to other published results for various shoulder interventions [8, 11, 12, 18, 19]. Our retrospective data analysis makes it however impossible to analyse the interesting question regarding the influence of peri- or immediate postoperative pain on the long-term outcome.

Furthermore the presence of *peri- or postoperative complications* affects patient satisfaction negatively, which is not unexpected, but to our knowledge so far unreported in the literature. In addition to that we analysed the influence of needed *revision surgery*, which negatively influenced patients satisfaction in the univariable analysis but showed only a trend ($p = 0.062$) in multivariable analysis.

Postoperative abduction was the only subvalue of the Constant Score, which turned out to independently positive influence patient satisfaction. This correlation seems to be unreported so far in orthopaedic literature and we should possibly focus even more on this determinant in postoperative rehabilitation.

The distinct correlation between patient satisfaction and the *postoperative subjective shoulder value* supports the validity of this analysis and clarifies the resemblance between these two subjective outcome parameters.

Conclusion

This investigation establishes that the absence of perioperative complication, excellent control of postoperative pain, surprisingly active abduction in the scapular plane (not elevation!) are associated with high patient satisfaction after rotator cuff repair or shoulder arthroplasty. It is, however, particularly important, that factors such as retirement, light physical work, private health insurance status, non-smoking, absence of chronic alcohol abuse, older age or receiving treatment by the chief of the department, were correlated with higher patient satisfaction independent of the pathology and type of surgery. On the other hand our results document that in view of patient satisfaction the patients' gender, marital status, dominance of the shoulder, nature of the injury, previous general operations, comorbidities, diabetes mellitus, psychotropic drugs or immunosuppressive medication are not associated with the ultimate subjective result. These findings may help to inform patients on their risks, to select patients for surgery and to focus peri- and postoperative treatment on the few modifiable factors identified to increase patient satisfaction.

Abbreviations

BMI: Body Mass Index; COPD: Chronic obstructive pulmonary disease; CS: Constant Shoulder Score; HIV: Human immunodeficiency virus; n.s.: Not significant; Pat: Patients; SD: Standard deviation; SSV: Subjective Shoulder Value

Acknowledgements

Prof. Dr. Burkhardt Seifert, statistical supervision.

Funding

No funding was obtained for this study.

Authors' contributions

SB participated in the design and conception of the study, coordination, data acquisition and interpretation of the results. He performed the statistical analysis and helped to draft the manuscript and it's publication. KW participated in the design and conception of the study, coordination and interpretation of the results. He helped to draft the manuscript and it's publication. CG participated in the design of the study and helped to draft the manuscript. The manuscript has been read and approved by all authors, which all believe it represents an honest work.

Competing interests
The authors declare that they have no competing interests.

References
1. Marks M, Herren DB, Vliet Vlieland TP, Simmen BR, Angst F, Goldhahn J. Determinants of patient satisfaction after orthopedic interventions to the hand: a review of the literature. J Hand Ther. 2011;24:303–12. doi: 10.1016/j.jht.2011.04.004.
2. Kowalski C, Ommen O, Steinhausen S, Pfaff H. Patientenzufriedenheit und ihre Determinanten. In: Pfaff H, editor. Lehrbuch Versorgungsforschung: Schattauer Verlag; 2011. p. 69–71(ISBN No. 978-3-7945-2797-7).
3. Haseborg F, Zastrau R. Qualität, Markenbildung und Krankenhauswahlentscheidung - Implikationen der neuen Qualitätstransparenz für das Krankenhausmarketing. In: Klauber J, editor. Krankenhausreport 2004 - Schwerpunkt Qualitätstransparenz: Schattauer Verlag; 2005. p.151–63 (ISBN No. 3-7945-2350-4).
4. Töpfer A. Erfolgreiches Changemanagement im Krankenhaus: Springer Berlin Heidelberg; 2006. p. 3–23 (ISBN No. 978-3-540-37208-0).
5. Wüthrich-Schneider DE. Patientenzufriedenheit - Wie verstehen? Schweizerische Ärztezeitung. 2000;81:1046–8.
6. Kowalski C, Ommen O, Steinhausen S, Pfaff H. Patientenzufriedenheit und ihre Determinanten. In: Pfaff H, editor. Lehrbuch Versorgungsforschung: Schattauer Verlag; 2011. p. 69. (ISBN No. 978-3-7945-2797-7).
7. Watson EM, Sonnabend DH. Outcome of rotator cuff repair. Journal of Shoulder Elbow Surgery. 2002;11:201–11. doi: 10.1067/mse.2002.122271.
8. Chen AL, Bain EB, Horan MP, Hawkins RJ. Determinants of patient satisfaction with outcome after shoulder arthroplasty. J Shoulder Elb Surg. 2007;16:25–30. doi: 10.1016/j.jse.2006.04.013.
9. Kim HM, Caldwell JM, Buza JA, Fink LA, Ahmad CS, Bigliani LU, et al. Factors affecting satisfaction and shoulder function in patients with a recurrent rotator cuff tear. J Bone Joint Surg Am. 2014;96:106–12. doi: 10.2106/jbjs.l.01649.
10. Muh SJ, Streit JJ, Wanner JP, Lenarz CJ, Shishani Y, Rowland DY, et al. Early follow-up of reverse total shoulder arthroplasty in patients sixty years of age or younger. J Bone Joint Surg Am. 2013;95:1877–83. doi: 10.2106/jbjs.l.10005.
11. Tashjian RZ, Bradley MP, Tocci S, Rey J, Henn RF, Green A. Factors influencing patient satisfaction after rotator cuff repair. J Shoulder Elb Surg. 2007;16:752–8. doi: 10.1016/j.jse.2007.02.136.
12. O'Holleran JD, Kocher MS, Horan MP, Briggs KK, Hawkins RJ. Determinants of patient satisfaction with outcome after rotator cuff surgery. J Bone Joint Surg Am. 2005;87:121–6. doi: 10.2106/jbjs.c.01316.
13. Morris BJ, Haigler RE, Laughlin MS, Elkousy HA, Gartsman GM, Edwards TB. Workers' compensation claims and outcomes after reverse shoulder arthroplasty. J Shoulder Elb Surg. 2015;24:453–9. doi: 10.1016/j.jse.2014.07.009.
14. Denard PJ, Ladermann A, Burkhart SS. Long-term outcome after arthroscopic repair of type II SLAP lesions: results according to age and workers' compensation status. Arthroscopy. 2012;28:451–7. doi: 10.1016/j.arthro.2011.09.005.
15. Henn RF, Tashjian RZ, Kang L, Green A. Patients with workers' compensation claims have worse outcomes after rotator cuff repair. J Bone Joint Surg Am. 2008;90:2105–13. doi: 10.2106/jbjs.f.00260.
16. Misamore GW, Ziegler DW, Rushton JL. Repair of the rotator cuff. A comparison of results in two populations of patients. J Bone Joint Surg Am. 1995;77:1335–9.
17. Viola RW, Boatright KC, Smith KL, Sidles JA, Matsen FA. Do shoulder patients insured by workers' compensation present with worse self-assessed function and health status? J Shoulder Elb Surg. 2000;9:368–72. doi: 10.1067/mse.2000.107391.
18. Jacobs CA, Morris BJ, Sciascia AD, Edwards TB. Comparison of satisfied and dissatisfied patients 2 to 5 years after anatomic total shoulder arthroplasty. J Shoulder Elb Surg. 2016; doi: 10.1016/j.jse.2015.12.001. [Epub ahead of print].
19. Yeargan SA, Briggs KK, Horan MP, Black AK, Hawkins RJ. Determinants of patient satisfaction following surgery for multidirectional instability. Orthopedics. 2008;31:647.
20. Choi YJ, Ra HJ. Patient satisfaction after Total knee arthroplasty. Knee Surg Relat Res. 2016;28(1):1–15. doi: 10.5792/ksrr.2016.28.1.1.
21. Maratt JD, Lee YY, Lyman S, Westrich GH. Predictors of satisfaction following Total knee arthroplasty. J Arthroplast. 2015;30(7):1142–5. doi: 10.1016/j.arth.2015.01.039.
22. Anderson P, Cremona A, Paton A, Turner C, Wallace P. The risk of alcohol. Addiction. 1993;88:1493–508.
23. J Jacobs CA, Christensen CP. Factors influencing patient satisfaction two to five years after primary total knee arthroplasty. J Arthroplast. 2014;29:1189–91. https://doi.org/10.1016/j.arth.2014.01.008.
24. JH O, Kim SH, Ji HM, Jo KH, Bin SW, Gong HS. Prognostic factors affecting anatomic outcome of rotator cuff repair and correlation with functional outcome. Arthroscopy. 2009;25:30–9. doi: 10.1016/j.arthro.2008.08.010.
25. Schroder CP, Skare O, Gjengedal E, Uppheim G, Reikeras O, Brox JI. Long-term results after SLAP repair: a 5-year follow-up study of 107 patients with comparison of patients aged over and under 40 years. Arthroscopy. 2012;28:1601–7. doi: 10.1016/j.arthro.2012.02.025.
26. Cho CH, Seo HJ, Bae KC, Lee KJ, Hwang I, Warner JJ. The impact of depression and anxiety on self-assessed pain, disability, and quality of life in patients scheduled for rotator cuff repair. J Shoulder Elb Surg. 2013;22:1160–6. doi: 10.1016/j.jse.2013.02.006.
27. Ackerman IN, Graves SE, Bennell KL, Osborne RH. Evaluating quality of life in hip and knee replacement: psychometric properties of the World Health Organization quality of life short version instrument. Arthritis Rheum. 2006;55:583–90. doi: 10.1002/art.22107.
28. Bot AG, Menendez ME, Neuhaus V, Ring D. The influence of psychiatric comorbidity on perioperative outcomes after shoulder arthroplasty. J Shoulder Elb Surg. 2014;23:519–27. doi: 10.1016/j.jse.2013.12.006.
29. McKee MD, Yoo DJ. The effect of surgery for rotator cuff disease on general health status. Results of a prospective trial. J Bone Joint Surg Am. 2000;82-A:970–9.
30. Balyk R, Luciak-Corea C, Otto D, Baysal D, Beaupre L. Do outcomes differ after rotator cuff repair for patients receiving workers' compensation? Clin Orthop Relat Res. 2008;466:3025–33. doi: 10.1007/s11999-008-0475-1.
31. Lee JJ, Patel R, Biermann JS, Dougherty PJ. The musculoskeletal effects of cigarette smoking. J Bone Joint Surg Am. 2013;95:850–9. doi: 10.2106/jbjs.l.00375.
32. Lovich SF, Arnold PG. The effect of smoking on muscle transposition. Plast Reconstr Surg. 1994;93:825–8.
33. Jorgensen LN, Kallehave F, Christensen E, Siana JE, Gottrup F. Less collagen production in smokers. Surgery. 1998;123:450–5.

13

Are paraspinous intramuscular injections of botulinum toxin a (BoNT-A) efficient in the treatment of chronic low-back pain? A randomised, double-blinded crossover trial

Mélanie Cogné[1,2,3]*, Hervé Petit[2], Alexandre Creuzé[2], Dominique Liguoro[4] and Mathieu de Seze[2,3]

Abstract

Background: Treatment for patients with chronic low-back pain (LBP) is a public health issue. Intramuscular injections of botulinum toxin A (BoNT-A) have shown an analgesic effect on LBP in two previous randomized controlled studies. The objective of the study was to verify the efficacy of paravertebral injections of BoNT-A in patients with LBP.

Methods: Patients were included in this phase 3 randomized double-blinded trial comparing the efficacy of BoNT-A versus placebo in a crossover study on LBP. Both groups received 200 units of BoNT-A in paravertebral muscles or a placebo, and vice versa at Day 120. The main judgment criterion was LBP intensity 1 month after the injections, evaluated by using a visual pain scale (VAS). Secondary assessment criteria included: LBP intensity 90 and 120 days after injection day; number of days when an allowed antalgic oral treatment was needed in between each evaluation; functional disability measured by the Quebec Back Pain Disability Scale; quality of life; inability to work; patient satisfaction in relation to the treatment's effect; spinal mobility; and strength of spinal muscles, measured by isokinetic technique.

Results: Nineteen patients completed the study. There was no significant difference between the groups' average LBP during the last 8 days at Day30 ($p = 0.97$). There was no significant difference between the two groups regarding the secondary assessment criteria ($p > 0.05$).

Conclusions: Injections of BoNT-A in the paravertebral muscles were not found to be effective to relieve chronic LBP. The limits of the study are that the dose of BoNT-A used was lower than in other studies, and that the limited number of patients included may explain the negative results.

Trial registrations: Identifiers: NCT03181802. Unique Protocol ID: CHUBX2003.

Keywords: Low-back pain, Botulinum toxin, Disability, Function, Quality of life, Work

Background

Chronic low-back pain (LBP) is a public health problem that concerns 5 to 7% of the general occidental population [1] and has a significant impact on the quality of life of its sufferers [2].

Since the significance of lumbar stiffness in relation to contraction of the erector spinae muscles has been linked to the level of intensity of LBP [3], the lumbar erector spinae muscles have become a therapeutic target. Many recent arguments purport that paravertebral muscles have a predominant pathogenic role in perpetuating chronic back pain. During spinal movements, paravertebral muscles' activity, recorded by electromyography, show abnormalities in subjects with low-back pain compared to subjects without LBP. A decrease in the power ratio between the erector spinae and flexor spinal muscles, measured by isokinetic techniques, is associated with chronic low-back pain. Finally, the significance of lumbar stiffness in relation to the erector spinae muscles contracting is linked to the level of intensity of low-back pain [3].

* Correspondence: melaniecogne@hotmail.fr
[1]Service de Médecine Physique et de Réadaptation, hôpital Raymond Poincaré, 92380 Garches, France
[2]Service de Médecine Physique et de Réadaptation, CHU de Bordeaux, 33076 Bordeaux, France
Full list of author information is available at the end of the article

Local muscular treatments have already been tried such as physiotherapy, massage, infrared therapy and botulinum toxin A (BoNT-A) [4–6].

In addition to its muscle-relaxing effect, local intramuscular injections of BoNT-A have also shown an analgesic effect on pain related to dystonia, tension headaches, myofascial pain syndrome and chronic neck pain [7–11]. This effect is usually reversible after 3 months. Foster et al. [4] used BoNT-A A for its peripheral muscle relaxant action as a local intramuscular treatment of chronic LBP. This double-blinded, placebo, controlled trial in 31 patients showed that paravertebral administration of BoNT-A in patients with chronic LBP relieved pain and improved function at 3 and 8 weeks after treatment. Machado et al. [6] showed also in a randomized controlled trial that BoNT-A injections relieved pain and improved quality of life of 19 patients at 4 weeks. Further open studies have been performed to value the efficacy of BoNT-A in patients with chronic LBP [12–15] but all of them aimed to establish predictive factors of pain relief, and the efficacy was limited to 3 months. A Cochrane meta-analysis [16] concluded that "there was low quality evidence in the short term, and very low quality in the intermediate term, that BoNT-A injections reduced pain intensity more effectively than saline injections in participants with LBP" and that "there was very low quality evidence that BoNT-A injections compared to corticosteroid injections could reduce chronic LBP intensity in the short term".

Studying the therapeutic effect of paravertebral injections of BoNT-A requires further studies to confirm the reported short-term therapeutic effect and to determine potential predictive factors of efficacy.

Objectives of this trial

Main objective: To evaluate the analgesic effect 1 month after a single injection of 200 IU of BoNT-A in 10 bilateral paravertebral intramuscular points for treating chronic LBP.

Secondary objectives

- To evaluate the analgesic effect of paravertebral injections of BoNT-A 3 months after its administration in chronic LBP sufferers.
- To measure the impact of paravertebral injections of 200 IU of BoNT-A in a single administration on lumbar stiffness and on spinal extensor muscle strength in patients with chronic LBP.
- To search for predictive factors of the analgesic effect of BoNT-A injections.

Materials and methods

This study was a randomized, double-blinded, placebo-controlled phase 3 trial comparing BoNT-A Type A

injections (Botox) to a placebo in patients with chronic LBP (Level 2, OCEBM Levels of Evidence Working Group*, "The Oxford 2011 Levels of Evidence"). This superiority trial obtained support from the French Hospital Clinical Research Project (PHRC).

The number of participants included in the study was similar as those included in the previous study (see [4]), that showed a strong positive effect of BoNT-A injections on LBP. Furthermore, the design of our study (i.e. a crossover) increased the power of the statistical analysis. In this context, 60 inclusions were planned (30 in each group). Nevertheless, regular intermediary analyses were planned by an independent scientific committee, to ensure that the trial did not present any secondary effect, or that we could conclude in an intermediary step that BoNT-A was inefficient in pain relief. After obtaining a similar number of injections than Foster, the study was stopped by the scientific committee, because there was no trend in pain relief.

Ethics, consent and permissions

This trial obtained the approval of a French ethics Committee (2003/02) and all participants received an information note and gave their written informed consent. The clinical trial registration number was: Identifiers: NCT03181802, Unique Protocol ID: CHUBX2003.

Population

The patients included were consulted by Physical and Rehabilitation Medicine spinal pathology specialists at the University Hospital of Bordeaux, met the eligibility criteria, and volunteered to participate in the study.

Inclusion criteria were: LBP defined as a pain located between the thoracic lumbar hinge and the gluteal sulcus, where pain had evolved over a period of 6 months despite well conducted medical treatment, self-assessed lumbar pain intensity over 50 mm long on a visual analogue scale of 100 mm (0 = no pain; 100 = maximal pain), having been on sick leave for 60 or more days in the year preceding the inclusion (in order to include patients with high consequences of chronic low-back pain on their work), the same long-term chronic pain treatment for at least 6 weeks, and a paravertebral painful point pressure.

Exclusion criteria were: age under 18 or over 55 years (to avoid secondary causes of low back pain, like spinal tumor), ongoing pregnancy or breast-feeding, a neuromuscular pathology (myasthenia gravis, amyotrophic lateral sclerosis, myopathy, polymyositis), aminoglycoside treatment at the time of inclusion, skin infection at injection points, diabetes and alcoholism (in order to avoid other etiologies of chronic pain), a history of injecting BoNT-A A, anticoagulation treatment, sciatica, suspected spinal inflammatory disorder (spondylitis, inflammatory rheumatism, tumoral pathology), a failed back surgery syndrome (when surgery failed to relieve low-back pain), incapacity to stand, cardiorespiratory deficiency which does not allow the isokinetic exploration of the spinal muscles, cognitive disorders limiting patient participation, conflicts of interest owing to existing pain (unconsolidated work accident, ongoing damage compensation). Spine infection, tumour or trauma had been specifically excluded by an MRI done by all patients before the inclusion in the present study. Some of risk factors associated with going from acute low-back pain to chronic low-back pain are linked to the socio-professional context, notably with the job dissatisfaction [17, 18]. Furthermore, 2 studies [17, 19] showed that there was a significant positive association between a damage compensation and chronic incapacity. In general, patients with unconsolidated work accident or ongoing damage compensation have a higher probability to be at risk of chronic disease; they also have a lower probability to positive response to treatment in general. That is why we excluded them from the study. We measured it by asking to each participant: "are you currently in an unconsolidated work accident?" and "are you currently ongoing a damage compensation?". As a High Authority of Health in France (l'Agence Nationale d'Accréditation et d'Evaluation en Santé, Diagnostic, Prise en charge et suivi des malades atteints de lombalgie chronique, Décembre 2000) classified the beginning of a LBP after the age of 55 as an « alert sign », we excluded them from the study.

No patient was allowed to take opiates during the time of the study, and facet joint injections were also not permitted during the study period. Physiotherapy programs offered during the study period were isometric exercises and core muscle strengthening exercises one or twice per week (usual physiotherapy in chronic low-back pain, that patients made before the study, and which was not modified during the study).

Experimental procedure
Task
The design of this study was a crossover. The subjects were randomized into two groups and successively received the two treatments of the study: patients in group 1 received intramuscular paravertebral injections of BoNT-A during the first sequence of treatment, then a placebo during the second sequence of treatment 120 days later; patients in group 2 received a placebo during the first sequence of treatment, then intramuscular paravertebral injections of BoNT-A during of the second sequence of treatment 120 days later. The crossover was performed 120 days after the inclusion in the study, because most patients with initial improvement induced by BoNT-A injections reported in previous studies [12] that the beneficial effect waned at four months.

A paper table of randomization was used by the pharmacist at the University Hospital of Bordeaux (block randomization with block size of 6). The pharmacist who performed the randomization was blinded to the patient's characteristics.

Therapeutic procedure: For each group, the injected solution was prepared by the hospital pharmacist in order that both the patients and the injectors were blinded to the nature of the injected solution. The treatments compared were: 200 IU of BoNT-A diluted in 4 ml of physiological saline injected intramuscularly in the paravertebral lumbar muscles, versus 4 ml of physiological saline injected intramuscularly in the paravertebral lumbar muscles (placebo). The injector administered the solution in 10 intramuscular puncture points (0.4 mL/point) equally distributed from L1 to L5, bilaterally. The site of injection was detected by electromyography using the injection needle. No complementary pain treatment was prescribed after the injections.

Follow-up: patients were examined at inclusion Days 0, 30, 90, 120 (Day of the crossover), 150, 210 and 240, i.e., D0, D30, D90 and D120 after both sessions of injection. The follow-up was done in person. Patients were blinded throughout the entire study.

Measures
The main judgment criterion was the level of LBP intensity at D30 (when the maximal effect of BoNT-A injections is anticipated). Pain intensity was measured on a horizontal visual analogue scale 100 mm long, with « no pain » written on one end and « maximum pain » on the other (0 = no pain; 100 = maximal pain). The question asked was: "How was the intensity of your LBP over the last 8 days?" To consider the pain decrease as clinically significant, we used the guidelines of Pham et al. [20], who suggested that a change of 40 mm could be clinically significant.

Secondary judgment criteria

– Initial pain was detailed as follows: Immediate average LBP was recorded on VAS at the first injection (D0). Average pain intensity over the last week and the last month were also recorded at D0, with the same horizontal visual analogue scale.
– Lumbar pain intensity at D90 and D120 was measured on a horizontal visual analogue scale 100 mm long, with « no pain » written on one end and "maximum pain" on the other. The question asked was: "How was the intensity of your LBP over the last 8 days?" (0 = no pain; 100 = maximal pain).
– The number of days when oral pain treatment (antalgic or non-steroid anti-inflammatory, opiates were not permitted) between evaluation times was

taken. Days when treatment was taken were noted as they occurred by the patient in a calendar, which was distributed at D0. We thought that a change of 25% would be significant.

- Functional disability related to LBP was measured by the Quebec Back Pain Disability Scale at each evaluation time. The higher the score (/100), the higher the disability. We considered as determined by Ostelo et al. [21] 20 points of change of the Quebec score as clinically significant.
- Quality of life was measured at each evaluation time on a horizontal visual analogue scale 100 mm long. The question asked was: "In your opinion, how was your quality of life over the last month?" (0 = no impact to 100 = major deterioration). We considered as clinically significant a change of 0.2 standard deviation (small change), 0.5 standard deviation (moderate change) and 0.8 standard deviation (large change) [22, 23].
- Inability to work was measured by a compendium of data indicating the number of sick leave days due to LBP in the 8 months preceding inclusion and during follow-up. A change of 25% was considered as clinically significant.
- Patient satisfaction regarding the effect of the treatment was measured on a horizontal visual analogue scale 100 mm long at each evaluation time. The question asked at each evaluation was: "In your opinion, how is the overall efficacy of the treatment that you have received?"(0 = no efficacy; 100 = high efficacy). A change superior than 50% was considered as clinically significant.
- Spinal mobility was measured at each evaluation time by using Schober & Macrae's test (Miller 1984). Two lines were drawn 10 cm above the postero superior iliac spine and 5 cm below the postero superior iliac spine. The distances in a standing position and in anteflexion were measured. A difference less than 4 cm was considered as a spine stiffness.
- Spinal muscle strength was measured by flexion and extension isokinetic technique at a speed of 60° per second before the injections, at D30, D120, D150 and D240. A variation of strength up to 20% or a reversal of the flexor/extensor ratio was considered as clinically significant.
- MODIC classification of discopathy and Hadar classification of the rector spinae muscles were based on MRI performed in the previous year. The MODIC measures are divided in 3 classes: [24]: there were type 1 (inflammatory phase), type 2 (fatty phase) and type 3 (marked sclerosis adjacent to the endplates). We collected the data in order to look for predictive factors for efficacy of BoNT-A.

- Tolerance to BoNT-A injections was studied by actively asking at each visit for possible side effects (pain at injection points, sensation of general weakness, falling, nausea, diplopia, dry mouth).

Statistical analysis

Comparisons were made by a paired Student t-test after verifying the conditions of validity of the test (normal distribution, homogeneous variances). The Chi square test was used in order to compare the gender distribution of the two groups. Paired t-tests and Chi square tests were performed on cumulative data from 19 patients following placebo (19 patients) and BoNT-A injections (19 patients) after a crossover. Linear regression analysis was also planned. Risk of type 1 error was $\alpha = 5\%$ at each statistical analysis. To run the statistical analyses, we used the Excel software, version 15.32. The statistician who decided the kind of statistics used was blinded. The author who made the statistical analyses was not blinded, but he/she did not compile the data into the statistical software.

Results

The group who began the injections with BoNT-A was named group 1; the group who began the injections with a placebo was named group 2. As planned, in order to increase the power of the statistical analysis of the crossover, we pooled post-BoNT-A follow-up and post-placebo follow-up. The group with BoNT-A injections was named group A and the group with placebo injections was named group B. The follow-up of groups A and B was performed at D30, D90 and D120 following each injection time.

Flow diagram (Figure 1)

In this study, 19 patients were approached and eligible to the study. No patient declined participation in the study. The inclusion period was about 23 months. All patients included were randomized in one of the two groups. Nine of them received BoNT-A at D0, 10 of them received placebo at D0. In the BoNT-A group (group 1), all patients were followed at D30, D90, all of them received placebo at D120, were followed at D150, D210 and D240 and completed the trial. In the placebo group (group 2), one patient was lost during the follow-up at D90 and one patient was lost during the follow-up at D210; 8 patients received BoNT-A at D120, all of them were followed at D150, D210 and D240 and completed the trial. We excluded the 2 lost patients from the statistical analysis, because they did not benefit from the 2 injections (BoNT-A and placebo). Patients' distribution is presented in Fig. 1.

Description of the population at baseline (standard deviations are noted in parentheses) (Table 1)

The group who initially received BoNT-A was named group 1; the group who initially received the placebo

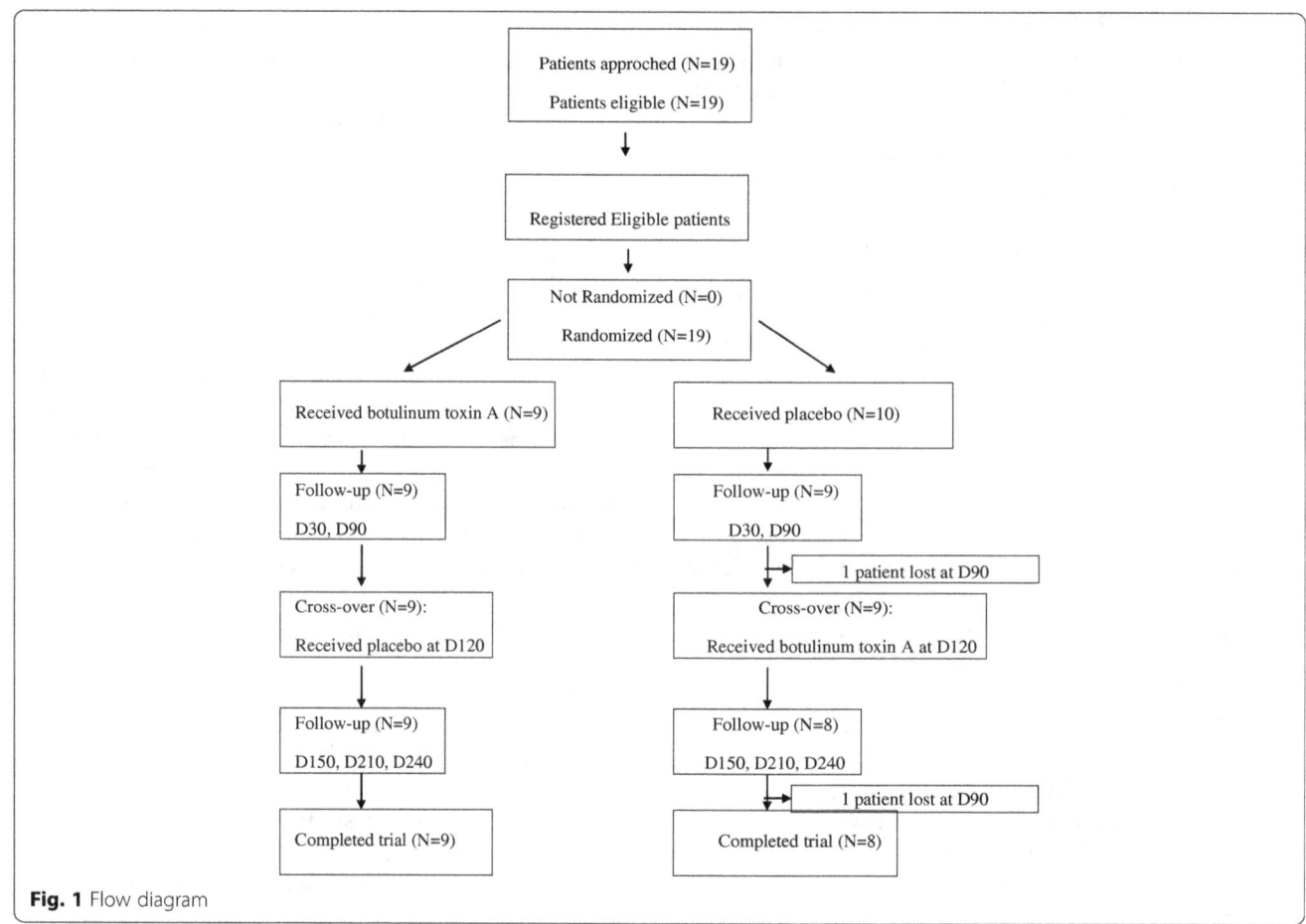

Fig. 1 Flow diagram

was named group 2. The group 1 contained 6 women and 3 men, and the group 2 contained 10 women (Chi square = 3.96, $p = 0.047$). There was no significant difference concerning the mean age of group 1 (38.1(±5.94)) and group 2 (38.2(±10.27)) ($p = 0.98$). The mean usual spinal pain intensity of group 1 was 59.33 mm (±15.71) and the one of group 2 was 58.70 (±15.89) ($p = 0.93$). The usual root pain intensity did not differ between groups either ($p = 0.26$) (mean pain intensity in group 1: 42.89 mm (±26.98); mean pain intensity in group 2: 28.40 mm (±27.16)). The mean pain intensity during the last month was 63.11 mm (±25.70) in group 1 and 66.70 mm (±24.50) in group 2 ($p = 0.76$); the mean pain intensity during the last 8 days was 67.67 mm (±22.37) in group 1 and 57.50 mm (±25.63) in group 2 ($p = 0.37$). There was no significant difference concerning the mean Quebec initial score between group 1 (52.56 mm (±11.64)) and group 2 (51.70 mm (±16.55)) ($p = 0.90$). There was no significant difference concerning the mean disability during the last month between group 1 (7.44 mm (±12.99)) and group 2 (13.4 mm (±14.55)) ($p = 0.36$); but the disability during the last 8 months was higher in the group 2 (151.6 mm (±96.56)) than in the group 1 (58.22 mm (±82.29)) ($p = 0.03$). The quality of life

at inclusion was estimated at 76.56 mm (±16.41) for group 1 and at 65.00 mm (±17.80) for group 2 ($p = 0.16$). There was no significant difference concerning the number of days with painkillers or anti-inflammatories between group 1 (19.67 days (±13.44)) and group 2 (14.1 days (±12.57)) ($p = 0.36$). In group 1, 4 patients had a right-, 3 had a left- and 2 had a bilateral paravertebral painful point pressure; in group 2, 4 patients had a right- and 6 patients had a bilateral paravertebral painful point pressure. In group 1, 8 patients and 6 patients of group 2 had a stiffness ($p = 0.17$). The Schober's test was measured at 4.22 cm (±1.30) for group 1 and 3.95 cm (±1.77) for group 2 ($p = 0.71$). The hand-ground distance was about 28.60 cm (±13.60) in group 1 and 20.60 (±15.60) for group 2 ($p = 0.25$). The mean number of localization of spinal pain was 3.13 (±1.46) in group 1 and 3.60 (±1.84) in group 2 ($p = 0.55$), and the mean number of localization of paravertebral pain was 5.00 (±1.51) in group 1 and 4.60 (±2.32) in group 2 ($p = 0.67$). No patients presented a Lasegue sign at the inclusion; 2 patients presented a pseudo-Lasegue sign in group 1 and 5 presented a pseudo-Lasegue sign in group 2 ($p = 0.30$). Only one patient in group 2 presented a disco-radicular conflict ($p = 0.34$). The isokinetic evaluation revealed a maximum

Table 1 Demographic data of 19 randomized patients (mean or number are noted, standard deviations are in parentheses) at Day 0 (D0)

Patients	Botulinum toxin	Placebo	t-test (p)
Sample size	$N = 9$	$N = 10$	
Men/Women	3/6	0/10	0.047
Age: mean (SD) in years	38.1 (5.94)	38.2 (10.27)	0.49
Spinal pain intensity: mean (SD) /100 mm	59.33 (15.71)	58.70 (15.89)	0.47
Radicular pain intensity: mean (SD) /100 mm	42.89 (26.98)	28.40 (27.16)	0.13
Pain intensity during last month: mean (SD) /100 mm	63.11 (25.70)	66.70 (24.50)	0.38
Pain intensity during last week: mean (SD) /100 mm	67.67 (22.37)	57.50 (25.63)	0.18
Quebec initial score mean (SD) /100 mm	52.56 (11.64)	51.70 (16.55)	0.45
Disability during last 8 months: mean (SD) /100 mm	58.22 (82.29)	151.6 (96.56)	0.018
Disability during last month: mean (SD) /100 mm	7.44 (12.99)	13.4 (14.55)	0.18
Quality of life at inclusion: mean (SD) /100 mm	76.56 (16.41)	65.00 (17.80)	0.08
Number of days with painkillers or anti-inflammatories: number (SD)	19.67 (13.44)	14.1 (12.57)	0.18
Paravertebral painful point pressure Right/Left/Bilateral	4/3/2	4/0/6	
Stiffness: number	8	6	0.08
Tendency to cough: number	5	7	0.27
Instability: number	9	8	0.08
Schober's test: centimeter (SD)	4.22 (1.30)	3.95 (1.77)	0.35
Hand-ground distance: centimeter (SD)	28.60 (13.60)	20.60 (15.60)	0.13
Spinal pain: mean (SD)	3.13 (1.46)	3.60 (1.84)	0.27
Paravertebral pain: number	2	5	0.33
Lasegue sign: number	0	0	
Pseudo-Lasegue sign: mean (SD)	0.25 (0.46)	0.5 (0.53)	0.15
Disco-radicular conflict: number	0	1	0.17
MODIC L1-L2 0/1/2/3	9/0/0/0	9/0/1/0	0.17
MODIC L2-L3 0/1/2/3	9/0/0/0	9/0/1/0	0.17
MODIC L3-L4 0/1/2/3	9/0/0/0	9/0/1/0	0.17
MODIC L4-L5 0/1/2/3	9/0/0/0	9/0/0/1	0.17
MODIC L5-S1 0/1/2/3	5/3/1/0	4/3/2/1	0.15
HADAR L1-L2 0/1/2/3	8/1/0/0	8/2/0/0	0.31
HADAR L2-L3 0/1/2/3	6/3/0/0	7/3/0/0	0.44
HADAR L3-L4 0/1/2/3	4/5/0/0	7/1/2/0	0.33
HADAR L4-L5 0/1/2/3	1/6/2/0	3/4/3/0	0.37
HADAR L5-S1 0/1/2/3	1/4/4/0	0/4/6/0	0.18
Isokinetic maximum strength: n/m (SD)	115.33 (58.63)	114.44 (37.63)	0.49
Isokinetic endurance: n/m (SD)	89.11 (62.50)	77.33 (53.86)	0.34
Flexors/extensors ratio at 60°: % (SD)	123.63 (37.56)	119.36 (49.51)	0.42

strength at 115.33n/m (±58.63) in group 1 and at 114.44n/m (±37.63) in group 2 ($p = 0.97$); the endurance was calculated at 89.11n/m (±62.50) in group 1 and 77.33n/m (±53.86) in group 2 ($p = 0.67$); the flexors/extensors ratio at 60° was calculated at 123.63% (±37.56) in group 1 and 119.36 (±49.51) in group 2 ($p = 0.84$). Population at baseline is described in Table 1.

Between-group comparisons (Table 2)
Level of LBP intensity
Between-group comparisons are presented in Table 2.

- LBP intensity during the last 8 days (Fig. 2):

There was no significant difference concerning the mean of the LBP intensity during the last 8 days between

Table 2 Presentation of averages, standard deviations and *p*-values of judgment criteria for group A and group B

		Number of patients (n) A/B	Mean group A	Standard deviation group A	Mean group B	Standard deviation group B	*p*-value
Average lumbar pain over last 8 days by visual analogue scale (/100 mm)	D0	18/19	67.70	24.64	60.35	28.07	*p* = 0.43
	D30	18/19	63.12	18.92	63.12	18.92	*p* = 0.75
	D90	15/16	62.60	27.39	58.43	24.66	*p* = 0.80
	D120	15/16	60.87	26.83	55.87	32.50	*p* = 0.70
Average root pain over last month by visual analogue scale (/100 mm)	D30	18/19	60.29	22.99	53.47	33.88	*p* = 0.45
	D90	15/16	42.07	37.40	27.57	33.05	*p* = 0.52
	D120	15/16	56.73	25.33	46.20	30.42	*p* = 0.70
Number of days with significant or very significant pain	D30	18/19	13.29	9.88	15.18	12.82	*p* = 0.55
	D90	15/16	11.43	10.45	11.71	16.94	*p* = 0.44
Functional disability related to low-back pain by Quebec Back Pain Disability Scale (/100)	D0	18/19	51.53	16.19	52.35	20.16	*p* = 0.89
	D30	18/19	53.76	13.18	52.29	20.74	*p* = 0.77
	D90	15/16	53.07	17.75	45.93	22.82	*p* = 0.47
	D120	16/16	52.87	21.69	42.93	23.70	*p* = 0.48
Inability to work during last 30 days (/30)	D0	18/19	11.00	14.56	11.06	14.55	*p* = 0.99
	D30	18/18	12.41	15.17	9.56	14.25	*p* = 0.35
	D90	15/16	12.41	14.59	9.69	17.93	*p* = 0.46
	D120	15/16	8.00	13.73	12.00	15.21	*p* = 0.34
Estimated impact of low-back pain on quality of life (/100)	D0	18/19	71.41	21.70	64.47	24.61	*p* = 0.37
	D30	18/19	68.71	18.85	64.06	23.33	*p* = 0.44
	D90	15/16	63.47	23.72	58.57	23.33	*p* = 0.38
	D120	15/16	61.00	30.01	60.67	29.63	*p* = 0.96
Number of days when pain medication or anti-inflammatories were necessary in last 30 days (/30)	D0	18/19	17.06	13.65	15.35	14.69	*p* = 0.71
	D30	18/19	16.06	13.21	13.41	13.44	*p* = 0.51
	D90	15/16	15.73	13.85	11.50	13.82	*p* = 0.79
	D120	15/16	14.80	14.87	13.53	14.54	*p* = 0.86
Patients' assessment of efficacy of treatment (/100)	D30	18/19	0.76	1.15	0.94	1.14	*p* = 0.62
	D90	15/16	1.33	1.80	1.43	1.60	*p* = 1.00
	D120	15/16	1.47	1.77	1.73	1.62	*p* = 1.00
Spinal flexibility measured by Schoeber Macrae's test (cm)	D0	18/19	5.00	2.34	4.21	1.86	*p* = 0.22
	D30	18/19	4.76	1.88	4.32	1.67	*p* = 0.48
	D90	15/16	4.00	1.18	4.54	1.31	*p* = 0.23
	D120	15/16	4.23	1.55	5.53	2.28	*p* = 0.18
Hand-ground distance (cm)	D0	18/19	26.17	13.32	25.64	14.03	*p* = 0.93
	D30	18/19	26.35	14.02	26.85	12.89	*p* = 0.92
	D90	15/16	24.87	14.51	16.79	10.17	*p* = 0.35
	D120	15/16	27.53	12.18	21.93	13.08	*p* = 0.25
Isokinetic maximum strength (n/m)	D0	16/17	116.00	45.53	126.40	63.41	*p* = 0.78
	D30	15/18	120.93	53.30	134.40	63.67	*p* = 0.70
	D120	13/14	126.69	67.20	135.07	50.35	*p* = 0.70
Isokinetic endurance (n/m)	D0	16/17	100.27	51.63	102.33	63.24	*p* = 0.81
	D30	15/17	96.07	53.38	108.73	69.00	*p* = 0.76
	D120	15/14	103.17	63.74	111.79	57.67	*p* = 0.65

Table 2 Presentation of averages, standard deviations and p-values of judgment criteria for group A and group B *(Continued)*

		Number of patients (n) A/B	Mean group A	Standard deviation group A	Mean group B	Standard deviation group B	p-value
Isokinetic maximum force ratio flexors/extensors (%)	D0	16/17	115.85	31.13	119.72	38.95	$p = 0.36$
	D30	15/17	122.93	33.83	107.86	24.41	$p = 0.16$
	D120	13/14	111.54	24.29	102.88	23.53	$p = 0.72$

Group A: all 17 patients assessed during 120 days after BoNT-A injections, group B: all 17 patients assessed during 120 days after placebo injections

group 1 and group 2 at D30 ($p = 0.59$), at D90 ($p = 0.94$), at D120 ($p = 0.73$), at D150 ($p = 0.92$), at D210 ($p = 0.80$) and at D240 ($p = 0.36$).

There was no significant difference concerning the mean of the LBP intensity during the last 8 days between group A and group B at D30 ($p = 0.75$), at D90 ($p = 0.80$) and at D120 ($p = 0.70$).

- Root pain intensity over the last month:

There was no significant difference concerning the mean root pain over last month between group 1 and group 2 at D30 ($p = 0.31$), at D90 ($p = 0.23$), at D120 ($p = 0.54$), at D150 ($p = 0.92$), at D210 ($p = 0.77$) and at D240 ($p = 0.46$).

There was no significant difference concerning the mean root pain over last month between group A and group B at D30 ($p = 0.45$), at D90 ($p = 0.51$) and at D120 ($p = 0.70$).

- Number of days with significant or very significant pain:

There was no significant difference concerning the number of days with significant or very significant pain between group 1 and group 2 at D30 ($p = 0.63$), at D90 ($p = 0.94$), at D120 ($p = 0.94$), at D150 ($p = 0.27$), at D210 ($p = 0.68$) and at D240 ($p = 0.64$).

There was no significant difference concerning the number of days with significant or very significant pain between group A and group B at D30 ($p = 0.55$), at D90 ($p = 0.44$) and at D120 ($p = 0.35$).

Functional disability related to LBP evaluated by Quebec back pain disability scale (figure 3)

There was no significant difference concerning the score of the Quebec scale between group 1 and group 2 at D30 ($p = 0.86$), at D90 ($p = 0.89$), at D120 ($p = 0.94$), at D150 ($p = 0.65$), at D210 ($p = 0.35$) and at D240 ($p = 0.13$).

There was no significant difference concerning the score of the Quebec scale between group A and group B at D30 ($p = 0.77$), at D90 ($p = 0.47$) and at D120 ($p = 0.48$).

Inability to work during the last 30 days

There was no significant difference concerning the number of days with inability to work during the last 30 days between group 1 and group 2 at D30 ($p = 0.35$), at D90 ($p = 0.46$), at D120 ($p = 0.27$), at D150 ($p = 0.10$), at D210 ($p = 0.47$) and at D240 ($p = 0.86$).

There was no significant difference concerning the number of days with inability to work during the last 30 days between group A and group B at D30 ($p = 0.35$), at D90 ($p = 0.46$) and at D120 ($p = 0.34$).

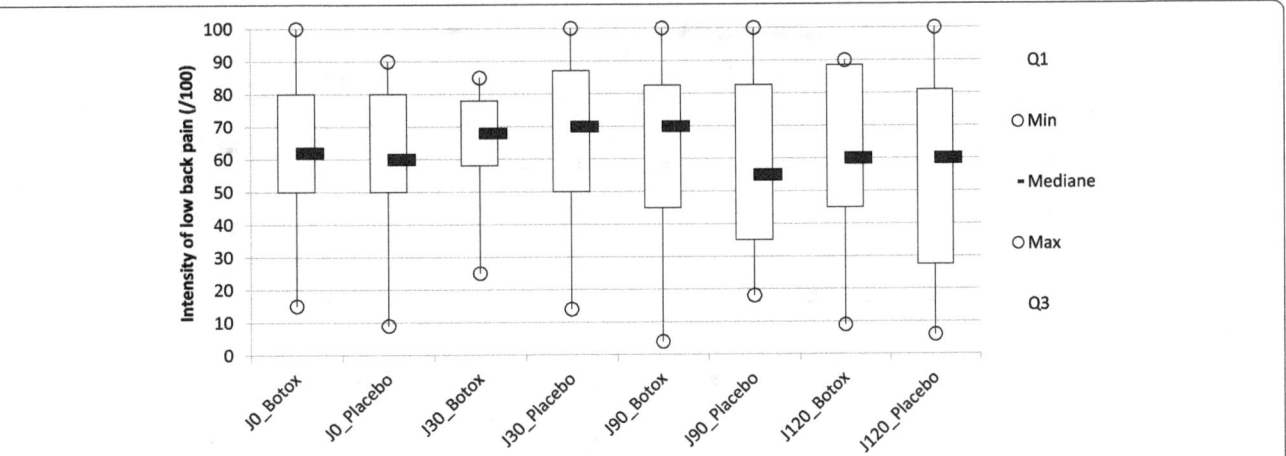

Fig. 2 Pain intensity at D0,30, 90 and 120 for patients treated by Botulinum toxin A (BoNT-A) (group A) or by placebo (group B). Pain intensity was measured on a horizontal visual analogue scale 100 mm long, with « no pain » written on one end and « maximum pain » on the other. The question asked was: "How was the intensity of your low-back pain over the last 8 days?"

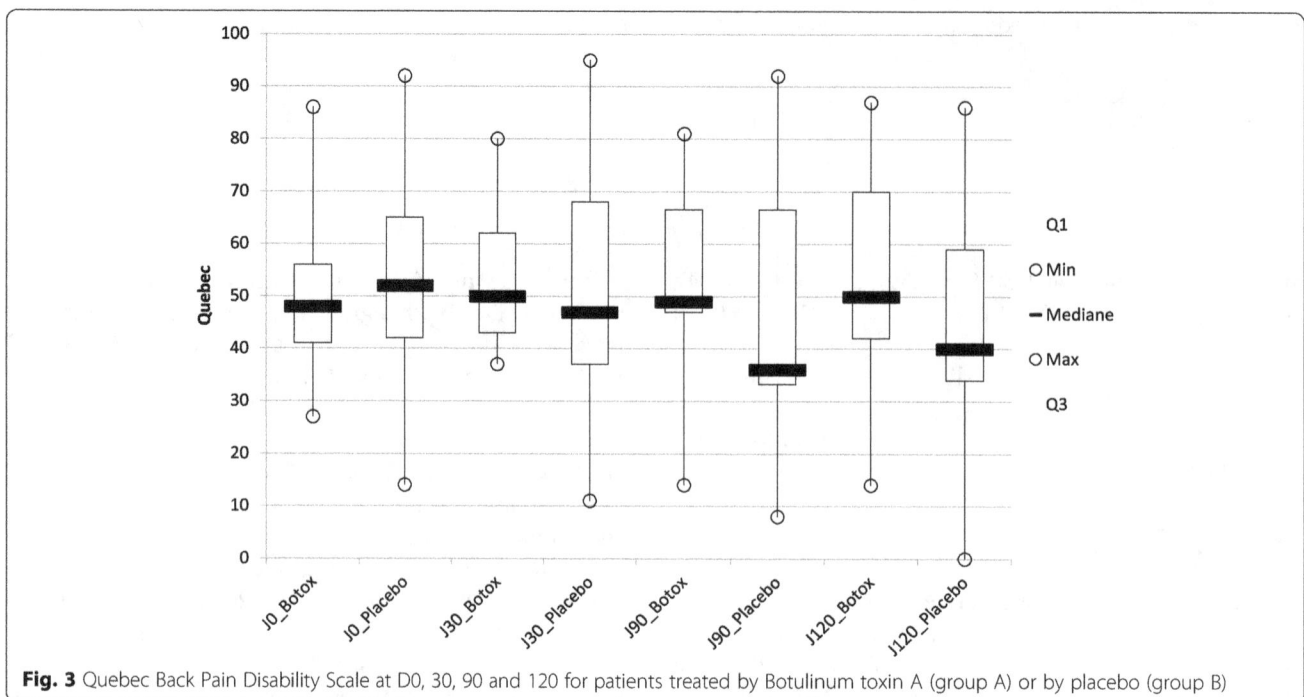

Fig. 3 Quebec Back Pain Disability Scale at D0, 30, 90 and 120 for patients treated by Botulinum toxin A (group A) or by placebo (group B)

Estimated impact of LBP on quality of life (figure 4)

There was no significant difference concerning the estimating impact of LBP on quality of life during the last month between group 1 and group 2 at D30 ($p = 0.38$), at D90 ($p = 0.56$), at D120 ($p = 0.90$), at D150 ($p = 0.98$), at D210 ($p = 0.98$) and at D240 ($p = 0.93$).

There was no significant difference concerning the estimating impact of LBP on quality of life during the last

month between group A and group B at D30 ($p = 0.44$), at D90 ($p = 0.38$) and at D120 ($p = 0.95$).

Number of days when pain medication or anti-inflammatories were necessary in last 30 days

There was no significant difference concerning the number of days when pain medication or anti-inflammatories were necessary in the last 30 days between group 1 and

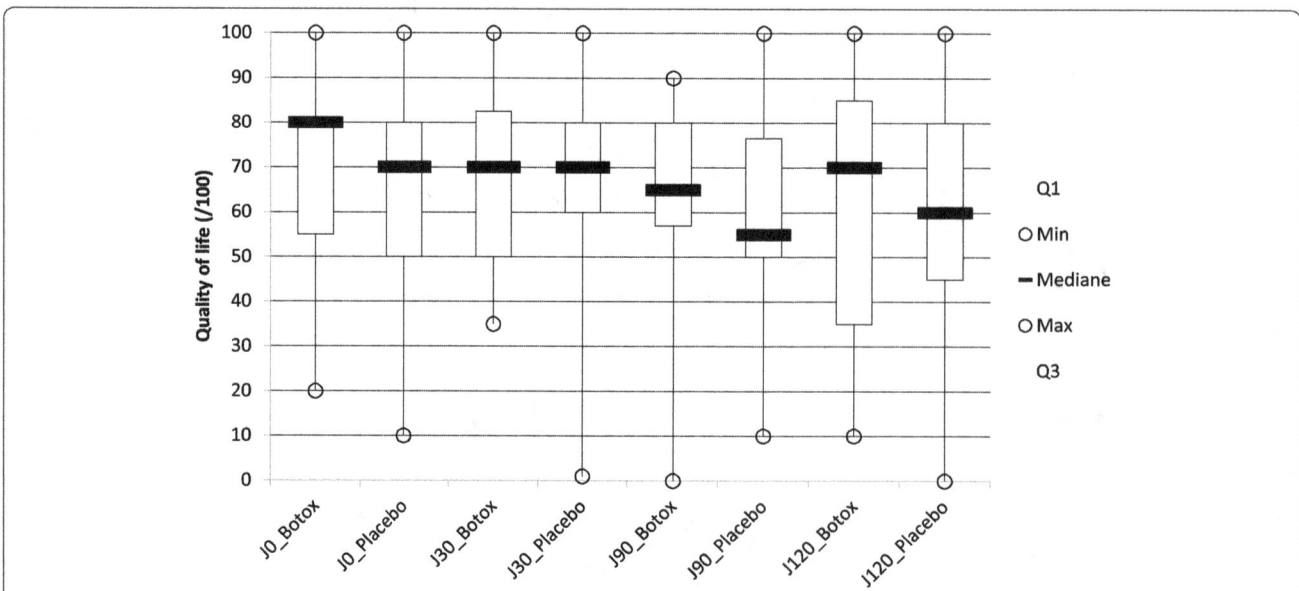

Fig. 4 Estimated impact of low-back pain on quality of life at D0, D30, D90 and D120 for patients treated by Botulinum toxin A (group A) or by placebo (group B). It was measured on a horizontal visual analogue scale 100 mm long. The question asked was: "in your opinion, how was your quality of life over the last month?" (0 = no impact to 100 = major deterioration)

group 2 at D30 ($p = 0.82$), at D90 ($p = 0.51$), at D120 ($p = 0.73$), at D150 ($p = 0.57$), at D210 ($p = 0.58$) and at D240 ($p = 0.92$).

There was no significant difference concerning the number of days when pain medication or anti-inflammatories were necessary in the last 30 days between group A and group B at D30 ($p = 0.51$), at D90 ($p = 0.79$) and at D120 ($p = 0.86$).

Patients' assessment of efficacy of treatment

There was no significant difference concerning the patients' assessment of efficacy of treatment between group 1 and group 2 at D30 ($p = 0.73$), at D90 ($p = 0.69$), at D120 ($p = 0.89$), at D150 ($p = 0.91$), at D210 ($p = 0.64$) and at D240 ($p = 0.51$).

There was no significant difference concerning the patients' assessment of efficacy of treatment between group A and group B at D30 ($p = 0.62$), at D90 ($p = 1.00$) and at D120 ($p = 1.00$).

Spinal flexibility measured by Schoeber Macrae's test

There was no significant difference concerning the spinal flexibility measured by Schoeber Macrae's test between group 1 and group 2 at D30 ($p = 0.49$), at D90 ($p = 0.06$), at D120 ($p = 0.30$), at D150 ($p = 0.64$), at D210 ($p = 0.47$). There was a significant difference between group 1 and group 2 concerning the spinal flexibility at D240 ($p = 0.04$).

There was no significant difference concerning the spinal flexibility measured by Schoeber Macrae's test between group A and group B at D30 ($p = 0.48$), at D90 ($p = 0.23$) and at D120 ($p = 0.18$).

Hand-ground distance

There was no significant difference concerning the hand-ground distance between group 1 and group 2 at D30 ($p = 0.64$), at D90 ($p = 0.10$), at D120 ($p = 0.33$), at D150 ($p = 0.41$) and at D210 ($p = 0.81$). There was a significant difference concerning the hand-ground distance between group 1 and group 2 at D240 ($p = 0.58$).

There was no significant difference concerning the hand-ground distance between group A and group B at D30 ($p = 0.92$), at D90 ($p = 35$) and at D120 ($p = 0.25$).

Isokinetic maximum strength

There was no significant difference concerning the isokinetic maximum strength between group 1 and group 2 at D30 ($p = 0.34$), at D120 ($p = 0.30$) and at D150 ($p = 0.11$). There was a significant difference concerning the isokinetic maximum strength between group 1 and group 2 at D240 ($p = 0.04$).

There was no significant difference concerning the isokinetic maximum strength between group A and group B at D30 ($p = 0.70$) and at D120 ($p = 0.70$).

Isokinetic endurance

There was no significant difference concerning the isokinetic endurance between group 1 and group 2 at D30 ($p = 0.26$), at D120 ($p = 0.21$) and at D150 (0.08). There was a significant difference between group 1 and group 2 concerning the isokinetic endurance between group 1 and group 2 at D240 ($p = 0.03$).

There was no significant difference concerning the isokinetic endurance between group A and group B at D30 ($p = 0.76$) and at D120 ($p = 0.65$).

Isokinetic maximum force ratio flexors/extensors

There was no significant difference concerning the isokinetic maximum force measured by the radio flexors/extensors at 60° between group 1 and group 2 at D30 ($p = 0.90$), at D120 (0.89), at D150 (0.08), at D240 (0.19).

There was no significant difference concerning the isokinetic maximum force measured by the radio flexors/extensors at 60° between group A and group B at D30 ($p = 0.16$) and at D120 ($p = 0.72$).

Within-group comparisons

There was no significant difference in group A and in group B concerning the pain intensity between D0 and D120 ($p = 0.58$ for group A and $p = 0.70$ for group B).

Symmetric carryover effect

There was a symmetric carryover effect between group 1 and group 2 concerning the main judgement criterion, i.e. pain intensity at D30.

Adverse effects

The adverse effects were actively asked at each visit. No patients declared an adverse effect during the present study. No complications were experienced in this study.

Discussion

This randomized controlled trial did not find any advantage for injections of BoNT-A versus placebo in the paravertebral muscles of patients with LBP at 30, 90 et 120 days with regard to pain relief, functional disability, sick leave, quality of life, consumption of oral antalgics, spinal flexibility and isokinetic strength or endurance. Indeed, there was no significant difference between the two groups regarding the main criterion, i.e., average lumbar pain over the last 8 days at D30 ($p = 0.97$), nor was there any significant difference between the two groups regarding secondary judgment criteria ($p > 0.05$, see Table 2).

Our results differ largely from those of two previous studies [4, 6]. Since LBP is a complex phenomenon involving heavy lifting, twisting and trauma which is sometimes work-related [25] psychological factors [26], smoking, alcoholism, biomechanical and psychosocial professional factors, the difference in results could be due to differences in the populations of the two studies. Indeed, in a previous study [4], 3 patients had a discectomy compared to none in our study. In addition, no patient had any MRI evidence of acute disc pathology in the two previous studies [4, 6], whereas 6 patients in our study had a MODIC 1. Furthermore, in our study, only 3 male patients were included. Nevertheless, there was no difference between groups concerning the gender. Furthermore, the present literature is not uniform about the role of the gender on the chronicity of low-back pain [27, 28].

In our study, we used 200 units of Botox for bilateral injections. But we assume that the negative results of our study could also be secondary to the lower dose of botulinum toxin A used on each injection point compared to Foster et al.'s study. Indeed, we decided to inject bilaterally the paravertebral muscles, because there is usually a bilateral injury in both paravertebral muscles after an acute low back-pain, which leads to chronic low-back pain [29]. More precisely, we think that LBP could be secondary to an over-activity of muscles compensating multifidus' atrophy. The dose used in Machado et al.'s study (1000UI of Dysport in case of bilateral injections) was also superior to ours, which could explain the difference between the results.

Reporting a negative study is still an interesting point, because the efficiency of BoNT-A on chronic low-back pain is still not proved at this time, and because it could make reconsider on one part in researchers' further studies about BoNT-A and LBP, and one the other part in clinicians using BoNT-A injections for chronic LBP.

The strength of this trial is its randomized, controlled crossover design. A limitation is the small sample. Nevertheless, the number of patients treated was similar to that in previous studies [4, 6, 14], which showed a strong positive effect of BoNT-A on LBP. While some differences between the groups became apparent before the crossover (hand-ground distance, Schober's test, isokinetic measures), they disappeared when the data were aggregated after the crossover (group A and group B), perhaps owing to variations due to the size of groups 1 and 2. Indeed, group 1 demonstrated more spine stiffness and less strength than group 2, a finding that was unexpected.

The main result of the study is the absence of any significant difference or trend to feel pain relief with injections of BoNT-A A compared to placebo injections. A larger sample of patients now needs to be studied in order to identify those who would benefit most from BoNT-A injections for LBP.

Conclusions

Botulinum toxin injections did not show any efficacy in relieving pain in patients with chronic low-back pain in this randomised controlled trial using a cross-over. Result is in contradiction with the existing literature. With 200UI of Botox injected bilaterally, we did not find any pain relief. But this negative result could also be explained by the lower dose used compared to other studies, and by the low number of patients included. Nevertheless, this negative result could be useful being included in a meta-analysis.

Abbreviations
BoNT-A: Botulinum Toxin A; LBP: Low-back pain

Acknowledgements
The authors thank Briane Marie Sheperd, Ray Cooke and Anna Moraitis for helping with the English syntax. The authors thank also Dr. Jean-François Knebel for his help with the statistical analyses.
This work was supported by the French Hospital Clinical Research Project (PHRC).

Funding
The authors thank the Allergan company for co-funding this study (co-financing with 13,700 euros) within the French Hospital Clinical Research (PHRC Project) framework (42,000 euros). The Allergan company did not interfere with the collection, the analysis and the interpretation of data, nor with the writing of the manuscript.

Authors' contributions
MC made the statistical analysis and wrote the paper. HP and AC included some patients, helped for the interpretation of the statistical analyses and were involved in drafting the manuscript. MDS helped for promoting the study, included the patients and helped for the statistical analysis. DL helped for designing and promoting the study. She was also involved in drafting the manuscript. All authors discussed the results and commented on the manuscript. All authors read and approved the final manuscript.

Competing interests
The authors declare that they have no competing interests.

Author details
[1]Service de Médecine Physique et de Réadaptation, hôpital Raymond Poincaré, 92380 Garches, France. [2]Service de Médecine Physique et de Réadaptation, CHU de Bordeaux, 33076 Bordeaux, France. [3]EA4136 Handicap, Activité, Cognition, Santé, Bordeaux University, Bordeaux, France. [4]Neurosurgical Unit, University Hospital, Bordeaux, France.

References
1. Andersson GB. Epidemiological features of chronic low-back pain. Lancet. 1999;354:581–5.
2. Rossignol M, Abenhaim L, Séguin P, Neveu A, Collet JP, Ducruet T, Shapiro S. Coordination of primary health care for back pain. Spine. 2000;25:251–9.
3. Mellin G. Decreased joint and spinal mobility associated with low back pain in young adults. J Spinal Disord. 1990;3:228–43.
4. Foster L, Clapp L, Erickson M, Jabbari B. BoNT-a A and chronic low back pain: a randomized, double blind study. Neurology. 2001;56:1290–993.
5. Jazayeri SM, Ashraf A, Fini HM, Karimian H, Nasab MV. Efficacy of botulinum toxin type a for treating chronic low back pain. Anesh Pain Med. 2011;1:77–80.
6. Machado D, Kumar A, Jabbari B. Abobotulinum toxin a in the treatment of chronic low back pain. Toxins. 2016;8:374.
7. Cheshire WP, Abashian SW, Mann JD. BoNT-A in the treatment of myofascial pain syndrome. Pain. 1994;59:65–9.
8. Dutton JJ. BoNT-A in treatment of crabiocervical muscle spasms short and long term, local and sistemic effects. Surv Ophthalmol. 1996;41:51–65.
9. Grazko MA, Polo KB, Jabbari B. BoNT-a A for spaticity muscle spasms, and rigidity. Neurology. 1995;45:712–7.

10. Greene P, Kang U, Fahn S, Brin M, Moskowitz C, Flaster E. Double blind, placebo controlled trial of botulinum injection for the treatment of spasmodic torticollis. Neurology. 1990;40:1213–8.

11. Wheeler A, Goelkusian PA, Gretz SS. Randomised double blind, prospective pilot study of boutilinum toxin injection for refractory unilateral, cervicothoracic, paraspinal, myofacial pain syndrome. Spine. 1998;23:1662–7.

12. Herskowitz A. BOTOX (BoNT-a type A) treatment of patients with sub-acute low back pain: a randomized, double blind, placebo-controlled study. *The journal of Pain* Supplement 1 2004; 5(1), S62.

13. Jabbari B, Ney J, Sichani A, Monacci W, Foster L, Difazio M. Treatment of refractory, chronic low back pain with botulinum neurotoxin a: an open-label, pilot study. Pain Med. 2006;7:260–4.

14. Ney JP, Difazio M, Sichani A, Monacci W, Foster L, Jabbari B. Treatment of chronic low back pain with successive injections of BoNT-a a over 6 months: a prospective trial of 60 patients. Clin J Pain. 2006;22:363–9.

15. Subin B, Saleemi S, Morgan GA, Zaviska F, Cork RC. Treatment of chronic low back pain by local injection of BoNT-a A. Internet Journal of Anesthesiology. 2003;6:8.

16. Waseem Z, Boulias C, Gordon A, Ismail F, Sheean G, Furlan AD. BoNT-A injections for low-back pain and sciatica. *Cochrane database syst Rev* 2011 19; Issue 1. Art no.CD008257.

17. Coste J, Delecoeuillerie G, De Lara AC, LeParc JM, Paolaggi JB. (1994). Clinical course and prognostic factors in acute low back pain: an inception cohort study in primary care practice. BMJ 1994; 308,577-580.

18. Williams RA, Pruitt SD, Doctor JN, Epping-Jordan JE, Wahlgren DR, Grant I, ... & Atkinson JH. (1998). The contribution of job satisfaction to the transition from acute to chronic low back pain. Arch Phys Med Rehabil 1998; 79, 366-374.

19. Gatchel RJ. (2004). Comorbidity of chronic pain and mental health disorders: the biopsychosocial perspective. Am Psychol 2004; 59, 795.

20. Pham T, Tubach F. Etat sympomatique acceptable ou Patient Acceptable Symptomatic State (PASS). Rev Rhum. 2009;76:602–4.

21. Ostelo RW, Deyo RA, Stratford P, Waddell G, Croft P, Von Korff M, Bouter LM, de Vet HC. Interpreting change scores for pain and functional status in low back pain: towards international consensus regarding minimal important change. Spine. 2008;33:90–4.

22. Cohen J. Statistical Power Analysis for the Behavioral Sciences. 1988. 2nd ed. Hillsdale, NJ: Lawrence Erlbaum Associates.

23. Guyatt GH, Osoba D, Wu AW, Wyrwich KW, Norman GR. Clinical Significance Consensus Meeting Group. Methods to explain the clinical significance of health status measures. Mayo Clin Proc. 2002;77:371–83.

24. Modic MT, Steinberg PM, Ross JS, Masaryk TJ, Carter JR. Degenerative disk disease: assessment of changes in vertebral body marrow with MR imaging. Radiology. 1988;166:193–9.

25. Biering-Sørensen F. A prospective study of low back pain in a general population. III. Medical service–work consequence. Scand J Rehabil Med. 1983;15:89–96.

26. Joukamaa M. Psychological factors in low back pain. Ann Clin Res. 1987;19:129–34.

27. Valat JP, Goupille P, Védere V. Low back pain: risk factors for chronicity. Rev Rhum Engl Ed. 1997;64:189–94.

28. Wáng YXJ, Wáng JQ, Káplár Z. Increased low back pain prevalence in females than in males after menopause age: evidences based on synthetic literature review. Quantitative imaging in medicine and surgery. 2016;6:199.

29. Danneels LA, Vanderstraeten GG, Cambier DC, Witvrouw EE, De Cuyper HJ. CT imaging of trunk muscles in chronic low back pain patients and healthy control subjects. Eur Spine J. 2000;9:266–72.

14

Influence of age on results following surgery for displaced acetabular fractures in the elderly

Guo-Chun Zha[1][*][†], Xue-Mei Yang[2][†], Shuo Feng[1], Xiang-Yang Chen[1], Kai-Jin Guo[1][*] and Jun-Ying Sun[3][*]

Abstract

Background: Elderly patients have more special medical needs when compared with young ones; thus, the results of open reduction and internal fixation (ORIF) for acetabular fractures should be stratified by age in these patients. This study seeks to determine whether the age of the patient influences the results of the ORIF for acetabular fractures.

Methods: We performed a retrospective analysis of prospectively collected data on 53 elderly patients with displaced acetabular fractures who underwent ORIF between May 2004 and May 2011. Patients were divided into two groups by age: young–old group (60–74 years) and old–old group (75–90 years). The number of patients in each group was 28 and 25. The reduction quality and clinical function was evaluated using the Matta criteria and modified Postel Merle D'Aubigne Score, respectively. Operative time, bleeding amount, and complications were recorded.

Results: Patients in old–old group had significantly lower anatomical reduction rate ($p = 0.024$), less operative time ($p = 0.021$), and less bleeding amount ($p = 0.016$) than those in the young–old group. The reduction quality in the young–old group was strongly associated with clinical function ($p < 0.05$). However, no difference in clinical function was detected among the different reduction qualities in the old–old group ($p > 0.05$). Moreover, no significant difference in clinical functions ($p = 0.787$) and complications ($p = 0.728$) was detected between the two groups.

Conclusions: Old–old patients may expect comparable clinical functions and complications with young–old patients. The reduction quality in old–old patients may be not significantly associated with clinical function. Different treatment strategies may be applied for acetabular fractures with ORIF in different age groups.

Keywords: Acetabular fracture, Elderly patients, Age, Outcomes

Background

The incidence of acetabular fractures in the elderly has increased [1]. However, the optimal management of displaced acetabular fractures in elderly patients remains controversial. Some surgeons prefer advocated conservative treatment for elderly patients with limited physiological reserves and medical comorbidity that may increase the risk of surgery [2, 3]. Other surgeons advise total hip arthroplasty (THA) for elderly patients with poor bone quality that may increase the risk of poor reduction and loss of reduction or failure of fixation or both [4–6]. Considering the limited life expectancy, low activity level, and low functional requirements of elderly patients, some authors believe that open reduction and internal fixation (ORIF) is suitable for these patients [1, 7, 8].

The inconsistent clinical results can be attributed in part to the following reasons: (1) previous studies included patients of a wide age variety, i.e., greater than 40 [9], 50 [10], 55 [11] to 60 [1] and 70 years old [8]; and

---

* Correspondence: 41049015@qq.com; xzgkj@sina.com; cgc85012@126.com
[†]Equal contributors
[1]Department of Orthopedic Surgery, the Affiliated Hospital of Xuzhou Medical University, No. 99 Huaihai West Road, Xuzhou, Jiangsu 221002, People's Republic of China
[3]Orthopaedic Department, the First Affiliated Hospital of Soochow University, 188 Shizi Street, Suzhou, Jiangsu 215006, People's Republic of China
Full list of author information is available at the end of the article

(2) the results of studies that classified elderly patients as a single population were not stratified by age. Elderly patients have more special medical needs when compared with young ones; thus, different age groups of elderly patients may present different physiological reserves, lifestyle qualities, and osteoporosis degrees. Accordingly, the results of acetabular fractures in the elderly should be stratified by age. Extracting practical conclusions about the relationship of age, reduction quality, and clinical function after ORIF is difficult without a comparator group.

To the best of our knowledge, none of studies have focused exclusively on the relationship of the age to clinical function, reduction quality, and complication of ORIF for acetabular fracture in elderly patients. Therefore, this study seeks to determine whether the age of the patient influences the results of the ORIF for acetabular fractures.

Methods

Patient source

We performed a retrospective analysis of prospectively collected data on 66 consecutive elderly patients with displaced acetabular fractures between May 2004 and May 2011. Four patients were conservative therapy, and 62 patients underwent ORIF. The 62 patients were divided into two groups by age: young–old group (60–74 years) and old–old group (75–90 years). This study received approval from the institutional review board. Informed consent was obtained from all patients included in the study.

Surgical technique

All surgeries were performed by the senior author (J.Y.S) at an average of 5.8 ± 2.5 days (range, 2–14 days) from the initial injury. Skeletal traction was selectively employed through the distal femoral pin. The medical conditions of the patients were optimized through a preoperative multidisciplinary approach. Despite the absence of specific intraoperative management criteria, the surgeon closely followed the principles that accurate reduction is attempted for young–old patients with an active and good physical state. Limited operative procedure was used for old–old patients with low activity and functional requirements to achieve the stable internal fixation of fractures and prevent anatomical reduction.

All patients were placed in floppy lateral position and then operated under general anesthesia. The approach (Kocher–Langenbeck, Ilioinguinal, or Kocher–Langenbeck + Ilioinguinal) was decided according to the nature of the acetabular fracture and the preference of orthopedic surgeon (J.Y.S).

Perioperative regimen

All patients received adequate pain control during the perioperative period. The drain was removed after 48 h, and three standard plain radiographs were obtained after 3 days. On the day after surgery, the patients were encouraged to sit up in bed and perform passive functional exercises to strengthen the hip joint, quadriceps, and hamstrings. The patients were allowed touch-toe weight-bearing a maximum of 20 kg for the first 12 weeks with a walker or crutches depending on physical state. After 12 weeks, full weight-bearing gradually progressed according to patient tolerance.

Follow-up

After discharge, the patients were traced using telephone, letter, or e-mail and were asked to return for completing the clinical and radiological postoperative evaluation at 6 weeks, 3 months, 1 year, and annually thereafter. Patients who refused or were unable to return were contacted by two surgeons (S.J.D and J.X.T) to obtain the information in their home.

Data collection

The information included comorbidity, mechanism of injury, fracture type, associated injury, operative time, bleeding amount (including operative blood loss and wound drainage), operative approach, complications, quality of reduction, clinical function, and radiological outcomes. The results from patients who were confirmed to have died from natural causes after 12 months follow-up was included in this study. By contrast, the results from patients who had been lost to follow-up or confirmed to have died from natural causes within 12 months follow-up were excluded. Data from the final follow-up visit were analyzed for this study.

Radiographic and clinical evaluation

Three standard plain preoperative radiographs (anteroposterior pelvis, obturator oblique, and iliac oblique views) were obtained along with computed tomography scans to classify fracture according to Letournel's classification system [12]. Reduction quality was evaluated on the three-standard plain post-operative radiographs and graded as anatomical (0 mm to 1 mm of displacement), imperfect (2 mm to 3 mm displacement), or poor (more than 3 mm displacement) on the basis of the residual displacement as defined by Matta [9].

Clinical function was categorized as excellent (18 points), good (15–17 points), fair (13–14 points), or poor (< 13 points) on the basis of the modified Postel Merle D'Aubigne Score, which includes degree of pain (0–6 points), degree of ambulation (0–6 points), and range of motion (0–6 points) components [9, 13]. Radiological outcome was evaluated on the follow-up postoperative radiographs and was graded as excellent, good, fair, and poor in accordance with Matta criteria [9].

The acetabular fracture types were classified by a senior author (J.Y.S). Reduction quality was evaluated by two surgeons (S.K.Z and Z.S.Z) who did not participate in any of the surgical procedures. Two other surgeons (S.J.D and J.X.T) who were blinded to reduction quality completed the clinical and radiological evaluation. The senior author (J.Y.S) made the final assessment when the results (reduction quality and radiological outcome) were inconsistent. We take the average of the clinical outcomes that were evaluated by the two surgeons.

Statistical analysis

Analysis was performed using STATA version 11.0 (StataCorp LP, College Station TX). Continuous data were expressed as mean ± standard deviation (SD) and were analyzed using t-test or one-way ANOVA. Tukey's test was performed for multiple comparisons. The ordinal data were analyzed with Kruscal–Wallis test. Statistical significance was considered at $p < 0.05$ unless otherwise specified.

Results

Patient characteristics

Of the 62 patients, 7 (11.3%) were lost to follow-up at a mean of 18 months (6–31 months) postoperatively and 2 (3.2%) had died from natural causes within 12 months follow-up, during which all patients had excellent or good clinical function. The nine patients were excluded from this study. The remaining 53 patients (44 males and 9 females) aged 60–90 (mean age: 72.8 ± 6.6 years) were enrolled. The mean follow-up was 52.5 ± 24.1 months (range: 18–110 months). Detailed distribution of patient demographics and characteristics, fracture types, mechanism of injury, and associated injury is shown in Table 1.

Operative variable

Operative approach, operative time, and bleeding amount are shown in Table 2. Anatomical reduction was observed in 28 patients (52.8%), imperfect in 19 (35.8%), and poor in 6 (11.3%). Compared with the old–old patients, the young–old patients were more likely to achieve anatomical reduction (67.9% vs. 36%, $p = 0.024$) (Table 2) but more blood loss (705 mL vs. 591 mL, $p = 0.016$) and longer operative time (145 min vs. 110 min, $p = 0.021$) (Table 2).

Clinical results at the final follow-up

Clinical function was excellent in 19 patients (35.8%), good in 20 (37.7%), fair in 4 (7.5%), and poor in 10 (18.9%). The average clinical score (modified Merle d'Aubigne-Postel score) was 15.6 ± 2.7 points (range:

Table 1 Demographics of both groups

Variable	Young-old group (n = 28)	Old-old group (n = 25)
Mean age (years)	67.8 ± 4.1 (60–74)	78.5 ± 3.5 (75–90)
Sex ratio (male:female)	25: 3	19: 6
Mean BMI (kg/m²)	22.3 ± 2.8 (17.9–25.5)	22.3 ± 2.1 (21.3–24.8)
Comorbidity (n)		
Hypertension	15	18
Anemia	6	9
Cardiopathy	2	4
Diabetes mellitus	3	2
Pulmonary	1	4
Cerebrovascular accident	1	3
Fracture types		
Associated both column	9	9
T-shaped	6	3
Transverse + posterior wall	5	2
Anterior column	1	4
Posterior wall	3	2
Anterior wall	0	4
Transverse	2	1
Posterior column	1	0
Posterior column + posterior wall	1	0
Mechanism of injury		
Fall at home	2	7
Pedestrian	1	10
Bike accident	2	1
Motorcyclist	4	0
Auto vs. Pedestrian	14	5
Fall from >2 m	5	2
Associated injury		
Splenic rupture	1	0
Sacroiliac joint dislocation	1	0
Thoracic spine and costal fracture	1	0
Head trauma	1	0
Mean follow-up (months)	60.7 ± 26.6 (24–110)	43.3 ± 17.2 (18–84)

9–18 points). Two patients in the young–old group (3.8%) underwent THA at 30 and 35 months after their initial injuries. One of the two patients have a femoral head injury and subsequent osteonecrosis of the femoral head (Fig. 1), and the other has a poor reduction and subsequent severely post-traumatic osteoarthritis.

Table 2 Operative parameters of both groups (n = 53)

Variable	Young-old group (n = 28)	Old-old group (n = 25)	p-value
Operative approach			0.022
Kocher-Langenbeck	7	4	
Ilioinguinal	1	8	
Kocher-Langenbeck + Ilioinguinal	20	13	
Mean operative time (min)	145 ± 53	110 ± 54	0.021
Mean bleeding amount (ml)	705 ± 308	591 ± 204	0.012
Quality of reduction			0.024
Anatomic	19	9	
Imperfect	7	12	
Poor	2	4	

Up to 75% of the young–old patients and 72% of the old–old patients can achieve good to excellent clinical function. The clinical scores were comparable in both groups (15.5 ± 3.2 vs. 15.7 ± 2.1, $p = 0.787$); however, comparison of the components of the modified Postel Merle D'Aubigne Score showed that the patients in the young–old group had lower pain scores (4.9 ± 1.2 vs. 5.5 ± 0.7, $p = 0.029$), higher ambulation scores (5.5 ± 1.0 vs. 4.9 ± 0.9, $p = 0.027$), and similar range of motion scores (5.1 ± 1.2 vs. 5.3 ± 0.7, $p = 0.457$) than those in the old-old group (Table 3).

The average clinical scores were significantly higher in the young–old patients with anatomical reduction (16.6 ± 2.4 points; range: 9–18 points) than in those with imperfect reduction (13.3 ± 1.9 points; range: 9–18 points) ($p = 0.015$) and poor reduction (12.0 ± 2.8 points; range: 10–14 points) ($p = 0.005$, Fig. 2).

The average clinical scores in the old–old patients with anatomical, imperfect, and poor reduction were 16.1 ± 2.1 (range: 12–18 points), 15.8 ± 2.1 (range: 12–18 points), and 14.8 ± 2.5 points (range: 12–18 points), respectively. No statistical difference in clinical scores was detected between the different grades in reduction quality ($p > 0.05$, Fig. 2, Fig. 3).

The rate of postoperative complication was slightly higher in the old–old group (44.0%) than in the young–old group (39.3%), but no difference was found between the groups ($p = 0.728$, Table 4). Nine (14.5%) of the 62

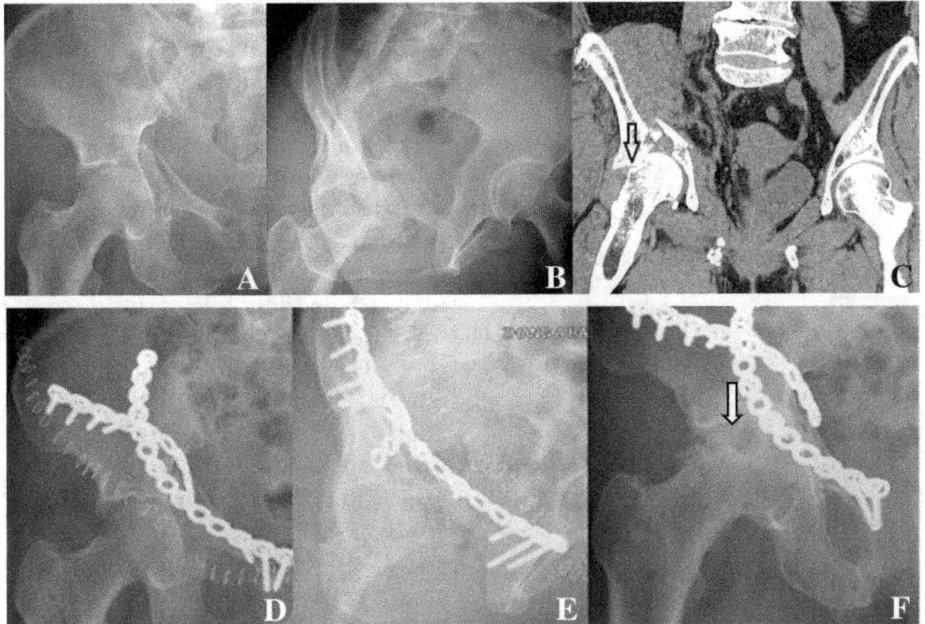

Fig. 1 Radiographs of a 66-year-old female patient with an anterior wall acetabular fracture. **a** Anteroposterior radiograph; **b** Obturator oblique radiograph; **c** CT scan, showing femoral head injury (arrow). **d, e** Immediately after surgery, showing a satisfactory reduction of fracture; **f** The radiograph taken at 30 months postoperatively, showing an osteonecrosis of the femoral head (arrow)

Table 3 Clinical outcomes of both groups at the final follow-up

Variable	Young-old group (n = 28)	Old-old group (n = 25)	p-value
Clinical scores (points)	15.5 ± 3.2	15.7 ± 2.1	0.787
Degree of pain	4.9 ± 1.2	5.5 ± 0.7	0.029
Degree of ambulation	5.5 ± 1.0	4.9 ± 0.9	0.027
Range of motion	5.1 ± 1.2	5.3 ± 0.7	0.457

patients died from natural causes during the follow-up period; of these nine patients, one died at 6 months, one at 9 months, and seven at 18–72 months postoperatively (average: 35 ± 19 months). The average age at the time of surgery of the nine patients was 78.4 ± 6.3 years (range: 68–85 years).

Radiological outcomes at the final follow-up

We found that better clinical function meant fewer patients willing to return for radiological evaluation. For example, only 16 patients have completed radiological evaluation. Of these patients, radiological outcomes were excellent in three patients, good in four patients, fair in three patients, and poor in six patients. The radiological outcomes do not reflect the real situation of all patients because most patients were not assessed. Thus, these outcomes were not included in this analysis.

Discussion

With the increased acetabular fractures in the elderly population, an understanding of how these patients respond to ORIF is important. We compared the postoperative clinical function and complication rates between old–old and young–old patients who underwent ORIF and investigated the influence of patient age on the association of reduction quality and clinical function.

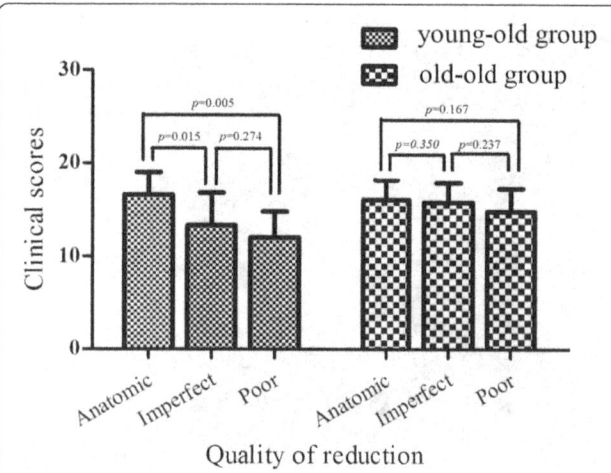

Fig. 2 The relationship between quality of reduction and clinical scores

The clinical scores were similar in both groups (15.5 points vs. 15.7 points, $p = 0.787$). By contrast, previous studies presented an inverse relationship between age and clinical function [4–6, 9]. This discrepancy in results may be attributed to the fact that previous studies [9–11] represent a wide age variety and compare the clinical function between young patients (< 40, 50, and 55 years old) and old patients (> 40, 50, or 55 years old), whereas the present study represents only elderly patients (60–90 years) and a comparator group (young–old patients vs. old–old patients). We also compared the component of clinical score between the two groups and found higher pain scores ($p = 0.029$) and lower ambulation scores ($p = 0.026$) in the old–old patients than in the young–old patients but a comparable range of motion scores ($p = 0.457$). This result may be related to the different pain tolerance levels of patients and the increased pain threshold in the old–old patients.

Although elderly patients often have comorbid medical conditions, few age-related complications were observed and no perioperative death occurred in this study. These findings may be attributed to the rational treatment strategy for elderly patients. This strategy includes optimization of preoperative patient's medical condition to improve surgery tolerance, as well as minimization of operative trauma and time and blood loss to achieve stable internal fixation of fractures rather than to strive for anatomical reduction. When a surgeon strives for an intraoperative anatomical reduction, this procedure often prolonged operative time and increased blood loss that may harm to the older population because older patients, especially those with medical conditions, have weaker blood loss tolerance than young patients. In the present study, the patients in the young–old group showed higher anatomical reduction (67.9% vs.36.0%, $p = 0.024$), blood loss (705 ml vs. 591 ml, $p = 0.016$), and operative time (145 min vs. 110 min, $p = 0.021$) compared with those in the old–old group. This finding may explain the similar complication rate in both groups ($p = 0.728$).

In this study, we found that reduction quality exerted an age-dependent influence on clinical function. The reduction quality in the young–old patients was significantly associated with clinical function ($p = 0.001$), and an anatomical reduction was associated with a good or excellent function. By contrast, no statistical difference

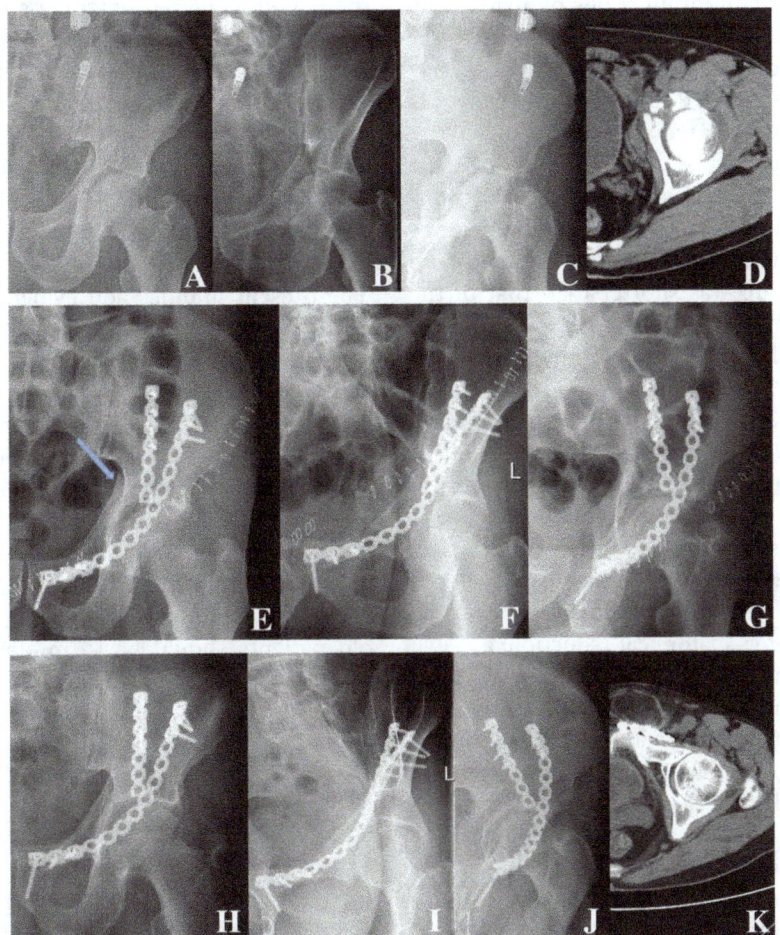

Fig. 3 Radiographs of a 75-year-old male patient with an anterior wall acetabular fracture. **a** Anteroposterior radiograph; **b** Obturator oblique radiograph; **c** Iliac oblique radiograph; **d** CT scan. Radiographs showing imperfect reduction (arrow) of the fracture immediately after the operation. **e** Anteroposterior radiograph; **f** Obturator oblique radiograph; **g** Iliac oblique radiograph. Radiographs showing an excellent radiological outcome at 84 months after the operation and the clinical score was 18 points. **h** Anteroposterior radiograph; **i** Obturator oblique radiograph; **j** iliac oblique radiograph; **k** CT scan

Table 4 Complications and natural death during the follow-up of both groups

Variable	Young-old group (n = 28)	Old-old group (n = 25)	p-value
Complications (n, %)	11 (39.3%)	11 (44.0%)	0.728
Lateral femoral cutaneous nerve palsy	0	2 (8.0%)	
Loss of reduction	0	2 (8.0%)	
Deep venous thrombosis	1 (3.6%)	1 (4.0%)	
Superficial infection	0	1 (4.0%)	
Heterotopic ossification	8 (28.6%)	4 (16.0%)	
Grade I	3	2	
Grade II	3	2	
Grade III	2	0	
Femoral head avascular necrosis	2 (7.1%)	0	
Incisional hernia	0	1 (4.0%)	
Death (n, %)	1 (3.6%)	6 (24.0%)	0.043

was detected among the clinical functions of anatomical, imperfect, and poor reduction in the old–old patients ($p = 0.587$). We speculated that the old–old patients may have characteristics (e.g., limited life expectancy, low activity level, low functional requirements, and weak muscle strength around the hip) that may reduce the wear and tear of the hip cartilage resulting from non-anatomical reduction and may increase their tolerance to non-anatomical reduction. In addition, the follow-up time of the old–old group was shorter than that of the young–old group (43 ± 17 months vs. 61 ± 27 months) because of the limited life expectancy of the old–old patients (the death rates in the old–old and young–old groups were respectively 24.0% and 3.6%, respectively), and this study included the patients who died. In addition, studies have reported that a precise anatomical reduction highly correlates with the best long-term clinical function rather than the short-term function [9, 14, 15]. Old–old patients with the above-mentioned characteristics may not necessarily need to sacrifice operative time and blood loss to strive for anatomical reduction; a stable fracture reduction that allows early postoperative ambulation may be accepted in old–old patients. In support to our findings, Archdeacon et al. [8] conducted a retrospective study of 26 patients older than 70 years with acetabular fracture and suggested that these patients can tolerate imperfect reduction.

We found that the age-dependent influence on the rate of anatomical reduction was higher in the young–old group than in the old–old group (67.9% vs. 36.0%, $p = 0.024$) and that the loss of reduction was more likely to occur in the old–old group than in the young–old group (8.0% vs. 0%). This result may be attributed to the fact that old–old patients often have a combination of osteoporosis and comminuted acetabular fractures, which complicate the completion of anatomical reduction and stability [9]. Moreover, accurate reduction was not attempted for some of the old–old patients in this study with the aforementioned characteristics.

Weakness of this study

This study has some limitations. First, the small sample size due to the relatively low incidence of acetabular fractures in elderly patients may compromise the robustness of the results. Second, the mean follow-up times of the young–old and old–old groups were 60.7 and 43.3 months, respectively, which may be too short to draw a definite conclusion on the association between reduction quality and clinical function, particularly in the old–old group. Third, all patients came from a single center, and the results of patients and treatment preferences from this center may not be applicable to other centers. Fourth, the clinical function was evaluated using the modified Postel Merle D'Aubigne Score instead of

the patient-centered outcome scores (e.g., EQ5D, SF-12, SMFA, and SF-36). The patient-centered outcome scores for elderly patients may be much helpful. However, the modified Postel Merle D'Aubigne Score is widely applied to assess the clinical function of patients with acetabular fractures, and this scoring system has been routinely used since 1990 [16, 17].

Conclusions

The present findings add evidence to justify performing ORIF in elderly patients with acetabular fractures. Our findings suggest that individuals older than 75 years may achieve similar clinical functions and complications to young–old patients. Moreover, unlike that in the young–old patients, the reduction quality in the old–old patients may be not affecting the clinical function. Therefore, the treatment strategy of acetabular fractures with ORIF may be different according to different age groups. In particular, the goal for young–old patients should be anatomical reduction, whereas that for old–old patients should be to minimize operative time and blood loss, and thus achieve a stable fixation that allows early post-operative ambulation.

Abbreviations
ORIF: Open reduction and internal fixation; THA: Total hip arthroplasty

Acknowledgements
The authors thank Sheng-Jie Dong, and Zhi Yang from the Department of Orthopedic Surgery, Affiliated Hospital of Xuzhou Medical University for the Working Environment for valuable technical assistance and support.

Funding
This work was supported by the Jiangsu Provincial Medical Youth Talent (QNRC2016800), the Science and Technology Planning Project of Xuzhou (KC16SL111), the Foundation of Jiangsu Province commission of Health and Family Planning (H2017081), and the Key Medical Subjects Foundation of Jiangsu Province (BE2015627).

Authors' contributions
ZGC, YXM did the study, analyzed the data, and wrote the manuscript. ZGC, YXM, SYJ, FS, CXY, GKJ was involved in the design, data management, and analysis of the study. SJY, FS, GKJ were involved in the study design, and data analysis. ZGC, YXM, FS, SJY, GKJ contributed to the study design and analysis. All authors read and approved the final manuscript.

Competing interests
The authors declare that they have no competing interests.

Author details
^{1}Department of Orthopedic Surgery, the Affiliated Hospital of Xuzhou Medical University, No. 99 Huaihai West Road, Xuzhou, Jiangsu 221002, People's Republic of China. ^{2}Hyperbaric Oxygen Treatment Center, the Affiliated Hospital of Xuzhou Medical University, No. 99 Huaihai West Road, Xuzhou, Jiangsu 221002, People's Republic of China. ^{3}Orthopaedic Department, the First Affiliated Hospital of Soochow University, 188 Shizi Street, Suzhou, Jiangsu 215006, People's Republic of China.

References

1. Ferguson TA, Patel R, Bhandari M, Matta JM. Fractures of the acetabulum in patients aged 60 years and older: an epidemiological and radiological study. J Bone Joint Surg Br. 2010;92(2):250–7.

2. Heeg M. Fractures of the acetabulum. Drukkerij van Denderen B.V: Groningen; 1990.

3. Tornetta P 3rd. Displaced acetabular fractures: indications for operative and nonoperative management. J Am Acad Orthop Surg 2001; 9(1):18–28.

4. Tidermark J, Blomfeldt R, Ponzer S, Söderqvist A, Törnkvist H. Primary total hip arthroplasty with a Burch-Schneider antiprotrusion cage and autologous bone grafting for acetabular fractures in elderly patients. J Orthop Trauma. 2003;17(3):193–7.

5. Mouhsine E, Garofalo R, Borens O, Blanc CH, Wettstein M, Leyvraz PF. Cable fixation and early total hip arthroplasty in the treatment of acetabular fractures in elderly patients. J Arthroplast. 2004;19(3):344–8.

6. Herscovici D Jr, Lindvall E, Bolhofner B, Scaduto JM. The combined hip procedure: open reduction internal fixation combined with total hip arthroplasty for the management of acetabular fractures in the elderly. J Orthop Trauma 2010; 24 (5):291–296.

7. Anglen JO, Burd TA, Hendricks KJ, Harrison P. The "Gull sign": a harbinger of failure for internal fixation of geriatric acetabular fractures. J Orthop Trauma. 2003;17(9):625–34.

8. Archdeacon MT, Kazemi N, Collinge C, Budde B, Schnell S. Treatment of protrusio fractures of the acetabulum in patients 70 years and older. J Orthop Trauma. 2013;27(5):256–61.

9. Matta JM. Fractures of the acetabulum: accuracy of reduction and clinical results in patients managed operatively within three weeks after the injury. J Bone Joint Surg Am. 1996;78(11):1632–45.

10. Kreder HJ, Rozen N, Borkhoff CM, Laflamme YG, McKee MD, Schemitsch EH, Stephen DJ. Determinants of functional outcome after simple and complex acetabular factures involving the posterior wall. J Bone Joint Surg Br. 2006; 88(6):776–82.

11. Moed BR, WillsonCarr SE, Watson JT. Results of operative treatment of fractures of the posterior wall of the acetabulum. J Bone Joint Surg Am. 2002;84(5):752–8.

12. Letournel E, Judet R. Fractures of the Acetabulum, 2nd ed. New York: Springer. pp 63–397(1993).

13. D'aubigne RM, Postel M. Functional results of hip arthroplasty with acrylic prosthesis. J Bone Joint Surg Am. 1954;36(3):451–75.

14. Mears DC, Velyvis JH, Chang CP. Displaced acetabular fractures managed operatively: indicators of outcome. Clin Orthop Relat Res. 2003;407:173–86.

15. Marsh JL, Buckwalter J, Gelberman R, Dirschl D, Olson S, Brown T, Llinias A. Articular fractures: does an anatomic reduction really change the result? J Bone Joint Surg Am. 2002;84(7):1259–71.

16. Zha GC, Sun JY, Chen L, Zheng HM, Wang Q, Jin Y. Late reconstruction of posterior acetabular wall fractures using iliac crest. J Trauma Acute Care Surg. 2012;72(5):1386–92.

17. Wei L, Sun JY, Wang Y, Yang X. Surgical treatment and prognosis of acetabular fractures associated with ipsilateral femoral neck fractures. Orthopedics. 2011;34(5):348.

15

Surgical treatment for diffused-type giant cell tumor (pigmented villonodular synovitis) about the ankle joint

Xingchen Li, Yang Xu, Yuan Zhu and Xiangyang Xu[*]

Abstract

Background: Diffused-type giant cell tumor(Dt-GCT) is a rare, aggressive disorder of the joint synovium, bursa and tendon sheaths. Osseous erosions and subchondral cysts may develop as the result of synovium infiltration in Dt-GCT. We present a retrospective study of a series of patients who are diagnosed with Dt-GCT about the ankle joint, there clinical outcome is evaluated in this study.

Material and method: Fifteen patients with radiologically and histologically confirmed Dt-GCT about the ankle joint were identified in our foot and ankle department. Patients were managed with open synovectomy for the tumor tissue and bone grafting for bony erosions. X-rays and MRI scans were used for evaluation of the tumor and bony erosions pre- and post-operatively. Pre- and post-operative ankle function was assessed using the American Orthopedic Foot and Ankle Society –Ankle and Hindfoot (AOFAS-AH) score and the Muscularskeletal Tumor Society (MSTS) score.

Results: The mean follow-up duration was 37.4 months (range 25 to 50 months). There were 6 males and 9 females, with a mean age of 35 years old (range 18 to 65 years). All patients had talar erosion with the average size of 10.1*9.1*8.2 mm, distal tibia was affected in 5 patients with the average size of 6.2*5.6*5.8 mm. 7 patients had tendon involvement, 2 patients had recurrence and progression of ankle osteoarthritis. Both of them underwent ankle fusion. At the time of last follow-up, the mean AOFAS-AH score increased from 49 to 80 points ($p < 0.05$), the MSTS score increased from 12 to 22 points ($p < 0.05$).

Conclusion: For Dt-GCT with bony erosions, open synovectomy combined with bone grafting seems to be a safe and effective operation for the salvage of ankle joint. Fusion is recommended for failed and severe cartilage destruction of the ankle joint.

Keywords: Giant cell tumors, Ankle joint, Joint preserving surgery, Bone transplantation

Background

Giant cell-rich tumors(GCT) that arise from tendons and synovium are now classified into two forms: localized and diffuse. In the World Health Organization(WHO) classification, the former is described as giant cell tumor of tendon sheath(GCT-TS), whereas the later is described as diffused-type giant cell tumor(Dt-GCT), also known as pigmented villonodular synovitis(PVNS) [1, 2].

GCT-TS is characterized by focal involvement of the synovium, tendon sheath or bursa, with nodular or pedunculated masses. While the Dt-GCT is relatively rare, benign and locally aggressive [3]. It is featured with the osseous erosions and subchondral cysts resulted from synovial infiltration [2, 4–7]. The etiology for Dt-GCT is still controversial and has not been well established in literature. Chronic inflammatory disease [8, 9] or a history of trauma [10] may cause Dt-GCT.

The most common joint involvement of Dt-GCT include knee, hand joints and hip, followed by ankle and shoulder [10–12]. Dt-GCT about the ankle joint accounts for approximately 2.5% of the cases [11]. Patients

* Correspondence: xu664531@126.com
Orthopaedic Department, Ruijin Hospital, Ruijin Er Road No.197, Shanghai 200025, China

may present with insidious pain, swollen and stiffness of the affected ankle joint which may has presented for months or years. Physical examination can find swollen and restricted range of motion of the ankle joint. Subtalar joint or even mid-foot joints can also be affected in several severe diffused cases.

Subchondral cysts and osseous erosions can present in Dt-GCT about the ankle joint. Loss of bony structure and volume is typical at sites of fracture and fusion. We hypothesis that for mild to moderate bony erosion of the ankle joint, open synovectomy combined with impaction bone grafting can be able to reduce symptoms and prevent further destruction of the talar cartilage and progression of the ankle osteoarthritis.

The aim of this study is to report our experience in the management of Dt-GCT about the ankle joint, and also to evaluate the clinical outcome of open synovectomy combined with bone grafting.

Methods

We retrospectively reviewed a total of 15 patients with radiologically and histologically confirmed Dt-GCT about the ankle joint (Fig. 1). Patient demographics include age, sex, side, symptom and follow-up duration, size of bony erosions, patient satisfaction were recorded (Table 1).

The diagnosis of Dt-GCT was made according to patient history, clinical manifestation, MRI findings and typical histological features. MRI scans were obtained under suspicion of Dt-GCT. The location and extent of involvement of the tumor were further evaluated by MRI, as well as the adjacent soft tissue, joints and tendon sheaths involvement.

MRI scans were also helpful to plan the appropriate surgical approach [13]. The surgical approach was carefully designed preoperatively based on the location of tumor tissue and bony erosions. Patients were managed with open synovectomy for the tumor tissue and bone

grafting for bony erosions. No radiotherapy was used for any patient.

Open synovectomy was performed for the treatment of Dt-GCT about the ankle joint. Based on the location of the tumor tissue and bony erosions, anterior or medial and lateral two incision approaches were used for exposure of the ankle joint. Bony erosions were identified and carefully debrided at the surgery, followed by impaction bone grafting to prevent the further fracture or collapse of the talar cartilage. Allogenic cancellous bone (Osteorad Ltd., Shanxi, China) was used for impaction bone grafting, while osteochondral autograft transplantation was considered when localized cartilage defect (greater than 10 mm in diameter) was identified at the surgery. Special instruments (osteochondral autograft transfer system, Arthrex, USA) were used for osteochondral autograft transplantation. Cylindrical autologous osteochondral plug, 8 or 10 mm in diameter taken from the ipsilateral knee joint was used for reconstruction of the talar defect. The medial upper part of the femoral chondyle was preferred as the donor site (Figs. 2, 3 and 4).

Functional outcome was evaluated using the American Orthopedic Foot and Ankle Society –Ankle and Hindfoot (AOFAS-AH) score and the Muscularskeletal Tumor Society (MSTS) score before and after surgery. The MSTS score was based on three general factors (pain, function, emotional acceptance) and three lower limb factors (use of supports, ability to walk and gait) [14]. Each category had a maximum score of 5 points and the total score was 30 points. The AOFAS-AH score was subdivided into pain (maximum 40 points), function (maximum 50 points), and alignment (maximum 10 points). Patient satisfaction level was graded as excellent, good, fair or poor.

SAS software (version 8.02, SAS Institute, USA) was used for statistical analysis. Paired student t-test was conducted for the evaluation of improvement in AOFAS-AH score and MSTS score. A P value less than 0.05 was considered to be statistically significant.

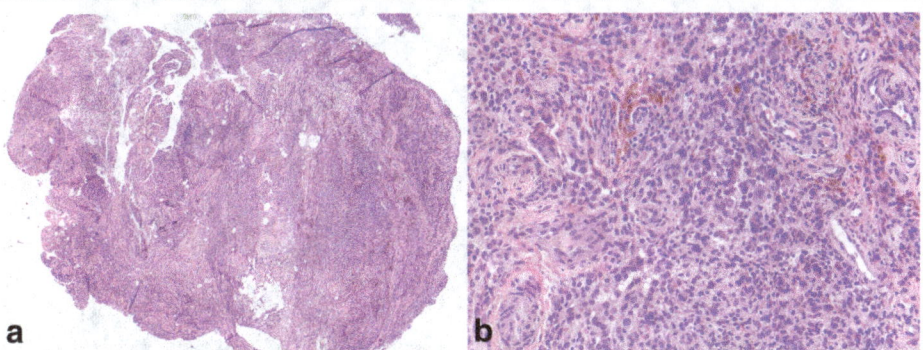

Fig. 1 The photomicrographs demonstrate the mixture of multinucleated giant cells, mononuclear cells, foam cells and hemosiderin deposits **a**, Low-power view (H&E stain, original magnification ×25); **b**, High-power view (H&E stain, original magnification ×200)

Table 1 Patient demographics

NO.	FU (M)	Side	Symptom Duration (M)	Bony Erosions (mm)	Talar Lesion Management	Additional Surgery	Patient Satisfaction
1	38	R	18	Talus: 10*13*8, 12*10*9, Distal Tibia: 5*5*7	OATS (Ø10mm, 2 plugs)	–	Good
2	26	R	24	Talus: 10*9*7, Distal Tibia: 11*8*10, Distal fibular: 8*12*8	Bone grafting (allogenic cancellous bone)	Modified Brostrom	Good
3	27	L	15	Talus: 7*6*6	Bone grafting (allogenic cancellous bone)	Modified Brostrom	Fair
4	43	R	12	Talus: 10*10*8, Distal Tibia: 4*4*3	OATS (Ø10mm,2 plugs)	Syndesmosis screw fixaion	Fair
5	25	L	10	Talus: 6*5*7	Bone grafting (allogenic cancellous bone)	Modified Brostrom	Excellent
6	44	R	16	Talus: 9*6*8	Bone grafting (allogenic cancellous bone)	Modified Brostrom	Good
7	30	R	15	Talus: 7*5*5	Bone grafting (allogenic cancellous bone)	–	Good
8	45	L	12	Talus: 5*9*7, Distal Tibia: 5*6*5	Bone grafting (allogenic cancellous bone)	–	Fair
9	37	L	10	Talus: 8*8*5	Bone grafting (allogenic cancellous bone)	Modified Brostrom	Bad
10	50	R	6	Talus: 14*9*11	OATS (Ø10mm, 2 plugs)	–	Bad
11	42	R	30	Talus: 6*7*8, Distal Tibia: 6*5*4	Bone grafting (allogenic cancellous bone)	–	Excellent
12	31	R	24	Talus: 10*11*9, Subtalar joint	Bone grafting (allogenic cancellous bone)	Modified Brostrom	Fair
13	49	L	12	Talus: 14*9*10	OATS (Ø10mm, 2 plugs)	–	Excellent
14	34	R	18	Talus: 9*8*8	Bone grafting (allogenic cancellous bone)	Modified Brostrom	Good
15	40	L	15	Talus: 14*12*7	OATS (Ø10mm, 2 plugs)	–	Fair

Results

The mean follow-up duration was 37.4 months (range 25 to 50 months). There were 6 males and 9 females in this study, with a mean age of 35 years old (range 18 to 65 years) at the time of surgery. The right ankle was involved in 9 patients (60%) and the remaining 6 patients (40%) had their left ankle got involved. 12 patients (80%) had a history of ankle trauma, while the remaining 3 patients (20%) denied any history of trauma. On average, symptoms presented for 15.8 months (range, 6 to 30 months) before the patient sought operative intervention. MRI scans were obtained pre-operatively for

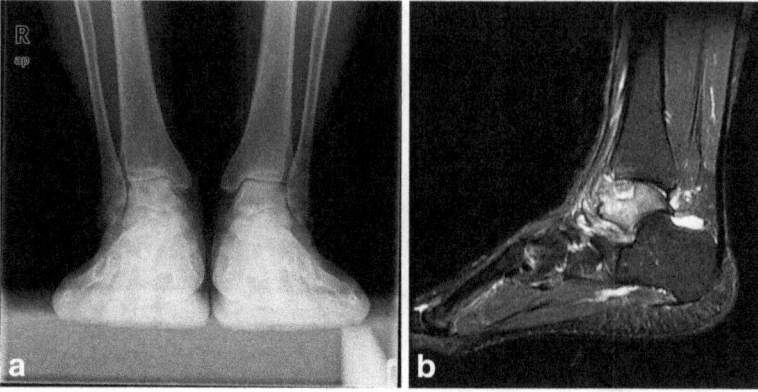

Fig. 2 a Weight bearing Anterioposterior view of the ankle joint showed a lucent area at the talus; **b** A large subchondral cyst wad identified with high signal on SIRT image

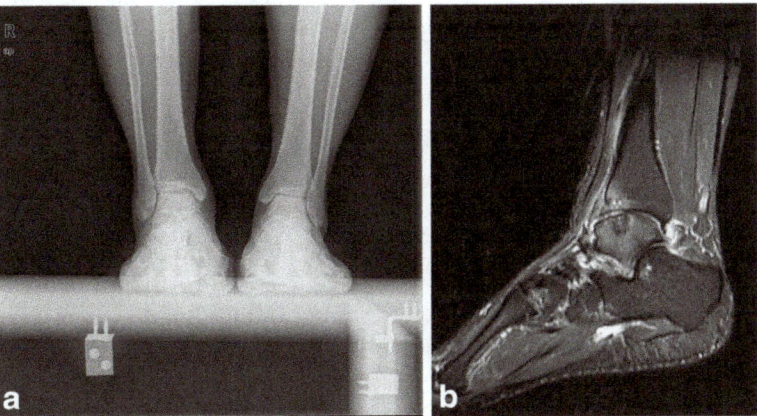

Fig. 3 a, an anteriomedial incision was made for the exposure of the tumor tissue and talus; **b**, two osteochondral autografts were used to fill the talar defects

further evaluation of the tumor and surrounding tissue infiltration. The posterior tibialis tendon was involved in 4 patients (26.7%), the flexor hallux longus tendon was involved in 2 patients (13.4%), the flexor digitorum longus tendon was involved in 1 patient (6.7%) and the peroneal tendons were involved in 2 patients (13.4%). The subtalar joint was involved in 1 patient (6.7%) and the syndesmosis was involved in 1 patient (6.7%). The mean size of talar erosion was 10.1*9.1*8.2 mm, the distal tibia was involved in 5 patients (33.3%) with the mean size of 6.2*5.6*5.8 mm.

Open synovectomy was performed for all patients. Anterior approach was preferred in 7 patients (46.7%), medial and lateral two incisions were used in 8 patients (53.3%). For bony erosions, allogenic cancellous bone grafting was performed in 10 patients (66.7%), and the remaining 5 patients (33.3%) were managed with osteochondral autograft transplantation. No donor site morbidity was reported at the time of last follow-up.

2 patients with large bony erosions refused to receive ankle fusion as a primary surgery. One of them was 35 years old and the other was 48 years old, both of them had a strong desire to preserve their ankle joints. So open synovectomy, debridement of the subchondral cysts and bone grafting were performed for salvage of the ankle joint. Though mild stiffness and pain of the ankle joint was noticed, both of them were satisfied with the surgery at the time of last follow-up,

1 patient underwent syndesmosis screw fixation as the result of bony erosion at the site of distal tibiofibular syndesmosis. In 7 patients (46.7%), the lateral ligament was thought to be inadequate to restore the stability of the ankle joint as the result of extensive open synovectomy, the additional modified Brostrom procedure were performed to restore the stability of the ankle joint.

The Muscularskeletal Tumor Society (MSTS) score and the AOFAS-AH questionnaires were used to assess the functional outcome of the surgery. The mean MSTS score increased from 12 pre-operatively to 22 points

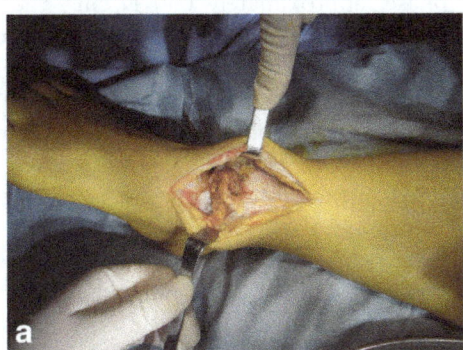
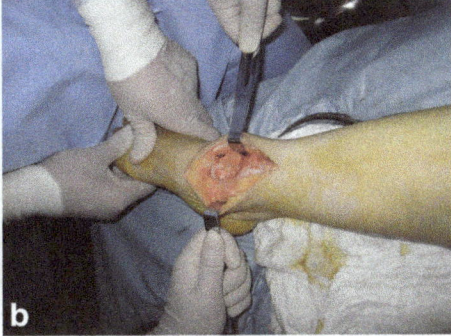

Fig. 4 a, Weight bearing Anterioposterior view of the ankle joint showed improvement of the subchondral cyst in talus at 31 months after surgery; **b**, The SIRT image displayed the healing of the autograft to the surrounding tissue, the improvement of the bone marrow edema

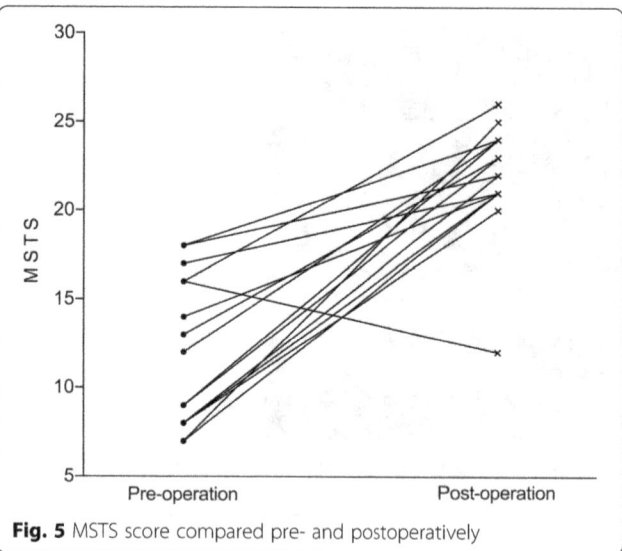

Fig. 5 MSTS score compared pre- and postoperatively

post-operatively at the time of last follow-up ($t = 6.8$, $p < 0.05$) (Fig. 5). The mean AOFAS-AH score increased from 49 pre-operatively to 80 points post-operatively ($t = 7.8$, $p < 0.05$) (Fig. 6). The AOFAS-AH pain subscale improved from 11 pre-operatively to 30 points post-operatively. The function subscale improved from 28 pre-operatively to 40 points post-operatively, and the alignment subscale remained the same at 10 points.

In regard to the overall satisfaction of the operation at the time of last follow-up, 8 patients (53.3%) rated the results as excellent or good, 5 (33.3%) were fair, and the remaining 2 (13.3%) were bad.

Magnetic resonance imaging scans were available for 8 patients (53.3%) at the time of last follow-up. The MRI findings showed at least 70% defect fill in 5 patients. 6 patients (75%) had normal or nearly normal signal at

repair sites, 5 patients (62.5%) had mild or no effusion and 4 patients (50%) showed mild or no underlying bone-marrow edema.

Discussion

GCT involving tendon sheaths and synovium can be subdivided into two types: the localized and the diffuse [1, 2]. The diagnosis is achieved by clinical evaluation, radiological and histological examinations. Dt-GCT is characterized by the insidious infiltration of the synovial lining and leading to osseous erosions [2, 6]. For patients with Dt-GCT about the ankle joint, tendon sheaths, talus, distal tibia and subtalar joint can be affected. In review of the literature, researches reporting the management of Dt-GCT about the ankle joint are quite limited.

The etiology of bony erosion is still controversial, increased joint pressure or pannus infiltration may be the reason for bony invasion [15, 16]. Efforts have been made to identify more detailed pathologies of Dt-GCT and bony involvement, like expression of an osteoclast phenotype [17, 18] or colony- stimulating factor 1 [19], and production of matrix metalloproteinases (MMP) [20, 21].

Despite the totally different pathologies between osteochondral lesion of the talus and bony erosion in Dt-GCT, cyclic loading of the ankle joint may be one of the contributors to subchondral cysts in both entities [22, 23]. Once the subchondral bone plate is broken as the result of trauma or synovial infiltration, ankle fluid can be forced into the subchondral bone during cyclic loading of the ankle joint. Subchondral cysts could occur as the result of cyclic loading of the joint and stimulating nerve endings in the subchondral bone, causing symptoms [22, 23]. To our knowledge, open synovectomy without the management of subchondral cysts will not be able to adequately relieve pain [24].

Meanwhile, early diagnosis and management for Dt-GCT and bony erosions are also essential for preventing further bone and cartilage damage [2, 25–28]. Ankle joint sustains extremely high pressure during the stance phase, approximately 650 N/cm^2, the pressure can be even much higher during running according the biomechanical tests [22, 29]. So loss of bony structure and volume is typical at the sites of fracture and fusion. Saxena A and his colleagues [25] reported their study of ten patients with Dt-GCT about the ankle joint, the mean follow-up duration was 4.5 years. 5 patients had bony involvement, they advocated that surgical management for these patients could include open synovectomy and bone grafting of the cystic areas, along with irrigation with hydrogen peroxide. In our study, all patients with bony erosions are also managed with bone grafting. The use of impaction bone grafting will reconstruct the bony defect and provide structural support to the surrounding

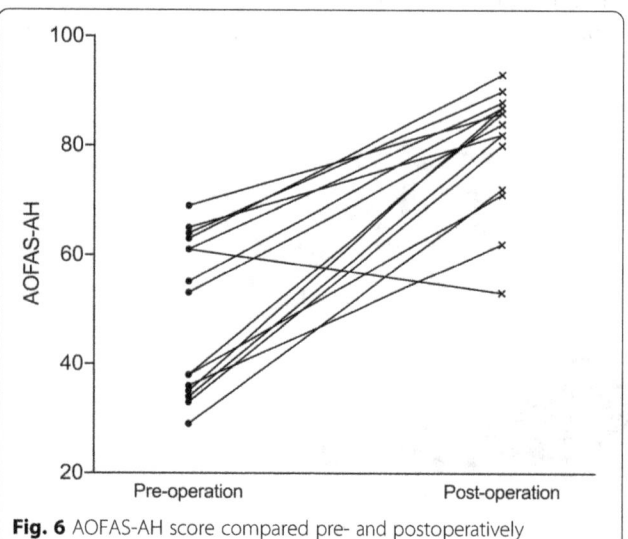

Fig. 6 AOFAS-AH score compared pre- and postoperatively

talar cartilage. Meanwhile, bone grafting also helps to improve the osteoinductive and osteoconductive processes. It is osteoinductive, bringing growth factors, signaling molecules that will facilitate bone growth and also osteoconductive, providing a mineral and collagen scaffold for native cells [30, 31]. Thus, Simultaneous treatment for the tumor tissue and bony erosion is warranted [25].

However, there is some disputes over the management for bony erosions of Dt-GCT in literature. Stvenson et al. [2] presented 13 patients with Dt-GCT about the foot and ankle simply underwent open total synovectomy, 5 patients who had ankle joint erosions, the periarticular erosions and cysts were curetted with no bone grafting. No radiotherapy was used after surgery. None of the 13 patients had recurrence and all of them achieved excellent ankle functions at final follow-up.

Recurrence is among the most common complications for GCT after operation. GCT-TS can be managed successfully with open total synovectomy. However, the recurrence rate can be high in Dt-GCT even after extensive excision of the tumor tissue. The reason for recurrence can be multifactorial, treatment strategies, surgeon's experience, the severity of the primary lesion and the involvement of the bony structures. Though Dt-GCT is usually managed with open synovectomy, while arthroscopic synovectomy is usually indicated in localized GCT, no consensus about the treatment strategies has been reached. Most recently, Noailles T and his colleagues [32] reviewed the literature about open surgery or arthroscopic synovectomy for GCT-TS in 2017, 33 articles were selected in this review, involving 1448 individuals. They concluded that arthroscopic excision was effective for localized GCT-TS for all four joints (shoulder, hip, knee, ankle). While the efficacy of arthroscopic synovectomy had only been shown for the knee joint for Dt-GCT.

2 patients (Patient No.9 and Patient No. 10) (13.3%) had recurrence and progressed to severe ankle osteoarthritis after primary open synovectomy in this study. Both of them complained continues ankle swelling, restricted range of motion of the ankle joint after surgery. And even unable to walk due to severe ankle pain during ambulation. X-rays or MRI showed severe articular destruction and bony erosions about the ankle joint. Ankle fusion was recommended for both of them. No recurrence was found after ankle fusion. None of the patients had wound problems after operation. Though 4 patients still had mild to moderate pain about the ankle joint with restricted range of motion of the ankle joint, they were satisfied with the surgery. We did not find any evidence of recurrence or progression of osteoarthritis on X-rays or MRI. Oral medication and functional rehabilitation was recommended for these patients.

Radiation has been advocated for Dt-GCT in postoperative setting after incomplete resection or failed primary surgery [33–35]. Mollon B and his colleagues [36] reported a meta-analysis about the effect of surgical synovectomy and radiotherapy on the rate of recurrence of Dt-GCT in 2015, very low-quality evidence found that the rate of recurrence of Dt-GCT was reduced by perioperative radiotherapy. And they suggested that open synovectomy or synovectomy combined with perioperative radiotherapy for Dt-GCT is associated with a reduced rate of recurrence.

Limitations of our study include the retrospective nature, limited patient number and follow-up duration and the use of self-reporting scores. Further prospective studies and longer term studies on larger patient population will be needed to ultimately determine the efficacy of this technique.

Conclusions

In conclusion, early diagnosis and management are essential for Dt-GCT about the ankle joint. Open synovectomy together with bone grafting seems to be a safe and effective operation for the salvage of the ankle joint. Fusion is recommended for failed and severe cartilage destruction of the ankle joint.

Abbreviations
AOFAS-AH: American Orthopaedic Foot and Ankle Society-Ankle and Hindfoot; Dt-GCT: Diffused-type Giant Cell Tumor; GCT: Giant Cell-rich Tumors; GCT-TS: Giant Cell Tumor of Tendon Sheath; MSTS: the Muscularskeletal Tumor Society; PVNS: Pigmented Villonodular Synovitis; WHO: World Health Organization

Acknowledgements
None.

Funding
This study was supported by a research grants from Medical Engineering Project of Shanghai Jiaotong University, Grand Number: YG2016MS61.

Authors' contributions
XL drafted the manuscript and performed the statistical analysis, YX and YZ helped to draft the manuscript and carried out the data collections, XX designed the study and helped to draft the manuscript. All authors read and approved the final manuscript.

Competing interests
The authors declare that they have no competing interests.

References
1. van der Heijden L, et al. The management of diffuse-type giant cell tumour (pigmented villonodular synovitis) and giant cell tumour of tendon sheath (nodular tenosynovitis). J Bone Joint Surg Br. 2012;94(7):882–8.
2. Stevenson JD, et al. Diffuse pigmented villonodular synovitis (diffuse-type giant cell tumour) of the foot and ankle. Bone Joint J. 2013;95-B(3):384–90.
3. Granowitz SP, D'Antonio J, Mankin HL. The pathogenesis and long-term end results of pigmented villonodular synovitis. Clin Orthop Relat Res. 1976;114: 335–51.

4. Sharma H, et al. Outcome of 17 pigmented villonodular synovitis (PVNS) of the knee at 6 years mean follow-up. Knee. 2007;14(5):390–4.

5. Sharma V, Cheng EY. Outcomes after excision of pigmented villonodular synovitis of the knee. Clin Orthop Relat Res. 2009;467(11):2852–8.

6. Lee M, et al. Diffuse pigmented villonodular synovitis of the foot and ankle treated with surgery and radiotherapy. Int Orthop. 2005;29(6):403–5.

7. Mori H, et al. Diffuse pigmented villonodular synovitis of the ankle with severe bony destruction: treatment of a case by surgical excision with limited arthrodesis. Am J Orthop (Belle Mead NJ). 2009;38(12):E187–9.

8. Galli M, et al. Localized pigmented villonodular synovitis of the anterior cruciate ligament of the knee: an exceptional presentation of a rare disease with neoplastic and inflammatory features. Int J Immunopathol Pharmacol. 2012;25(4):1131–6.

9. Sakkers RJ, de Jong D, van der Heul RO. X-chromosome inactivation in patients who have pigmented villonodular synovitis. J Bone Joint Surg Am. 1991;73(10):1532–6.

10. Myers BW, Masi AT. Pigmented villonodular synovitis and tenosynovitis: a clinical epidemiologic study of 166 cases and literature review. Medicine (Baltimore). 1980;59(3):223–38.

11. Rao AS, Vigorita VJ. Pigmented villonodular synovitis (giant-cell tumor of the tendon sheath and synovial membrane). A review of eighty-one cases. J Bone Joint Surg Am. 1984;66(1):76–94.

12. Korim MT, et al. Clinical and oncological outcomes after surgical excision of pigmented villonodular synovitis at the foot and ankle. Foot Ankle Surg. 2014;20(2):130–4.

13. Konrath GA, Shifrin LZ, Nahigian K. Magnetic resonance imaging in the diagnosis of localized pigmented villonodular synovitis of the ankle: a case report. Foot Ankle Int. 1994;15(2):84–7.

14. Enneking WF, et al. A system for the functional evaluation of reconstructive procedures after surgical treatment of tumors of the musculoskeletal system. Clin Orthop Relat Res. 1993;286:241–6.

15. Pandey S, Pandey AK. Pigmented villonodular synovitis with bone involvement. Arch Orthop Trauma Surg. 1981;98(3):217–23.

16. Heller SL, et al. Pigmented villonodular synovitis about the ankle: two case reports. Foot Ankle Int. 2008;29(5):527–33.

17. Darling JM, et al. Multinucleated cells in pigmented villonodular synovitis and giant cell tumor of tendon sheath express features of osteoclasts. Am J Pathol. 1997;150(4):1383–93.

18. Neale SD, et al. Giant cells in pigmented villo nodular synovitis express an osteoclast phenotype. J Clin Pathol. 1997;50(7):605–8.

19. Ota T, et al. Expression of colony-stimulating factor 1 is associated with occurrence of osteochondral change in pigmented villonodular synovitis. Tumour Biol. 2015;36(7):5361–7.

20. Uchibori M, et al. Expression of matrix metalloproteinases and tissue inhibitors of metalloproteinases in pigmented villonodular synovitis suggests their potential role for joint destruction. J Rheumatol. 2004;31(1):110–9.

21. Yoshida W, et al. Cell characterization of mononuclear and giant cells constituting pigmented villonodular synovitis. Hum Pathol. 2003;34(1):65–73.

22. van Dijk CN, et al. Osteochondral defects in the ankle: why painful? Knee Surg Sports Traumatol Arthrosc. 2010;18(5):570–80.

23. Zengerink M, et al. Current concepts: treatment of osteochondral ankle defects. Foot Ankle Clin. 2006;11(2):331–59. vi

24. Easley ME, Vineyard JC. Varus ankle and osteochondral lesions of the talus. Foot Ankle Clin. 2012;17(1):21–38.

25. Saxena A, Perez H. Pigmented villonodular synovitis about the ankle: a review of the literature and presentation in 10 athletic patients. Foot Ankle Int. 2004;25(11):819–26.

26. Brien EW, Sacoman DM, Mirra JM. Pigmented villonodular synovitis of the foot and ankle. Foot Ankle Int. 2004;25(12):908–13.

27. Sung KS, Ko KR. Surgical outcomes after excision of pigmented villonodular synovitis localized to the ankle and hindfoot without adjuvant therapy. J Foot Ankle Surg. 2015;54(2):160–3.

28. Goldman AB, DiCarlo EF. Pigmented villonodular synovitis. Diagnosis and differential diagnosis. Radiol Clin N Am. 1988;26(6):1327–47.

29. Ramsey PL, Hamilton W. Changes in tibiotalar area of contact caused by lateral talar shift. J Bone Joint Surg Am. 1976;58(3):356–7.

30. Miller CP, Chiodo CP. Autologous Bone Graft in Foot and Ankle Surgery. Foot Ankle Clin. 2016;21(4):825–37.

31. Khan SN, et al. The biology of bone grafting. J Am Acad Orthop Surg. 2005;13(1):77–86.

32. Noailles T, et al. Giant cell tumor of tendon sheath: open surgery or arthroscopic synovectomy? A systematic review of the literature. Orthop Traumatol Surg Res. 2017;103(5):809–14.

33. Heyd R, et al. Radiation therapy for treatment of pigmented villonodular synovitis: results of a national patterns of care study. Int J Radiat Oncol Biol Phys. 2010;78(1):199–204.

34. Horoschak M, et al. External beam radiation therapy enhances local control in pigmented villonodular synovitis. Int J Radiat Oncol Biol Phys. 2009;75(1):183–7.

35. Wu CC, et al. Two incision synovectomy and radiation treatment for diffuse pigmented villonodular synovitis of the knee with extra-articular component. Knee. 2007;14(2):99–106.

36. Mollon B, et al. The effect of surgical synovectomy and radiotherapy on the rate of recurrence of pigmented villonodular synovitis of the knee: an individual patient meta-analysis. Bone Joint J. 2015;97-B(4):550–7.

16

Biomechanical study of isolated radial head dislocation

Naoki Hayami[1], Shohei Omokawa[2*], Akio Iida[1], Jirachart Kraisarin[3], Hisao Moritomo[4], Pasuk Mahakkanukrauh[5,6], Takamasa Shimizu[1], Kenji Kawamura[1] and Yasuhito Tanaka[1]

Abstract

Background: Isolated radial head dislocation is a rare injury with an unclear pathomechanism, and the treatment is controversial. The purpose of the present study was to investigate the biomechanical contributions of the annular ligament, quadrate ligament, interosseous membrane, and annular ligament reconstructions to proximal radioulnar joint stability.

Methods: Five fresh frozen cadaveric upper extremities were amputated above the elbow and solidly fixed on a customized jig. Radial head dislocation was reproduced by sequential sectioning of ligamentous structures and passive mobility testing. Radial head displacement during mobility testing was measured with an electromagnetic tracking device in three forearm rotation positions. The data were compared among different sectioning stages and between two types of simulated ligamentous reconstruction.

Results: Lateral displacement of the radial head significantly increased in the neutral forearm rotation after annular ligament sectioning ($46 \pm 10\%$, $p < 0.05$). After quadrate ligament sectioning, we found significant posterior ($67 \pm 36\%$, $p < 0.05$) and lateral ($74 \pm 24\%$, $p < 0.01$) displacement in neutral forearm rotation and pronation. Significant radial head displacement was found in all directions and in all forearm positions after sequential sectioning of the proximal half of the interosseous membrane. Anatomical annular ligament reconstruction stabilized the proximal radioulnar joint except for anterior laxity in neutral forearm rotation ($15 \pm 6\%$, $p < 0.05$). The radial head with Bell Tawse procedure was significantly displaced in all directions.

Conclusion: The direction of radial head instability varied depending on the degree of soft tissue sectioning and specific forearm rotation. Anterior radial head dislocation may involve more severe ligament damage than other types of dislocation. Anatomical annular ligament reconstruction provided multidirectional radial head stability.

Keywords: Radial head dislocation, Biomechanical study, Annular ligament, Quadrate ligament, Interosseous membrane, Ligament reconstruction

Background

Traumatic dislocation of the radial head is usually associated with fractures of the forearm; isolated dislocation is a rare injury [1]. Anterior radial head dislocation is the most common form, but its pathomechanism remains obscure. Although the annular ligament is the primary stabilizer of the proximal radioulnar joint [2, 3], the contributions of other stabilizing structures such as the quadrate ligament and interosseous membrane (IOM) are not completely understood. A biomechanical study investigating the relative contributions of the annular ligament and the IOM (proximal, central, and distal bands) to preventing radial head dislocation [4] found that no single structure provided a significantly different percentage of static stability. Although those authors demonstrated the importance of the central band of the IOM in providing dynamic stability during forearm rotation, few specimens showed radial head dislocation, and there was minimal displacement (2–3 mm) in their motion simulation experiment. Moreover, it remains unclear how the quadrate ligament contributes to radial head stability [5, 6].

* Correspondence: omokawa@gaia.eonet.ne.jp
[2]Department of Hand Surgery, Nara Medical University, 840 Shijo-cho, Kashihara City, Nara Prefecture, Japan
Full list of author information is available at the end of the article

When radial head dislocation is neglected at the time of injury, surgical intervention is frequently needed. Resection or open reduction of the radial head with either annular ligament reconstruction [7, 8] or ulnar corrective osteotomy is generally performed. One of the most popular techniques for ligament reconstruction is the Bell Tawse procedure, where a slip of the triceps tendon is passed around the radial neck and secures it through a drill hole in the ulna. However, there is no single preferred procedure.

The present study aimed to investigate the contributions of the annular ligament, quadrate ligament, and IOM to the stability of the proximal radioulnar joint in a simulated radial head dislocation model using cadaveric specimens. Furthermore, restoration of joint stability was evaluated following both anatomic and non-anatomic (Bell Tawse procedure) ligamentous reconstructions.

We hypothesized that isolated radial head dislocation would be reproduced not by sectioning of the annular ligament alone but would require additional sectioning of the quadrate ligament and IOM and that the direction and degree of radial head instability would vary depending on the severity of ligament sectioning and on forearm position. Determining the key stabilizer to prevent each direction of radial head dislocation and the optimal forearm position to ensure post-reduction stability would provide useful information in the management of patients with radial head dislocation.

Methods
(specimen preparation)
We used five fresh frozen cadaver upper extremities (from three males and two females; average age, 63 years). None of the specimens had any skeletal or articular pathology of the elbow joint or forearm bones. All specimens were amputated above the elbow, and the wrists were also disarticulated at room temperature before use and were kept moist by spraying with normal saline during the experiment. Skin, muscle, and tendons were removed; ligaments around the elbow joint and the IOM were preserved.

(experimental setup)
The humerus and ulna were solidly fixed on a customized wooden jig with the elbow flexed at 90°. The radius was kept in one of three forearm positions (full pronation, neutral rotation, or full supination) with a 2.0-mm K-wire inserted in the distal radius from radial aspect (Fig. 1). We regarded as neutral rotation when this K-wire and long axis of humerus became parallel. We used an electromagnetic tracking device (trakSTAR™; Ascension Technology Corporation, Shelburne, VT, USA) to measure the displacement of the radial head relative to the proximal ulna. Sensors were inserted into the radial head and the proximal ulna. A cord was positioned around the neck of the radial head to apply load for passive mobility testing.

(passive mobility testing and data acquisition)
We performed passive mobility testing by loading the radial head with 20 N in the anterior, lateral, and posterior

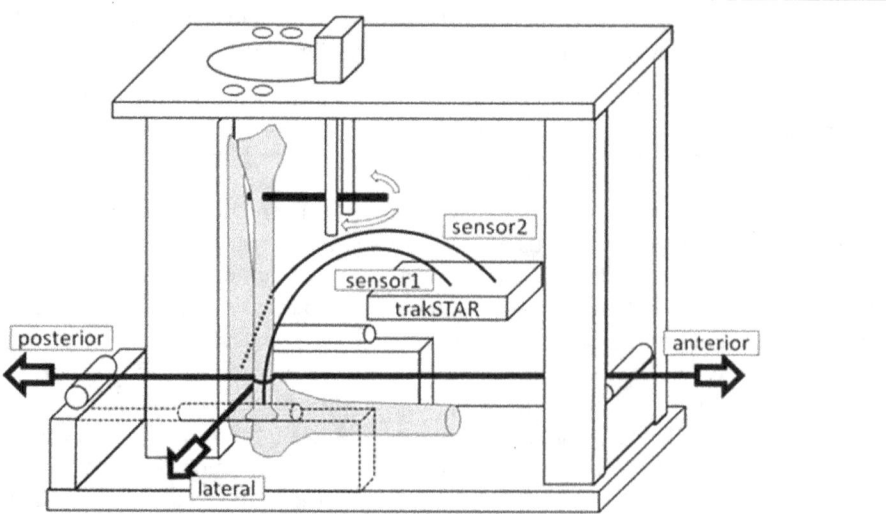

Fig. 1 Experimental setup. The humerus and ulna were solidly fixed on a customized wooden jig with the elbow flexed at 90°. The humerus was set horizontally and ulna was set perpendicularly to the ground. The radius was kept in one of three forearm positions (full pronation, neutral rotation, or full supination) with a 2.0-mm K-wire inserted in the distal radius only to keep forearm rotation. The displacement of the radial head relative to the proximal ulna was measured by an electromagnetic tracking device (trak STAR™; Ascension Technology Corporation, Shelburne, VT, USA). Sensors were inserted into the radial head and the proximal ulna. A cord was positioned around the neck of the radial head to apply load for passive mobility testing

directions. A custom-made device prevented forearm rotation during passive mobility testing. We calculated the radial head displacement as a percentage of the radial head diameter by measuring position before and after loading the radial head in full pronation, neutral rotation, and full supination. The displacement ratio of the radial head was calculated from these data. These procedures were repeated at each sectioning stage and reconstruction stage as indicated below.

(sectioning of radial head stabilizers)

We simulated radial head instability with the ligaments intact and with sequential sectioning of the elbow ligaments and IOM (Fig. 2). Sectioning stages were defined as follows: stage 0, elbow with anterior joint capsule sectioned; stage 1, elbow with annular ligament sectioned; stage 2, elbow with annular and quadrate ligaments sectioned; stage 3, elbow with annular and quadrate ligaments and proximal half of the IOM sectioned.

(annular ligament reconstruction)

After sectioning the ligaments and the IOM, we reconstructed the annular ligament with the following two procedures: stage R1, annular ligament reconstruction according to Bell Tawse procedure [9]; stage R2, anatomical annular ligament reconstruction with a triceps tendon slip passed around the radial neck through a bony tunnel created at the original ligamentous attachment sites on the ulna parallel to the proximal radioulnar joint and just distal to the radial notch. This is a modification of the procedure described by Itadera [10], in which a palmaris longus tendon graft is used. We used a distally based central one-third (4 mm in width)

triceps tendon slip for each reconstruction and evaluated radial head instability in neutral forearm rotation.

(statistical analysis)

Statistical analysis was performed with SPSS version 22 for Windows (SPSS Inc., Chicago, IL, USA). The radial head displacement ratio was analyzed with two-way repeated measures analysis of variance. After confirming the statistical significance of stages, forearm positions and their interaction, the data among sectioning stages were analyzed by Dunnett's multiple comparison test to compare with stage 0. Displacement ratios were compared among different forearm positions with Tukey's multiple comparison test. To evaluate the significance of annular ligament reconstruction, Tukey's test was also used to compare the data among intact and two reconstruction stages.

Results

(incidence of radial head dislocation)

We defined dislocation as more than 50% displacement (Fig. 3). At stage 0, no radial head dislocation was observed. At stage 1, in neutral forearm rotation three radial heads (60%) dislocated laterally and one (20%) dislocated posteriorly. In supination, one radial head (20%) dislocated laterally. At stage 2, in neutral rotation there were four (80%) dislocations laterally and 4 (80%) posteriorly; during both supination and pronation, one radial head dislocated posteriorly and two dislocated laterally. No anterior dislocation was observed at stage 2, regardless of forearm position. At stage 3, four to five radial heads dislocated (80–100%) in each direction and in each forearm position except in the anterior direction in neutral forearm rotation (only one radial head, 20%).

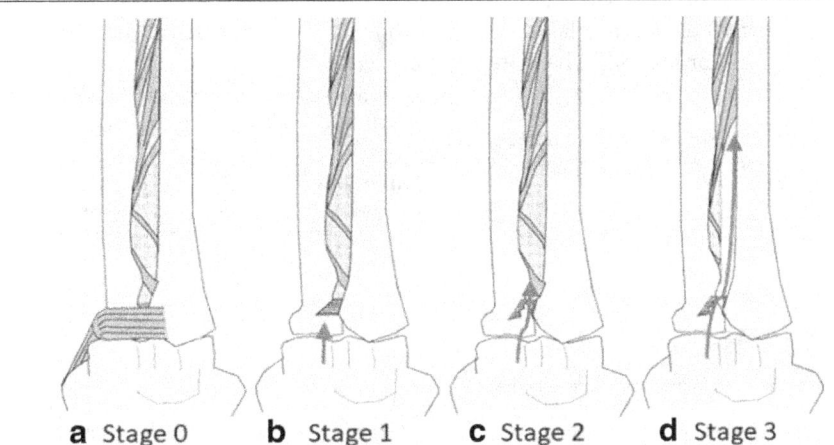

a Stage 0   **b** Stage 1   **c** Stage 2   **d** Stage 3

Fig. 2 Sectioning stages of radial head stabilizers. **a** Stage 0: elbow with anterior joint capsule sectioned. **b** Stage 1: elbow with annular ligament sectioned. **c** Stage 2: elbow with annular and quadrate ligaments sectioned. **d** Stage 3: elbow with annular and quadrate ligaments and proximal half of the IOM sectioned

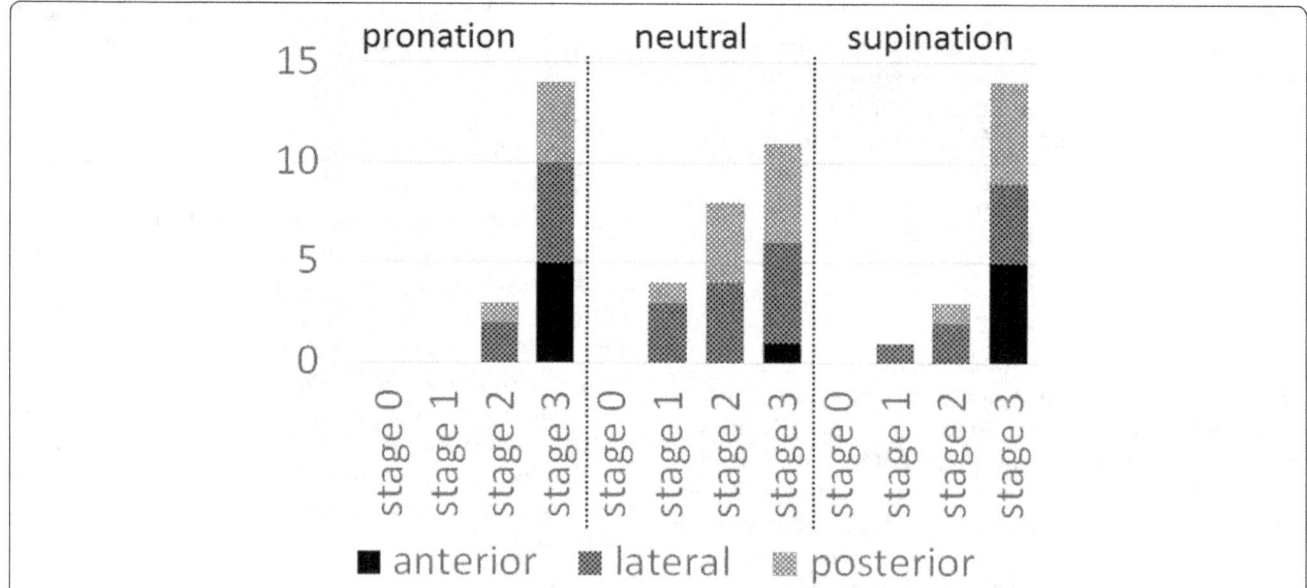

Fig. 3 Incidence of radial head dislocation. According to ligament sectioning, the incidence of radial head dislocation increased. Radial head began to dislocate laterally after annular ligament sectioned. And next, posterior radial head dislocation was observed after quadrate ligament sectioned especially in neutral position. Anterior radial head dislocation was occurred after proximal half of IOM sectioned

(displacement ratio of the radial head at each stage)

Stage 0 (elbow with joint capsule sectioned)
The displacement ratio was less than 10% in all directions and in all forearm positions.

Stage 1 (elbow with annular ligament sectioned)
The radial head displacement ratio was significantly greater in the lateral direction in neutral rotation than at stage 0 (Table 1). The displacement ratio in the other tests was not significantly greater than at stage 0.

Stage 2 (elbow with annular and quadrate ligaments sectioned)
In neutral rotation, the posterior displacement ratio was significantly greater than at stage 0 as was the lateral displacement ratio (Table 2). In pronation, the lateral displacement ratio was significantly greater than at stage 0 (Table 1). In supination, there was no significant increase in displacement ratio compared with stage 0 in any direction. The anterior displacement ratio was not significantly greater than at other stages in any forearm rotation (Table 3).

Stage 3 (elbow with annular and quadrate ligaments and proximal IOM sectioned)
The radial head was significantly displaced in all directions in all forearm rotations (Tables 1, 2 and 3). The anterior displacement ratio was only significantly greater at this stage than at stage 0 (Table 3).

Stage R1 (ligament reconstruction with bell Tawse procedure)
The anterior displacement ratio of the radial head averaged less than 20% in all forearm rotations. The

Table 1 Lateral radial head displacement ratio according to sectioning stage and forearm rotation (percentage; mean ± SD)

	pronation	neutral	supination
Stage 0	2 ± 1[a]	4 ± 1	3 ± 1
Stage 1	5 ± 3[a]	46 ± 10*	21 ± 25
Stage 2	41 ± 38*	74 ± 24**	42 ± 42
Stage 3	158 ± 22**	154 ± 30**	70 ± 42**,b

*: Indicates a value that is significantly different from that of stage 0 in the same column, with $p < 0.05$
**: Indicates a value that is significantly different from that of stage 0 in the same column, with $p < 0.01$
[a]Indicates a value that is significantly different from neutral rotation in the same row
[b]Indicates a value that is significantly different from the other positions in the same row

Table 2 Posterior radial head displacement ratio according to sectioning stage and forearm rotation (percentage; mean ± SD)

	pronation	neutral	supination
Stage 0	2 ± 1	3 ± 1	2 ± 0
Stage 1	5 ± 2[a]	37 ± 17	7 ± 2
Stage 2	24 ± 37	67 ± 36*	34 ± 49
Stage 3	68 ± 33**,a	200 ± 40**	123 ± 56**,a

*: Indicates a value that is significantly different from that of stage 0 in the same column, with $p < 0.05$
**: Indicates a value that is significantly different from that of stage 0 in the same column, with $p < 0.01$
[a]Indicates a value that is significantly different from neutral rotation in the same row

Table 3 Anterior radial head displacement ratio according to sectioning stage and forearm rotation (percentage; mean ± SD)

	pronation	neutral	supination
Stage 0	3 ± 0	5 ± 2	4 ± 1
Stage 1	7 ± 3	8 ± 4	8 ± 4
Stage 2	12 ± 6	9 ± 3	12 ± 6
Stage 3	95 ± 31**	39 ± 14**,a	109 ± 35**

**: Indicates a value that is significantly different from that of stage 0 in the same column, with $p < 0.01$
aIndicates a value that is significantly different from the other positions in the same row

displacement ratio tended to become larger in lateral and posterior directions. The radial head was significantly displaced in all directions (Table 4).

Stage R2 (anatomical annular ligament reconstruction)

Anterior, lateral, and posterior displacement ratios averaged less than 15%, 20%, and 30%, respectively, in all forearm rotations. The radial head was stabilized multidirectionally except in the anterior direction in neutral forearm rotation (Table 4).

(comparison of displacement ratio among three forearm positions)

Comparing the anterior displacement, the displacement ratio was significantly smaller in neutral rotation than in pronation or supination at stage 3 (Table 3). Comparing the lateral displacement, the displacement ratio in neutral rotation was significantly larger than in pronation at stage 1. The displacement ratio in supination was significantly smaller than in the other positions at stage 3 (Table 1). Comparing the posterior displacement, the displacement ratio in pronation was significantly smaller than in neutral rotation at stages 1 and 3 (Table 2).

Discussion

Numerous studies have examined distal radioulnar joint instability, but a paucity of information exists regarding the biomechanics of the proximal radioulnar joint. Although isolated radial head dislocation is a rare injury, understanding the stabilizing mechanism of the proximal radioulnar joint may help in the management of acute

Table 4 Radial head displacement ratio in different directions according to reconstruction stage (percentage; mean ± SD)

	anterior	lateral	posterior
Stage 0	5 ± 2	4 ± 1	3 ± 1
Stage R1	15 ± 5**	70 ± 26**	118 ± 31**
Stage R2	15 ± 6*	20 ± 3	28 ± 26

*: Indicates a value that is significantly different from that of stage 0 in the same column, with $p < 0.05$
**: Indicates a value that is significantly different from that of stage 0 in the same column, with $p < 0.01$

and chronic radial head dislocation. The current study revealed increasing displacement of the radial head during passive mobility testing with sequential sectioning of the proximal radioulnar joint-stabilizing structures from the proximal to distal direction. The radial head was dislocated in a lateral, posterior, and anterior direction depending on the degree of ligament sectioning; there were specific forearm positions in which the radial head was stabilized at each sectioning stage.

When the annular ligament was sectioned, lateral mobility of the radial head increased significantly in neutral forearm rotation; two of the five specimens dislocated laterally in this position. These results indicate that the annular ligament is a primary stabilizer in preventing lateral radial head dislocation.

After the additional sectioning of the quadrate ligament, significant posterior and lateral displacement of the radial head occurred. Posterior dislocation was found in two of the five specimens in neutral rotation. These results indicate that the quadrate ligament prevents posterior dislocation of the radial head. Spinner [5] and Wiley [3] described the functional anatomy of the quadrate ligament and reported that the ligament has a check–rein effect on the proximal radioulnar joint, tightening during pronation and supination and loosening in neutral forearm rotation. The current results support this check–rein effect of the quadrate ligament from a biomechanical point of view.

Significant anterior displacement occurred only after sequential sectioning of the proximal half of the IOM. These results indicate that the IOM is an important stabilizer in preventing anterior radial head dislocation, regardless of forearm position. In previous studies, the central band of the IOM was reported to be the stiffest stabilizing structure of the forearm [11, 12], contributing more to radial head stability than the annular ligament and proximal band of the IOM [4] during forearm pronation and supination. Thus, the presence of anterior radial head dislocation in clinical practice may suggest more severe soft tissue damage than that present with lateral and posterior dislocation.

There is no consensus on which position of forearm rotation is best for stabilization of the radial head. Several authors have recommended that the forearm be immobilized in supination rather than in neutral rotation or pronation, while others have recommend the neutral rotation after manual reduction of the radial head [8, 13–16]. The current results comparing stability among different forearm positions indicate that the ideal stabilizing position may differ depending on the direction of radial head dislocation. In patients with lateral radial head dislocation, supination may be recommended during post-reduction immobilization. In contrast, immobilization in pronation is recommended following

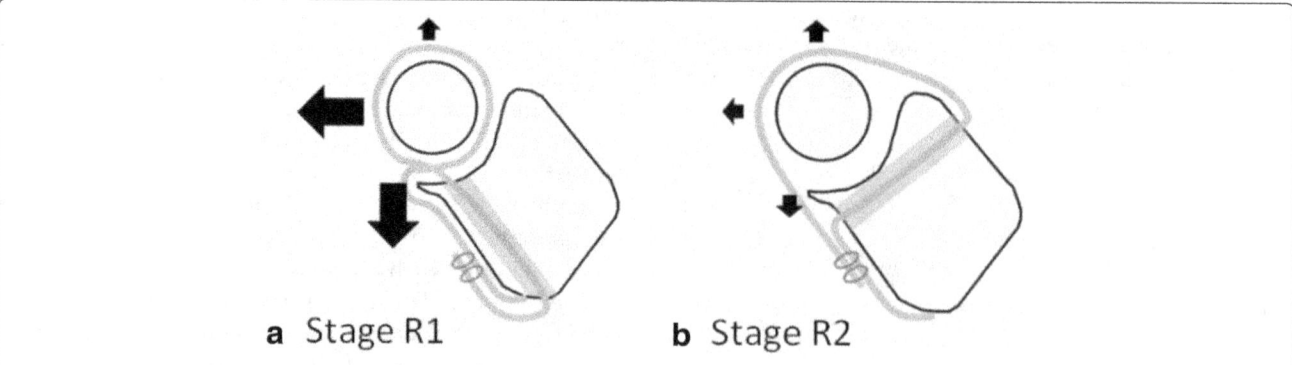

Fig. 4 Schema of annular ligament reconstructions. **a** Stage R1: Bell Tawse procedure reduced anterior radial head dislocation; however, it was difficult to stabilize the radial head in the posterolateral direction with this technique because of the non-anatomical nature of the procedure. **b** Stage R2: Anatomical reconstruction stabilized the radial head in all directions

closed reduction of posterior radial head dislocation [17]. The radius and ulna are crossed in pronation, and this bony contact may prevent posterior migration of the radial head. A neutral forearm rotation is recommended to stabilize the radial head following reduction of anterior dislocation with severe IOM injury, because the remaining distal IOM is tight in this position [18].

There are several surgical procedures available for the treatment of chronic radial head dislocation, including osteotomy of the ulna [19–22] with or without annular ligament reconstruction [16, 23–25]. Annular ligament reconstruction according to the Bell Tawse procedure is one popular technique, in which a slip of the triceps tendon is looped around the radial neck to stabilize the radial head. Although this procedure reduces anterior radial head dislocation, it is difficult to stabilize the radial head in the lateral and posterior directions with this technique because of the non-anatomical nature of the procedure (Fig. 4). Several clinical reports using this procedure for chronic radial head dislocation showed fair results with restricted forearm rotation and elbow flexion/extension [2, 26]. In the current study, the Bell Tawse procedure allowed posterolateral radial head instability, whereas anatomical reconstruction stabilized the radial head in all directions. Anatomical annular ligament reconstruction may provide multi-directional stability of the proximal radioulnar joint in patients with gross instability of the radial head. Thus, despite the rarity of the condition in clinical practice, the authors recommend performing anatomical annular ligament reconstruction rather than non-anatomical reconstruction procedures for patients with chronic radial head dislocation.

This study has several limitations. First, the soft tissue perhaps cannot tolerate repeated load and stretched during the experiment. To minimize this error, the load should not be too high, so 20 N of force was chosen.

The same load was used previously in biomechanical studies of the wrist [27, 28]. Second, the sequence of ligament sectioning may differ from the clinical scenario in radial head dislocation. We modified the sequence of ligament sectioning from a previous biomechanical study [29], sectioning the stabilizing structures from the proximal to distal direction. A randomized or different sequence of ligamentous and IOM sectioning would provide additional information. Third, we did not assess the dynamic effects of the muscles around the radial head. Salama et al. reported anterior dislocation of the radial head after biceps contraction caused by electric shock [30]. The dynamic effect of the biceps muscle may increase anterior displacement.

Conclusion

Isolated radial head dislocation is extremely rare. Nevertheless, the current study provided useful information related to the contributions of the annular ligament, the quadrate ligament, and the proximal half of IOM to radial head stability. Our findings may help with appropriate choice of post-reduction forearm position in acute injury and choice of reconstruction technique for chronic injury.

Abbreviation
IOM: Interosseous membrane

Acknowledgments
The authors thank the staff of the Department of Anatomy, Orthopedics and Surgical Training Center, Faculty of Medicine, Chiang Mai University, for their assistance in this study.

Funding
This work received financial support from JSPS KAKENHI Grant Number JP17K18021 to purchase and prepare the experimental materials.

Authors' contributions

NH: acquisition, analysis, and interpretation of data, drafting the paper. SO: research design, interpretation of data, revising the paper critically. AI: research design, acquisition of data, revising the paper critically. JK: acquisition, analysis, and interpretation of data, coordinating laboratory instrument. HM: research design, analysis, and interpretation of data. PM: acquisition, analysis, and interpretation of data, interpretation of data, preparing the cadavers. TS: acquisition, analysis of data, revising the paper critically. KK: analysis, and interpretation of data, revising the paper critically. YT: research design, revising the paper critically, approval of the submitted and final versions. All authors have read and approved the final submitted manuscript.

Competing interests

The authors declare that they have no competing interests.

Author details

[1]Department of Orthopedic Surgery, Nara Medical University, 840 Shijo-cho, Kashihara City, Nara Prefecture, Japan. [2]Department of Hand Surgery, Nara Medical University, 840 Shijo-cho, Kashihara City, Nara Prefecture, Japan. [3]Department of Orthopedic Surgery, Faculty of Medicine, Chiang Mai University, Chiang Mai 50200, Thailand. [4]Department of Physiotherapy, Osaka Yukioka College of Health Science, 41,1,1, Soujiji, Ibaraki City, Osaka, Japan. [5]Department of Anatomy, Faculty of Medicine, Chiang Mai University, Chiang Mai 50200, Thailand. [6]Excellence in Osteology Research and Training Center (ORTC), Chiang Mai University, Chiang Mai 50200, Thailand.

References

1. Hamilton W, Parkes JC 2nd. Isolated dislocation of the radial head without fracture of the ulna. Clin Orthop Relat Res. 1973;97:94–6.
2. Hudson DA, De Beer JD. Isolated traumatic dislocation of the radial head in children. J Bone Joint Surg Br. 1986;68:378–81.
3. Wiley JJ, Pegington J, Horwich JP. Traumatic dislocation of the radius at the elbow. J Bone Joint Surg Br. 1974;56B:501–7.
4. Anderson A, Werner FW, Tucci ER, Harley BJ. Role of the interosseous membrane and annular ligament in stabilizing the proximal radial head. J Shoulder Elb Surg. 2015;24:1926–33.
5. Spinner M, Kaplan EB. The quadrate ligament of the elbow–its relationship to the stability of the proximal radio-ulnar joint. Acta Orthop Scand. 1970;41: 632–47.
6. Tubbs RS, Shoja MM, Khaki AA, Lyerly M, Loukas M, O'neil JT, Salter EG, Oakes WJ. The morphology and function of the quadrate ligament. Folia Morphol (Warsz). 2006;65:225–7.
7. Oner FC, Diepstraten AF. Treatment of chronic post-traumatic dislocation of the radial head in children. J Bone Joint Surg Br. 1993;75:577–81.
8. Horii E, Nakamura R, Koh S, Inagaki H, Yajima H, Nakao E. Surgical treatment for chronic radial head dislocation. J Bone Joint Surg Am. 2002;84-A:1183–8.
9. Bell Tawse AJ. The treatment of malunited anterior Monteggia fractures in children. J Bone Joint Surg Br. 1965;47:718–23.
10. Itadera E, Ueno K. Recurrent anterior instability of the radial head: case report. J Hand Surg Am. 2014;39:206–8.
11. Moritomo H, Noda K, Goto A, Murase T, Yoshikawa H, Sugamoto K. Interosseous membrane of the forearm: length change of ligaments during forearm rotation. J Hand Surg Am. 2009;34:685–91.
12. Werner FW, Taormina JL, Sutton LG, Harley BJ. Structural properties of 6 forearm ligaments. J Hand Surg Am. 2011;36:1981–7.
13. Aversano F, Kepler CK, Blanco JS, Green DW. Rare cause of block to reduction after radial head dislocation in children. J Orthop Trauma. 2011;25:e38–41.
14. Oka K, Murase T, Moritomo H, Sugamoto K, Yoshikawa H. Morphologic evaluation of chronic radial head dislocation: three-dimensional and quantitative analyses. Clin Orthop Relat Res. 2010;468:2410–8.
15. Sasaki K, Miura H, Iwamoto Y. Unusual anterior radial head dislocation associated with transposed biceps tendon: a case report. J Shoulder Elb Surg. 2006;15:e15–9.
16. Wang MN, Chang WN. Chronic posttraumatic anterior dislocation of the radial head in children: thirteen cases treated by open reduction, ulnar osteotomy, and annular ligament reconstruction through a Boyd incision. J Orthop Trauma. 2006;20:1–5.
17. Dhawan A, Hospodar PP. Isolated posttraumatic posterior dislocation of the radial head in an adult. Am J Orthop (Belle Mead NJ). 2002;31:83–6.
18. Malone PS, Cooley J, Morris J, Terenghi G, Lees VC. The biomechanical and functional relationships of the proximal radioulnar joint, distal radioulnar joint, and interosseous ligament. J Hand Surg Eur Vol. 2015;40:485–93.
19. Hasler CC, Von Laer L, Hell AK. Open reduction, ulnar osteotomy and external fixation for chronic anterior dislocation of the head of the radius. J Bone Joint Surg Br. 2005;87:88–94.
20. Exner GU. Missed chronic anterior Monteggia lesion. Closed reduction by gradual lengthening and angulation of the ulna. J Bone Joint Surg Br. 2001; 83:547–50.
21. Bhaskar A. Missed Monteggia fracture in children: is annular ligament reconstruction always required? Indian J Orthop. 2009;43:389–95.
22. Gyr BM, Stevens PM, Smith JT. Chronic Monteggia fractures in children: outcome after treatment with the bell-Tawse procedure. J Pediatr Orthop B. 2004;13:402–6.
23. Datta T, Chatterjee N, Pal AK, Das SK. Evaluation of outcome of corrective ulnar osteotomy with bone grafting and annular ligament reconstruction in neglected monteggia fracture dislocation in children. J Clin Diagn Res. 2014; 8:LC01–4.
24. Tan L, Li YH, Sun DH, Zhu D, Ning SY. Modified technique for correction of isolated radial head dislocation without apparent ulnar bowing: a retrospective case study. Int J Clin Exp Med. 2015;15:18197–202.
25. Garg P, Baid P, Sinha S, Ranjan R, Bandyopadhyay U, Mitra S. Outcome of radial head preserving operations in missed Monteggia fracture in children. Indian J Orthop. 2011;45:404–9.
26. Lloyd-Roberts GC, Bucknill TM. Anterior dislocation of the radial head in children: aetiology, natural history and management. J Bone Joint Surg Br. 1977;59-B:402–7.
27. Iida A, Omokawa S, Moritomo H, Omori S, Kataoka T, Aoki M, Wada T, Fujimiya M, Tanaka Y. Effect of wrist position on distal radioulnar joint stability: a biomechanical study. J Orthop Res. 2014;32:1247–51.
28. Miyamura S, Shigi A, Kraisarin J, Omokawa S, Murase T, Yoshikawa H, Moritomo H. Impact of Distal Ulnar Fracture Malunion on Distal Radioulnar Joint Instability: A Biomechanical Study of the Distal Interosseous Membrane Using a Cadaver Model. J Hand Surg Am. 2017;42:e185–91.
29. Weiss AP. Hastings H 2nd.V. The anatomy of the proximal radioulnar joint. J Shoulder Elb Surg. 1992;1:193–9.
30. Salama R, Wientroub S, Weissman SL. Recurrent dislocation of the head of the radius. Clin Orthop Relat Res. 1977;125:156–8.

17

Quadriceps force and anterior tibial force occur obviously later than vertical ground reaction force: a simulation study

Ryo Ueno[1], Tomoya Ishida[1], Masanori Yamanaka[1*], Shohei Taniguchi[1], Ryohei Ikuta[2], Mina Samukawa[1], Hiroshi Saito[1] and Harukazu Tohyama[1]

Abstract

Background: Although it is well known that quadriceps force generates anterior tibial force, it has been unclear whether quadriceps force causes great anterior tibial force during the early phase of a landing task. The purpose of the present study was to examine whether the quadriceps force induced great anterior tibial force during the early phase of a landing task.

Methods: Fourteen young, healthy, female subjects performed a single-leg landing task. Muscle force and anterior tibial force were estimated from motion capture data and synchronized force data from the force plate. One-way repeated measures analysis of variance and the post hoc Bonferroni test were conducted to compare the peak time of the vertical ground reaction force, quadriceps force and anterior tibial force during the single-leg landing. In addition, we examined the contribution of vertical and posterior ground reaction force, knee flexion angle and moment to peak quadriceps force using multiple linear regression.

Results: The peak times of the estimated quadriceps force (96.0 ± 23.0 ms) and anterior tibial force (111.9 ± 18.9 ms) were significantly later than that of the vertical ground reaction force (63.5 ± 6.8 ms) during the single-leg landing. The peak quadriceps force was positively correlated with the peak anterior tibial force ($R = 0.953$, $P < 0.001$). Multiple linear regression analysis showed that the peak knee flexion moment contributed significantly to the peak quadriceps force ($R^2 = 0.778$, $P < 0.001$).

Conclusion: The peak times of the quadriceps force and the anterior tibial force were obviously later than that of the vertical ground reaction force for the female athletes during successful single-leg landings. Studies have reported that the peak time of the vertical ground reaction force was close to the time of anterior cruciate ligament (ACL) disruption in ACL injury cases. It is possible that early contraction of the quadriceps during landing might induce ACL disruption as a result of excessive anterior tibial force in unanticipated situations in ACL injury cases.

Keywords: Anterior cruciate ligament, Biomechanics, Musculoskeletal model, Quadriceps

Background

Anterior cruciate ligament (ACL) injury is the most serious, common, and costly injury in young athletes [1]. It is estimated that 80,000 to more than 250,000 ACL injuries occur each year in the U.S. [2]. ACL reconstruction is a common treatment, and approximately 100,000 reconstructions are performed annually in the U.S. [2].

The direct cost of an ACL reconstruction in the U.S. was almost $12,000–17,000, making ACL reconstruction responsible for over $1 billion of the national health care costs [3, 4]. Furthermore, 67% of patients cannot return to competitive sports by 12 months post surgery [5]. Patients also require a long postoperative rehabilitation period after their ACL reconstruction. Therefore, effective ACL prevention programs are urgently needed. To resolve this problem, it is necessary to understand the ACL injury mechanism in more detail.

Seventy percent of ACL injuries result from a non-contact situation, such as jump landings and cutting

* Correspondence: yamanaka@hs.hokudai.ac.jp
[1]Faculty of Health Sciences, Hokkaido University, North 12, West 5, Kitaku, Sapporo 060-0812, Japan
Full list of author information is available at the end of the article

tasks [6]. Previous in vitro studies have shown the effect of the external load and muscle force on the ACL force and strain [7–15]. Quadriceps force is commonly known to induce anterior tibial drawer and increase the ACL load [8, 9]. DeMorat et al. [10] reported that 4500 N of isolated quadriceps force produced significant anterior tibial translation with ACL rupture. It has been considered that high quadriceps force is a mechanism of ACL injury [10, 16].

Under anterior tibial force, the tension of the ACL is higher in the low angle of knee flexion [8, 17]. Therefore, an immediate increase in anterior tibial force after foot contact would present a greater risk of ACL injury. Kiapour et al. [14] suggested that peak ACL strain occurred at approximately 45 ms with maximum anterior tibial translation during a simulated single-leg drop landing using a cadaveric biomechanical testing apparatus. Although it is well known that quadriceps force generates anterior tibial force in the low angle of knee flexion [18], it is unclear whether quadriceps force causes great anterior tibial force during the early phase of a landing task [19]. Quadriceps force generates the internal knee extension moment to resist the external knee flexion moment during a landing task. The knee flexion moment is likely greater during the late phase because of the increase in knee flexion angle during landing [20]. Therefore, it is possible that the quadriceps force is greater during the late phase of landing. However, in vivo case studies and in vitro biomechanical studies have suggested greater vertical ground reaction force also causes a greater ACL load [11, 15, 21]. In their video research, Koga et al. [22] indicated that ACL injury occurred with a peak ground reaction force based on the estimated center of mass accelerations after initial foot contact with the ground. However, while the video research provided an estimation of the knee kinematics of ACL injury, it has not been shown how muscle force induces ACL injury [22–26].

A musculoskeletal modeling approach has been used to examine the effect of muscle force on ACL loading during landing tasks [27–31]. This approach is useful for estimating the muscle force during in vivo dynamic motions, which was not revealed in the video research or in vitro biomechanical testing. Focusing on the muscle force provides new insight into how the muscle force around the knee contributes to knee joint force, such as anterior tibial force, during landing tasks. Previous studies have been validated by comparisons with surface electromyography (EMG) and muscle activation (MA) estimated using the musculoskeletal model [27–30]. Therefore, this numerical model may suggest new insights regarding whether quadriceps contraction generates great anterior tibial force during the early phase of a landing task.

The purposes of the present study were (i) to compare the peak time of the vertical ground reaction force, quadriceps force and anterior tibial force during a landing task; (ii) to examine the relationship between peak quadriceps force and anterior tibial force; and (iii) to examine the contribution of experimental variables to the peak quadriceps force during the landing. The hypothesis of this study was that (i) the peak times of the quadriceps force and anterior tibial force were later than that of the vertical ground reaction force, (ii) the quadriceps force was correlated with the anterior tibial force and (iii) the knee flexion moment and knee flexion angle significantly contributed to quadriceps force.

Methods
Subjects and experimental task

Fourteen young, healthy, female subjects (age 21.5 ± 0.8 years, height 162.1 ± 5.9 cm, mass 53.2 ± 6.6 kg) participated in the present study. Each participant performed three trials of single-leg landing after sufficient instruction. The participants were instructed to stand on a 30-cm-high box with their preferred leg and drop off the box onto a force plate (Type 9286, Kistler AG, Winterthur, Switzerland), landing on the same leg (right leg for all, Fig. 1). Institutional review board approval and informed consent were obtained before the present study was conducted. The participants were accepted into the study if they had no history of lower extremity injury requiring surgical repair and had not suffered a knee injury within the previous 6 months. No subjects had any history of intrinsic bone disorders, metabolic disease, hormonal abnormalities or myogenic abnormalities, nor were they taking any medications. In addition, no subjects had excessively high or low muscle mass, and they did not demonstrate evident laxity or stiffness based on clinical orthopedic testing (e.g., Lachman test, pivot shift test and valgus stress test).

Study procedure overview

The overall data collecting and processing procedure is shown in Fig. 2. This study involved two distinct parts: the first comprised motion analysis trials in which the 14 female subjects performed the single-leg landing to obtain the marker trajectories, ground reaction force and EMG data. The second part was the numerical simulation of each trial with OpenSim 3.2, an open-source software [32], using kinematic and kinetic data from the motion analysis. To obtain the joint kinematics, muscle force and joint reaction force, a sequence of processes including anatomic scaling, inverse kinematics (IK), residual reduction algorism (RRA), static optimization (SO) and joint reaction analysis was performed. Finally, to validate the simulation, the wave patterns of the MA of quadriceps

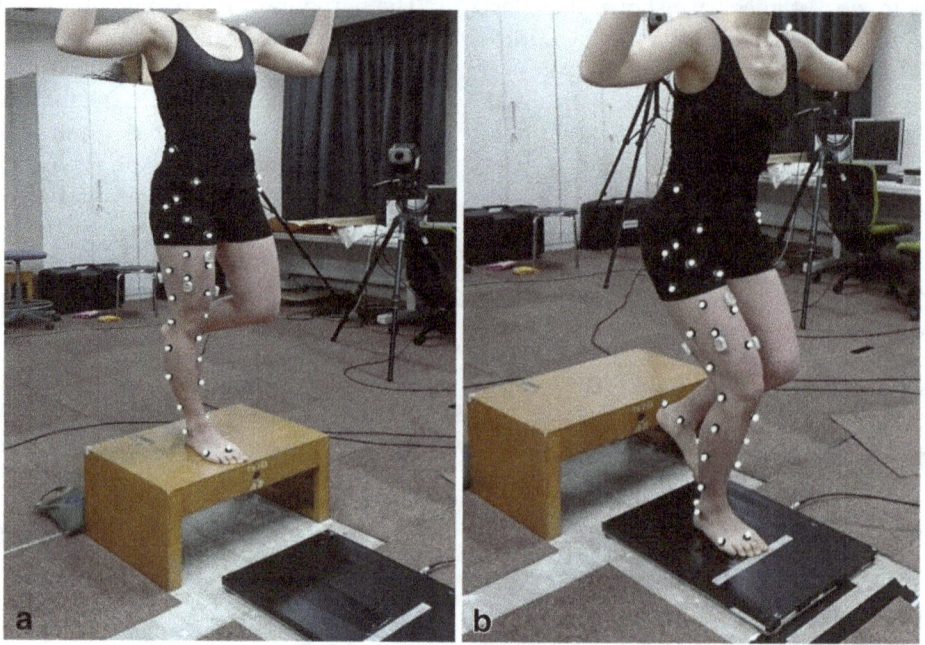

Fig. 1 Motion capture during the single-leg landing trial. The subjects stood on their right leg on a 30-cm-high box (**a**) and dropped off on to a force plate, landing on their right leg (**b**)

estimated with OpenSim were compared to those of the EMG from the motion analysis.

Data collection

Thirty-nine reflective markers were placed at strategic anatomical locations to obtain the knee kinematics (Fig. 3) [33]. The markers' trajectories were collected using the EvaRT 4.4 motion capture system (Motion Analysis Corporation, Santa Rosa, CA, USA) and six digital cameras (Hawk cameras; Motion Analysis Corporation) at 200 Hz. Ground reaction forces were synchronously recorded at 1000 Hz using the force plate. Both kinematic and ground reaction force data ware low-pass filtered using a zero-lag fourth order Butterworth filter at 12 Hz.

The EMG data were measured using a wireless surface EMG system (WEB-1000; Nihon Kohden Corporation, Tokyo, Japan) with a sampling rate of 1000 Hz. The electrodes were placed on the rectus femoris, vastus medialis, and vastus lateralis of each participant's right leg. All electrode positionings and related procedures were performed according to the SENIAM recommendations [34]. The raw experimental EMG data were band-pass filtered using a zero-lag fourth order Butterworth filter at cutoff frequency of 20 to 500 Hz and then full-wave rectified and low-pass filtered using a zero-lag fourth order Butterworth filter at a cutoff frequency of 12 Hz. Finally, peak EMG magnitudes for each trial were used to normalize the smoothed EMG data.

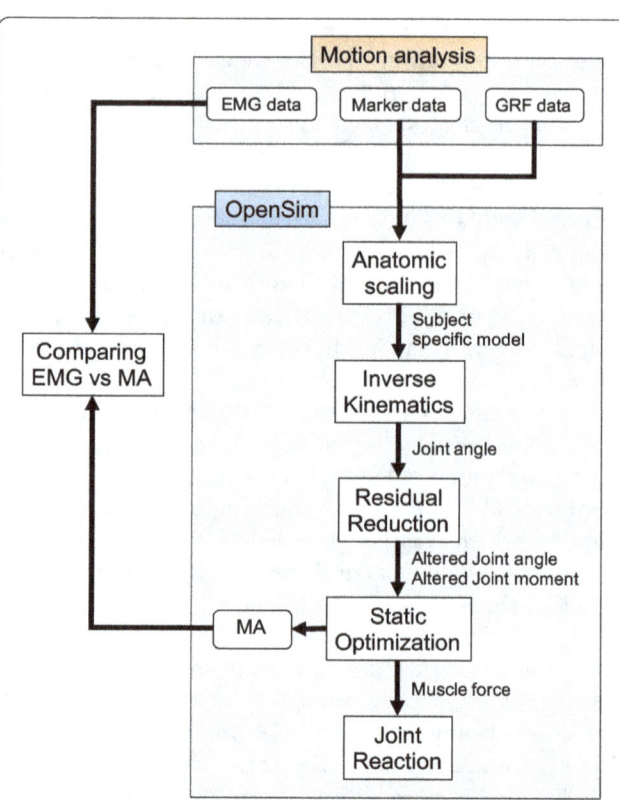

Fig. 2 Flow chart for data processing, from motion capture to OpenSim analyses. GRF: ground reaction force, EMG: electromyography, MA: muscle activation

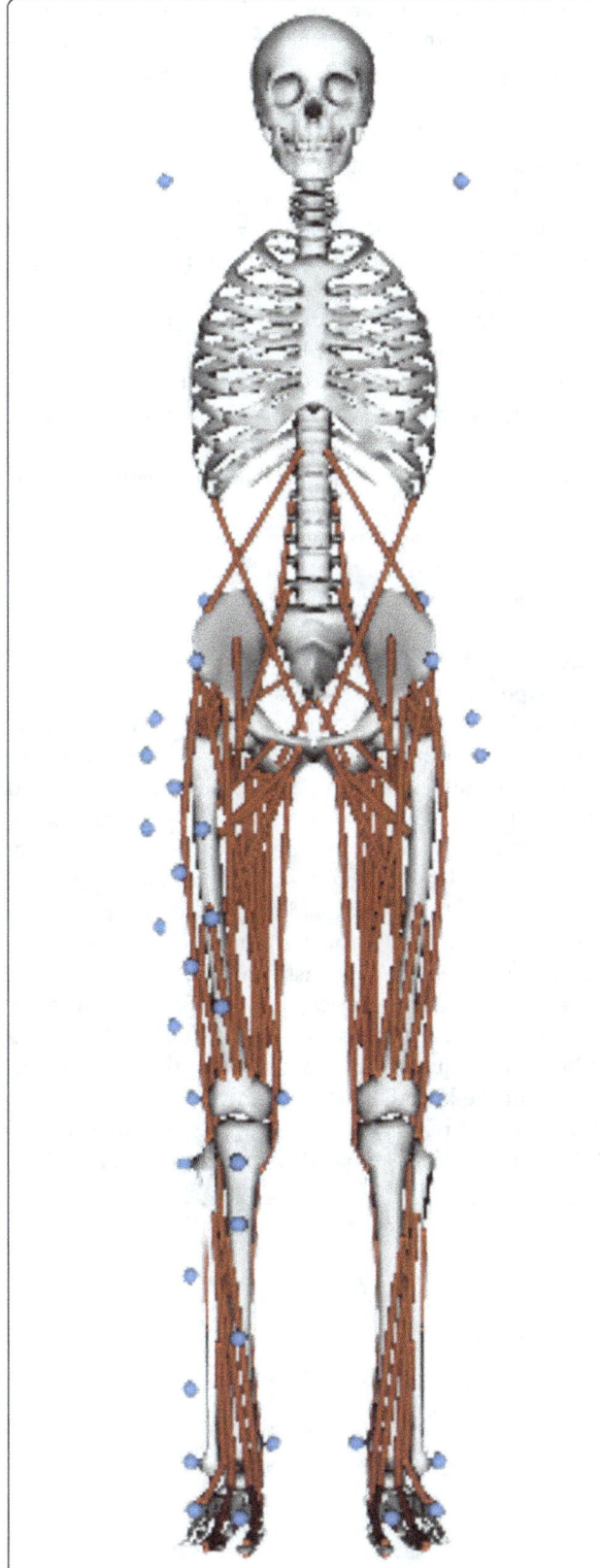

Fig. 3 Generic musculoskeletal model and marker placements

Musculoskeletal models

Subject-specific musculoskeletal models were created by scaling the generic model, gait 2392, in OpenSim (Fig. 3). In the scaling process, the size, weight and inertial property of the subject-specific model were adjusted to those of the participants. The participants' anthropometric measurements based on the marker positions and body weight measured during their static trial were used to scale the generic model. The generic model, gait 2392, had 23 degrees of freedom and 92 muscle-tendon actuators without any ligaments or upper extremity segments. According to previous studies [27, 28, 31], the maximum isometric forces for all muscles were scaled to twice those used by Delp et al. [35] to enable the muscle to resist the large external knee flexion moment during a single-leg landing. The strength of isometric muscle force of the subject-specific model was not scaled to that of each subject in the scaling process. After the model scaling, sequential IK, RRA, SO and joint reaction analyses were conducted.

The IK tool defined the joint kinematics using marker trajectories obtained from the motion capture system during the single-leg landing task. There were dynamical inconsistencies between the experimental joint kinematics from the IK and ground reaction force, an effect of modeling and marker data processing. RRA was conducted to alter the joint kinematics and the torso mass center of the subject-specific model to increase its consistency with the ground reaction force. Using the joint kinematics from RRA and ground reaction force data, the SO tool estimated the muscle force and activation. SO resolves the net joint moment into individual muscle forces by minimizing the sum of the squared MA at each time step. The step-driven Hill-type muscle model considers the force-length-velocity properties. Quadriceps force was defined as the combination of the rectus femoris and vasti muscle forces. Finally, a joint reaction analysis computed the internal joint force results using muscle force and external loads. The anterior component of the knee joint force in the tibial frame was defined as the anterior tibial force. All variables, EMG and MA were averaged using data from three successful trials.

Data reduction

Foot strike was defined as the moment at which vertical ground reaction force reached just above 10 N. The landing phase was defined as the period from foot strike to peak knee flexion. The peak values for the vertical and posterior ground reaction force, altered knee flexion angle and knee flexion moment from the RRA, quadriceps force and anterior tibial force during the landing phase were used for the following statistical analysis.

Statistical analysis

The sample size for one-way repeated measures of analysis of variance (ANOVA) was calculated with a combined effect size f of 0.25 (medium), an α-level of 0.05 and a power of 0.8 in a priori power calculation. The calculated sample size was 12, and 14 subjects were recruited for this study. One-way repeated measures ANOVA and a post hoc Bonferroni test were conducted to compare the peak time of the vertical ground reaction force, anterior tibial force and quadriceps force during the single-leg landing.

Pearson's correlation coefficients were calculated to reveal the relationships of the peak values of vertical and posterior ground reaction force, knee flexion angle, knee flexion moment and anterior tibial force with the peak quadriceps force. A stepwise multiple linear regression analysis was performed to predict the peak quadriceps force using vertical and posterior ground reaction force, knee flexion angle and knee flexion moment as independent variables. Statistical significance was set at $P < 0.05$ for all analyses using the IBM SPSS Statistics 19 software program (IBM, Chicago, IL, USA).

Results

The computationally estimated MA of the quadriceps showed fairly good consistency with collected experimental EMG findings (Fig. 4). Some delays of MA compared with EMG results were consistent with the electromechanical delay observed between EMG measurements and force production [36].

The time-history graph of normalized vertical and posterior ground reaction force, quadriceps force, anterior tibial force, knee flexion angle and knee flexion moment for all subjects is shown in Fig. 5, and the peak values of the variables are shown in Table 1. The mean values of the peak time for each force were 63.5 (6.8) ms, 96.0 (23.0) ms and 111.9 (18.9) ms after the initial foot contact for vertical ground reaction force, quadriceps force and anterior tibial force, respectively. The peak times of the estimated

quadriceps force and anterior tibial force were significantly later than that of vertical ground reaction force during the single-leg landing ($P < 0.001$). The peak time of the anterior tibial force was also later than the peak quadriceps force ($P < 0.001$) (Fig. 6).

The Pearson's correlation coefficient and the associated P-value for experimental variables and peak quadriceps force are given in Table 2. Peak quadriceps force was positively correlated with the peak anterior tibial force ($R = 0.953$, $P < 0.001$; Fig. 7).

The multiple regression model showed that the peak knee flexion moment contributed significantly to maximum quadriceps force ($P < 0.001$, $R^2 = 0.778$). The estimated regression model for peak quadriceps force was

$$\text{Peak quadriceps force} = 360.8 + 23.69 \,(\text{peak knee flexion moment})$$

The P value of the variables included in the regression model was $P = 0.510$. For the intercept and peak knee flexion moment, we calculated $P < 0.001$.

Discussion

The purposes of the present study were to determine whether the peak time of the quadriceps force and anterior tibial force occur immediately after landing, to examine the relationship between quadriceps force and anterior tibial force and to examine the contribution of experimental variables to the peak quadriceps force during the single-leg landing task. The results supported our hypothesis that peak quadriceps force occurred at a later phase than peak vertical ground reaction force during the single-leg landing task. In addition, the results indicated that the quadriceps force generates greater anterior tibial force in the late phase during single-leg landing. The quadriceps force was predicted by an increase in the knee flexion moment.

EMG data were collected to compare the experimental EMG and the MA estimated using the musculoskeletal

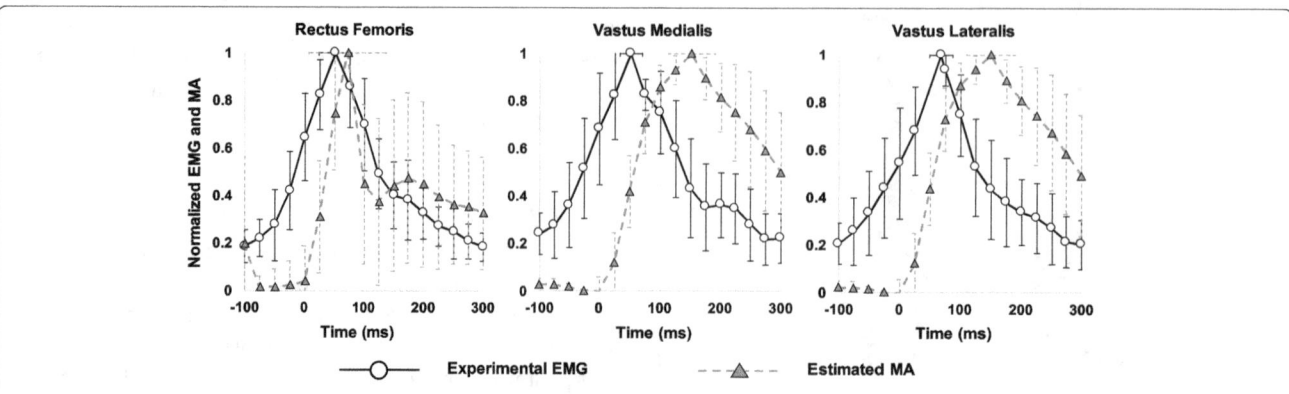

Fig. 4 Comparisons of mean ± 1 standard deviation for experimental electromyography (EMG: circle and solid black line) and estimated muscle activation (MA: triangle and dashed gray line) during single-leg landing for all subjects. Both EMG and MA data were normalized by their peak values during landing. The horizontal error bar at the peak of the plot represents ±1 standard deviation for the peak time of the EMG and MA

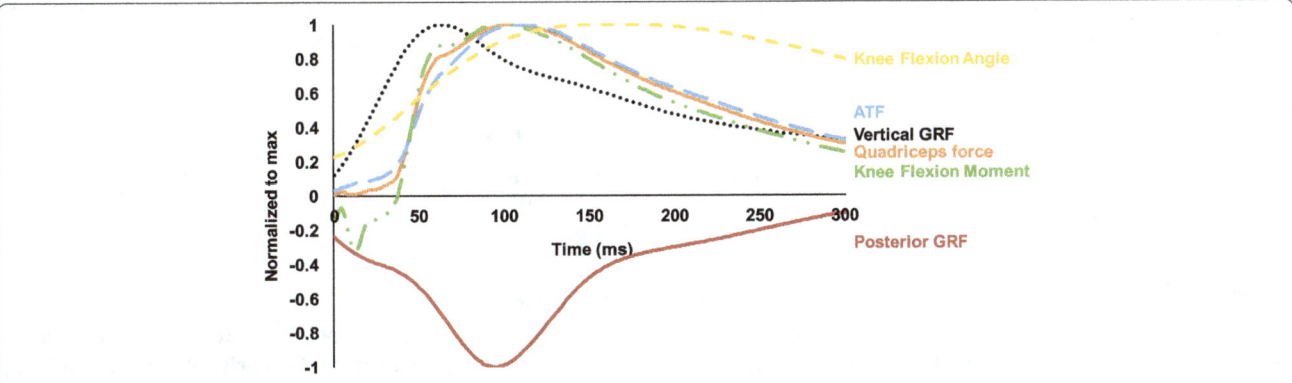

Fig. 5 Time-history graph of the vertical and posterior ground reaction force (GRF), knee flexion angle and moment, quadriceps force and anterior tibial force

modeling approach. Fairly good consistencies between the EMG and MA were found. The comparison of the EMG and MA suggested that the simulation would be complete. In addition, wave patterns of the knee flexion moment, which contribute significantly to quadriceps force, and the other kinetic, kinematic data (knee flexion angle, vertical and posterior ground reaction force) were consistent with those previously reported for single-leg landing [20, 27, 28, 31, 37]. Therefore, the predicted muscle force could be reasonably used to examine the peak time of the quadriceps force for landing.

The present study showed that the peak times of the estimated quadriceps force and anterior tibial force were significantly later than that of vertical ground reaction force during successful single-leg landings for the young female athletes. The peak time of the anterior tibial force was significantly later but close to the peak time of the quadriceps force. The peak time of the quadriceps force and anterior tibial force were also obviously later than the time of maximum anterior tibial translation during in vitro simulated single-leg landing, as Kiapour et al. [14] previously reported, while the peak time of the vertical ground reaction force was close to the time of ACL disruption in ACL injury cases [22]. Therefore, it is possible that earlier and greater activation of the quadriceps during landing might induce ACL disruption via excessive anterior tibial force under unanticipated circumstances in ACL injury cases. Further studies should be conducted to clarify the time-sequence of quadriceps

muscle forces and the ACL disruption during landing in ACL injury cases.

The regression analysis showed that the peak knee flexion moment contributed significantly to the peak quadriceps force. Although peak knee flexion angle was included in the regression model with stepwise selection, it was not significant. Thus, the peak flexion angle was excluded from the regression model. The wave pattern of the knee flexion moment was close to that of quadriceps force (Fig. 5). One key finding of this study is that quadriceps force is necessary to resist the greater external knee flexion moment during the late phase of landing. Shimokochi et al. [20] researched the effect of the several sagittal plane body postures - the trunk leaning forward with landing on the toes, upright trunk position with landing on the heel and a participant-selected position – on the knee extensor moment during single-leg landing. No significant differences in peak internal knee extensor moment were detected among the postures. In addition, there were likely minimal differences in the

Table 1 Mean (SD) values of the kinetic and kinematic variables

Variables	Mean (SD)
Vertical ground reaction force (N)	1619 (148)
Posterior ground reaction force (N)	−218 (33)
Quadriceps force (N)	3741 (774)
Anterior tibial force (N)	3613 (836)
Knee flexion moment (Nm)	143 (29)
Knee flexion angle (deg)	55.6 (5.2)

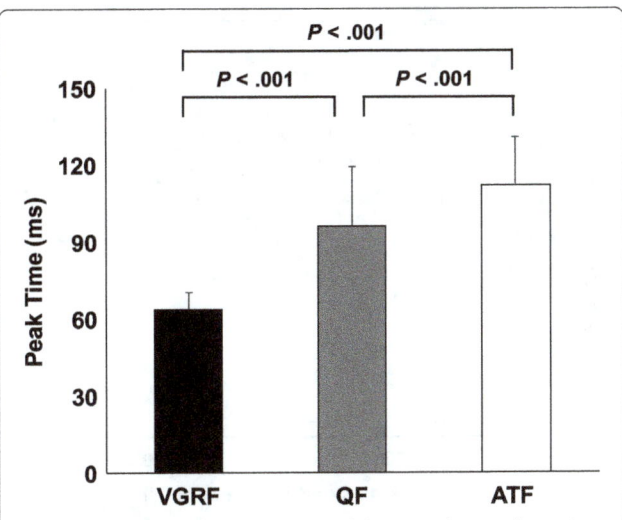

Fig. 6 Comparison of the peak time of the vertical ground reaction force (VGRF), quadriceps force (QF) and anterior tibial force (ATF)

Table 2 Correlations between kinetic and kinematic variables and peak quadriceps force

Variables	Peak quadriceps force	
	R^a	P value
Vertical ground reaction force (N)	0.519	0.057
Posterior ground reaction force (N)	−0.551	0.041
Knee flexion moment (Nm)	0.882	< 0.001
Knee flexion angle (deg)	0.505	0.065

[a]Pearson's correlation coefficients

time to peak knee extensor moment. The previous results and the present findings suggest that the peak quadriceps force will occur during the late phase even if trunk and ankle postures are altered during single-leg landing. Therefore, quadriceps force may not be greater at the time of the ACL rupture during an anticipated landing.

There were several limitations of this study. First, the load of the ACL and the other ligaments were not estimated in the manner reported in previous studies [27–30, 38]. Estimating the ACL load is useful for evaluating the injury risk directly, but we focused on the peak time of the quadriceps force, and that depended on the knee flexion moment. The purposes of the present study were well addressed without evaluating the ACL load. Second, a posterior tibial slope was not included in the generic model. The posterior tibial slope induces an anterior tibial force, altering the vector of the compressive load anteriorly on the tibial plateau. The effect of the vertical ground reaction force on the anterior tibial force would have been greater if the posterior tibial slope had been modeled, as Shimokochi et al. suggested [20]. Third, the same strength of muscles was used for all subject-specific models without adjusting to that of each individual participant. Finally, it is unclear how the quadriceps is activated in ACL injury situations when the peak

muscle force occurred during the late phase of successful single-leg landings. The knee flexion moment or muscle activation and the other kinetics have never been reported for ACL injury situations, with the exception of the estimated vertical ground reaction force [22]. In future studies, researching the knee flexion moment in cases of ACL injury may be useful to predict the quadriceps force contribution to ACL injury.

Conclusions

We examined whether quadriceps force generates great anterior tibial force during the early phase of single-leg landing. The peak time of the quadriceps force during the single-leg landing is obviously later than the time at which ACL injury occurred in previous reports. In addition, the knee flexion moment contributed significantly to the quadriceps force in a linear regression model.

Abbreviations

ACL: Anterior cruciate ligament; EMG: Electromyography; IK: Inverse kinematics; MA: Muscle activation; RRA: Residual reduction algorism; SO: Static optimization

Acknowledgements

Not applicable.

Funding

There was no external funding for this study.

Authors' contributions

All authors were involved in the design of the study and in the analysis and discussion of the results. RU performed most of the data processing, created the figures and graphs, and wrote the first draft of the manuscript. TI provided practical advice and participated in writing the manuscript. MY supervised the entire study process and helped to draft and review the manuscript. ST collected the data and performed the measurements. RI collected the data and performed the measurements. MS participated in the study design and helped to draft and review the manuscript. HS participated in the study design and helped to draft and review the manuscript. HT participated in the manuscript writing and provided final approval of the manuscript. All authors read and approved the final manuscript.

Competing interests

The authors declare that they have no competing interests.

Author details

[1]Faculty of Health Sciences, Hokkaido University, North 12, West 5, Kitaku, Sapporo 060-0812, Japan. [2]Hachioji Sports Orthopaedic Clinic, Hachioji-Nakacho-Bldg3, 5-1, Nakacho, Hachioji, Tokyo 192-0085, Japan.

References

1. Flynn RK, Pedersen CL, Birmingham TB, Kirkley A, Jackowski D, Fowler PJ. The familial predisposition toward tearing the anterior cruciate ligament: a case control study. Am J Sports Med. 2005;33:23–8.
2. Griffin LY, Albohm MJ, Arendt EA, Bahr R, Beynnon BD, Demaio M, et al. Understanding and preventing noncontact anterior cruciate ligament injuries: a review of the Hunt Valley II meeting, January 2005. Am J Sports Med. 2006;34:1512–32.
3. Griffin LY, Agel J, Albohm MJ, Arendt EA, Dick RW, Garrett WE, et al. Noncontact anterior cruciate ligament injuries: risk factors and prevention strategies. J Am Acad Orthop Surg. 2000;8:141–50.

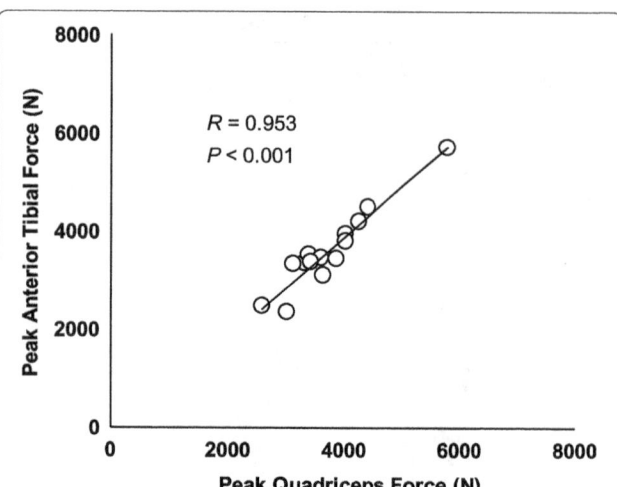

Fig. 7 Correlation between the peak quadriceps force and anterior tibial force for all subjects

4. Paxton ES, Kymes SM, Brophy RH. Cost-effectiveness of anterior cruciate ligament reconstruction: a preliminary comparison of single-bundle and double-bundle techniques. Am J Sports Med. 2010;38:2417–25.

5. Ardern CL, Webster KE, Taylor NF, Feller JA. Return to the preinjury level of competitive sport after anterior cruciate ligament reconstruction surgery: two-thirds of patients have not returned by 12 months after surgery. Am J Sports Med. 2011;39:538–43.

6. Boden BP, Dean GS, Feagin JA Jr, Garrett WE Jr. Mechanisms of anterior cruciate ligament injury. Orthopedics. 2000;23:573–8.

7. Markolf KL, Gorek JF, Kabo JM, Shapiro MS. Direct measurement of resultant forces in the anterior cruciate ligament. An in vitro study performed with a new experimental technique. J Bone Joint Surg Am. 1990;72:557–67.

8. Markolf KL, Burchfield DM, Shapiro MM, Shepard MF, Finerman GA, Slauterbeck JL. Combined knee loading states that generate high anterior cruciate ligament forces. J Orthop Res. 1995;13:930–5.

9. Li G, Rudy TW, Sakane M, Kanamori A, Ma CB, Woo SL. The importance of quadriceps and hamstring muscle loading on knee kinematics and in-situ forces in the ACL. J Biomech. 1999;32:395–400.

10. DeMorat G, Weinhold P, Blackburn T, Chudik S, Garrett W. Aggressive quadriceps loading can induce noncontact anterior cruciate ligament injury. Am J Sports Med. 2004;32:477–83.

11. Meyer EG, Haut RC. Excessive compression of the human tibio-femoral joint causes ACL rupture. J Biomech. 2005;38:2311–6.

12. YK O, Kreinbrink JL, Wojtys EM, Ashton-Miller JA. Effect of axial tibial torque direction on ACL relative strain and strain rate in an in vitro simulated pivot landing. J Orthop Res. 2012;30:528–34.

13. Levine JW, Kiapour AM, Quatman CE, Wordeman SC, Goel VK, Hewett TE, et al. Clinically relevant injury patterns after an anterior cruciate ligament injury provide insight into injury mechanisms. Am J Sports Med. 2013;41:385–95.

14. Kiapour AM, Quatman CE, Goel VK, Wordeman SC, Hewett TE, Demetropoulos CK. Timing sequence of multi-planar knee kinematics revealed by physiologic cadaveric simulation of landing: implications for ACL injury mechanism. Clin Biomech. Elsevier Ltd. 2014;29:75–82.

15. Quatman CE, Kiapour AM, Demetropoulos CK, Kiapour A, Wordeman SC, Levine JW, et al. Preferential loading of the ACL compared with the MCL during landing: a novel in sim approach yields the multiplanar mechanism of dynamic valgus during ACL injuries. Am J Sports Med. 2014;42:177–86.

16. Wall SJ, Rose DM, Sutter EG, Belkoff SM, Boden BP. The role of axial compressive and quadriceps forces in noncontact anterior cruciate ligament injury: a cadaveric study. Am J Sports Med. 2012;40:568–73.

17. Sakane M, Livesay GA, Fox RJ, Rudy TW, Runco TJ, Woo SL-Y. Relative contribution of the ACL, MCL, and bony contact to the anterior stability of the knee. Knee Surg Sports Traumatol Arthrosc. 1999;7:93–7.

18. Yasuda K, Sasaki T. Exercise after anterior cruciate ligament reconstruction. The force exerted on the tibia by the separate isometric contractions of the quadriceps or the hamstrings. Clin Orthop Relat Res. 1987;220:275–83.

19. Quatman CE, Hewett TE. The anterior cruciate ligament injury controversy: is "valgus collapse" a sex-specific mechanism? Br J Sports Med. 2009;43:328–35.

20. Shimokochi Y, Ambegaonkar JP, Meyer EG. Changing Sagittal-plane landing styles to modulate impact and tibiofemoral force magnitude and directions relative to the tibia. J Athl Train. 2016;51:669–81.

21. Cerulli G, Benoit DL, Lamontagne M, Caraffa A, Liti A. In vivo anterior cruciate ligament strain behaviour during a rapid deceleration movement: case report. Knee Surg Sports Traumatol Arthrosc. 2003;11:307–11.

22. Koga H, Nakamae A, Shima Y, Iwasa J, Myklebust G, Engebretsen L, et al. Mechanisms for noncontact anterior cruciate ligament injuries: knee joint kinematics in 10 injury situations from female team handball and basketball. Am J Sports Med. 2010;38:2218–25.

23. Olsen OE, Myklebust G, Engebretsen L, Bahr R. Injury mechanisms for anterior cruciate ligament injuries in team handball: a systematic video analysis. Am J Sports Med. 2004;32:1002–12.

24. Cochrane JL, Lloyd DG, Buttfield A, Seward H, McGivern J. Characteristics of anterior cruciate ligament injuries in Australian football. J Sci Med Sport. 2007;10:96–104.

25. Krosshaug T, Nakamae A, Boden BP, Engebretsen L, Smith G, Slauterbeck JR, et al. Mechanisms of anterior cruciate ligament injury in basketball: video analysis of 39 cases. Am J Sports Med. 2007;35:359–67.

26. Hewett TE, Torg JS, Boden BP. Video analysis of trunk and knee motion during non-contact anterior cruciate ligament injury in female athletes: lateral trunk and knee abduction motion are combined components of the injury mechanism. Br J Sports Med. 2009;43:417–22.

27. Laughlin WA, Weinhandl JT, Kernozek TW, Cobb SC, Keenan KG, O'Connor KM. The effects of single-leg landing technique on ACL loading. J Biomech. 2011;44:1845–51.

28. Mokhtarzadeh H, Yeow CH, Hong Goh JC, Oetomo D, Malekipour F, Lee PV-S. Contributions of the soleus and gastrocnemius muscles to the anterior cruciate ligament loading during single-leg landing. J Biomech. 2013;46:1913–20.

29. Kar J, Quesada PM. A musculoskeletal modeling approach for estimating anterior cruciate ligament strains and knee anterior-posterior shear forces in stop-jumps performed by young recreational female athletes. Ann Biomed Eng. 2013;41:338–48.

30. Morgan KD, Donnelly CJ, Reinbolt JA. Elevated gastrocnemius forces compensate for decreased hamstrings forces during the weight-acceptance phase of single-leg jump landing: implications for anterior cruciate ligament injury risk. J Biomech. 2014;47:3295–302.

31. Bakker R, Tomescu S, Brenneman E, Hangalur G, Laing A, Chandrashekar N. Effect of sagittal plane mechanics on ACL strain during jump landing. J Orthop Res. 2016;34:1636–44.

32. Delp SL, Anderson FC, Arnold AS, Loan P, Habib A, John CT, et al. OpenSim: open-source software to create and analyze dynamic simulations of movement. IEEE Trans Biomed Eng. 2007;54:1940–50.

33. Ishida T, Yamanaka M, Takeda N, Homan K, Koshino Y, Kobayashi T, et al. The effect of changing toe direction on knee kinematics during drop vertical jump: a possible risk factor for anterior cruciate ligament injury. Knee Surg Sports Traumatol Arthrosc. 2015;23:1004–9.

34. Hermens HJ, Freriks B, Disselhorst-Klug C, Rau G. Development of recommendations for SEMG sensors and sensor placement procedures. J Electromyogr Kinesiol. 2000;10:361–74.

35. Delp SL, Loan JP, Hoy MG, Zajac FE, Topp EL, Rosen JM. An interactive graphics-based model of the lower extremity to study orthopaedic surgical procedures. IEEE Trans Biomed Eng. 1990;37:757–67.

36. Corcos DM, Gottlieb GL, Latash ML, Almeida GL, Agarwal GC. Electromechanical delay: An experimental artifact. J Electromyogr Kinesiol. 1992;2:59–68.

37. Brown TN, McLean SG, Palmieri-Smith RM. Associations between lower limb muscle activation strategies and resultant multi-planar knee kinetics during single leg landings. J Sci Med Sport. Sports Medicine Australia. 2014;17:408–13.

38. Weinhandl JT, Earl-Boehm JE, Ebersole KT, Huddleston WE, Armstrong BSR, O'Connor KM. Anticipatory effects on anterior cruciate ligament loading during sidestep cutting. Clin Biomech. Elsevier Ltd. 2013;28:655–63.

18

Percutaneous medial hemi-epiphysiodesis using a transphyseal screw for caput valgum associated with developmental dysplasia of the hip

Chang Ho Shin[1], Wan Kee Hong[1], Doo Jae Lee[1], Won Joon Yoo[1], In Ho Choi[1] and Tae-Joon Cho[1,2]* ⓘ

Abstract

Background: The purpose of this study was to evaluate the radiologic outcome of percutaneous medial hemi-epiphysiodesis using a transphyseal screw for the management of caput valgum associated with developmental dysplasia of the hip (DDH).

Methods: Eighteen hips (18 patients) having caput valgum treated with screw hemi-epiphysiodesis were followed for more than 2 years, and were included in this study. The mean age at the time of the index operation was 8.3 years (range, 4.3 to 10.7 years) and age at the latest follow-up was 12.2 years (range, 9.4 to 16.4 years). The screw in 5 hips was changed into a longer one at postoperative 21.8 months (range, 14 to 29 months) because the proximal femur outgrew the screw. The screws in 11 hips were removed at the mean age of 10.9 years (range, 8.0 to 14.5 years). We retrospectively analyzed the change in various radiologic parameters over time.

Results: The mean Hilgenreiner-epiphyseal angle (HEA) of the operated side was $5.1 \pm 11.3°$ preoperatively, and increased to $20.6 \pm 11.3°$ at the latest follow-up ($p = 0.001$). The mean difference of the HEA between the operated and contralateral sides was $16.9 \pm 15.1°$ preoperatively, which decreased to $2.4 \pm 12.4°$ at the latest follow-up ($p = 0.008$). The mean articulo-trochanteric distance of the operated side, which was 3.2 ± 5.5 mm longer than that of the contralateral side preoperatively, became 5.6 ± 9.1 mm shorter at the latest follow-up ($p = 0.001$). The ratio of femoral neck length of the operated side to that of the contralateral side decreased over the follow-up period. Acetabular shape as measured by the Sharp angle and acetabular roof angle and femoral head coverage as measured by lateral center-edge angle did not change significantly by the index operation. The ratio of medial joint space width of the operated side to that of the contralateral side did not change significantly.

Conclusions: Screw medial hemi-epiphysiodesis can effectively correct caput valgum associated with DDH. However, this technique remains coxa brevis and does not seem to significantly affect acetabular morphology or reduce subluxation.

Keywords: Developmental dysplasia of the hip, Caput valgum, Hemi-epiphysiodesis, Transphyseal screw

* Correspondence: tjcho@snu.ac.kr
[1]Department of Orthopaedic Surgery, Seoul National University College of Medicine, Seoul, Republic of Korea
[2]Division of Pediatric Orthopaedics, Seoul National University Children's Hospital, 101 Daehak-ro Jongno-gu, Seoul 03080, Republic of Korea

Background

Osteonecrosis of the capital femoral epiphysis, resulting in growth disturbance of the proximal femur, is a common and major complication secondary to treatment of developmental dysplasia of the hip (DDH) [1–5]. Of four types of growth disturbance classified by Kalamchi and MacEwen, type II or lateral growth disturbance, which causes valgus tilt appearance of the femoral head on the neck, is the most common [6]. As a result of continued normal medial growth, the femoral head and longitudinal growth plate tilt laterally [7].

Although Kim et al. reported that lateral growth disturbance was not necessarily associated with poor acetabular remodeling [8], caput valgum could induce compromised acetabular index, increase uncovered portion of the femoral head, and promote subsequent acetabular labral tears and early-onset osteoarthritis [8–11]. In addition, it positions the fovea capitis femoris, with no hyaline cartilage, more superior and lateral to its original position, that was previously positioned slightly posterior and inferior to the center of the articular surface [12]. In the severe case of caput valgum, the femoral head could change to "cocked hat" deformity and be laterally subluxated [7].

Proximal femoral varus osteotomy (PFVO) could be a treatment option to correct caput valgum deformity caused by lateral growth disturbance. However, because PFVO is usually performed at the level of the lesser trochanter, away from the center of rotation of angulation, it occasionally requires a great amount of varization to correct deformity and leads to greater trochanter overriding. In addition, it is sometimes difficult to decide on the amount of varus when performing PFVO because it is hard to predict whether further deformity develops until skeletal maturity [13].

Guided growth of the proximal femur using a transphyseal screw across the inferomedial aspect of the proximal femoral epiphyseal plate is an alternative treatment option for caput valgum. Although guided growth using a transphyseal screw has been widely used after introduced by Métaizeau in 1998, a few animal studies reported the effect of medial hemi-epiphysiodesis using a transphyseal screw in skeletally immature hips [14–16]. To the best of our knowledge, there have been only two studies involving screw medial hemi-epiphysiodesis for lateral growth disturbance of the proximal femur followed by treatment of DDH [13, 17]. One of these studies mainly focused on a technique of deformity measurement and not on treatment outcome [17].

The purpose of this study was to evaluate the radiologic outcome of percutaneous medial hemi-epiphysiodesis using a transphyseal screw for caput valgum associated with DDH.

Methods

We collected cases of proximal femoral lateral growth disturbance associated with DDH presenting with progressive caput valgum that were treated with percutaneous medial hemi-epiphysiodesis using a transphyseal screw. Between August 2009 and December 2014, they were treated in a tertiary-care children's hospital and followed for more than 2 years. Hips associated with neuromuscular disease, skeletal dysplasia or congenital anomaly of other organs/systems were excluded. There was no teratologic hip dislocation or hip dislocation combined with arthrogryposis. Based on these criteria, 18 hips (18 patients) became the subjects of this study and medical records and serial radiographs were reviewed and analyzed.

There were 14 female (78%) and 4 male (22%) patients. Fourteen hips (78%) were unilateral DDH, and three hips (17%) were bilateral DDH with only one hip developing caput valgum. The remaining patient had bilateral DDH, whose both hips developed caput valgum and were treated with screw medial hemi-epiphysiodesis. One side was randomly selected and included in the study. Of 14 unilateral cases, 9 (64%) were right hips and 5 (36%) were left hips. The mean age ($\pm$ standard deviation) was 8.3 ± 1.9 years (range, 4.3 to 10.7) at the time of screw placement, and 12.2 ± 2.0 years (9.4 to 16.4) at the time of the latest follow-up. The duration of follow-up averaged 3.9 ± 1.4 years (2.0 to 6.9).

Surgical procedures which were performed before, concurrent with, or after screw medial hemi-epiphysiodesis, are listed in Table 1. No proximal femoral osteotomy or pelvic osteotomy, that can alter acetabular or femoral morphology, was performed after hemi-epiphysiodesis. Applied surgical

Table 1 Treatment history of the hips

	$N = 18^a$
Reduction method	
Closed reduction under general anesthesia	2 (11%)
Open reduction	16 (89%)
Procedures performed before hemi-epiphysiodesis	
Femoral varus osteotomy	3 (17%)
Salter innominate osteotomy	1 (6%)
Dega osteotomy	5 (28%)
Femoral varus osteotomy and Dega osteotomy[b]	5 (28%)
Femoral varus osteotomy and shelf aectabuloplasty[c]	1 (6%)
Femoral varus osteotomy, Dega osteotomy, and triple innominate osteotomy[c]	1 (6%)
Procedures concurrent with hemi-epiphysiodesis	
Dega osteotomy	1 (6%)
Shelf acetabuloplasty	1 (6%)
Epiphysiodesis, distal femur	2 (11%)
Procedures performed after hemi-epiphysiodesis	
Epiphysiodesis, distal femur	1 (6%)
Greater trochanter apophyisodesis	1 (6%)

[a]The values are given as the number of hips
[b]Procedures were performed at the same time in 4 hips and in sequence in 1 hip
[c]In sequence

technique was similar to Lee et al.'s method [18]. A screw was placed through inferomedial one third to one fourth of the proximal femoral physis on the anteroposterior (AP) view and through the center of the physis on lateral view. The number of the threads of the screw that were placed across the physis was more than three, and we stopped advancing the screw when the tip of the screw reached the subchondral bone. After inserting a screw, intraoperative arthrogram was routinely performed to confirm the position of the screw tip.

Anteroposterior radiographs of the pelvis were taken with the hip positioned in neutral rotation and neutral abduction/adduction at each visit. We measured indicators of pelvic alignment in all radiographs. The quotient of pelvic rotation indicating pelvis position in the horizontal plane was 1.01 ± 0.18 (0.68 to 1.46) and the symphysis os-ischium angle, indicating the pelvis position in the sagittal plane, was $99.9° \pm 8.7°$ (90.0° to 115.1°), which was considered acceptable [19, 20].

For evaluating proximal femoral morphology, the Hilgenreiner epiphyseal angle (HEA) [21], head-shaft angle (HSA) [22], and neck-shaft angle (NSA) [14] were measured (Fig. 1). For evaluating femoral neck length, the articulo-trochanteric distance (ATD) [23] and femoral neck length ratio [24] was measured and calculated, respectively. For evaluating acetabular morphology and subluxation, Sharp angle [25], acetabular roof angle [26], lateral center-edge angle (LCEA) [27], medial joint space (MJS) width ratio [28], and center-head distance discrepancy (CHDD) [29] were measured. Femoral neck length ratio and MJS width ratio were calculated by dividing the value of the operated side by the value of the contralateral side. Femoral neck length ratio and CHDD were measured only in the unilaterally affected 14 hips. The difference of radiologic parameters between

the operated and contralateral sides in unilaterally affected hips were also calculated. Changes in the parameters from time of screw placement to the time of latest follow-up, as well as changes of the differences of those values between both hips, were obtained. Two hips, which underwent pelvic osteotomy concurrent with hemi-epiphysiodesis, were excluded from the analysis reflecting changes in parameters in acetabular morphology and subluxation. Skeletal maturity at the time of screw removal was determined based on the closure of the proximal femoral growth plate and triradiate cartilage.

Leg-length-discrepancy (LLD) was evaluated by iliac crest height difference measured on standing AP radiograph of the pelvis. Four patients with bilateral DDH and two patients who underwent epiphysiodesis of the distal femur concurrent with screw medial hemi-epiphysiodesis of the proximal femur were excluded from the analysis of LLD. The patient who underwent epiphysiodesis of the distal femur at the latest follow-up was included in the analysis.

To determine intra-observer reliability, measurements were made by one of the authors (W.K.H.) on two different days, 2 weeks apart. To determine the inter-observer reliability, the same measurements were made by another author (C.H.S.) after a consensus building session to define the radiographic measurements. Intra-observer and inter-observer reliability were evaluated by intraclass correlation coefficients (ICCs), which were calculated assuming absolute agreement and a single measurement with a 2-way-random-effects-model. In the intra-observer reliability test, ICCs were 0.988 (95% confidence interval [CI], 0.967, 0.995) for HEA, 0.957 (0.890, 0.984) for HSA, 0.917 (0.796, 0.968) for NSA, 0.909 (0.766, 0.965) for Sharp angle, 0.973 (0.946, 0.986) for acetabular roof angle, 0.780 (0.511, 0.911) for LCEA, and 0.961 (0.919, 0.982) for MJS width ratio. In the inter-observer reliability test, the ICCs for the

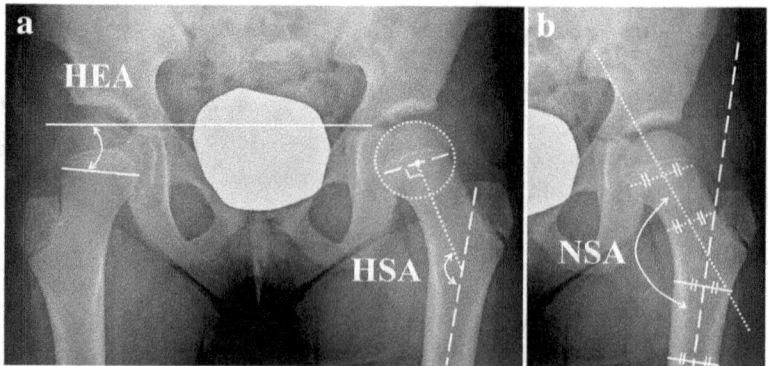

Fig. 1 a Hilgenreiner-epiphyseal angle is the angle between the Hilgenreiner line and a line connecting the medial and lateral end of the proximal femoral physis on the hip anteroposterior radiograph. Head-shaft angle is the angle between the proximal femoral shaft axis and a line which is drawn though the center of the proximal femoral epiphysis and perpendicular to the proximal femoral growth plate. Hilgenreiner-epiphyseal angle of the right hip is 6 degrees, and head-shaft angle of the left hip is 152 degrees on this radiograph. **b** Neck-shaft angle is the angle between the axis of the proximal femoral shaft and the axis of the femoral neck, which links the midpoints of neck diameter at both levels of the subcapital and the base of neck areas. Neck-shaft angle of the left hip is 140.5 degrees in this radiograph

same parameters were 0.871 (0.694, 0.950), 0.830 (0.607, 0.932), 0.903 (0.759, 0.963), 0.919 (0.799, 0.969), 0.826 (0.597, 0.931), 0.715 (0.510, 0.844), 0.762 (0.466, 0.904), and 0.886 (0.769, 0.945), respectively.

The Mann-Whitney U test was used to evaluate the significance of the difference between mean values between operated and contralateral sides. The Wilcoxon signed-rank test was used to evaluate the significance of change of parameters over time. P values <0.05 were considered significant.

Results

The changes of radiologic parameters between operated and contralateral hips from the index operation to the latest follow-up are presented in Tables 2 and 3. In the proximal femoral morphologic domain, mean HEA of the operated hips increased significantly since the index operation ($p = 0.001$). The change of HEA ranged from −6.1° to 34.6°. However, that of the contralateral hips did not change significantly. The difference of HEA between the operated and contralateral sides decreased significantly ($p = 0.008$) (Table 4), of which the respective average became close to zero degrees at latest follow-up.

Preoperatively, the operated side had significantly larger HSA than the contralateral side ($p < 0.001$), while the NSA was not significantly different between the sides ($p = 0.085$). The HSA of the operated side significantly decreased after

Table 2 Preoperative and postoperative data of the operated hips

$N = 18$	Preoperative status[a]	Latest follow-up[a]	P value[†]
Proximal femur			
Hilgenreiner-epiphyseal angle (°)	5.1 ± 11.3	20.6 ± 11.3	0.001
Head-shaft angle (°)	169.5 ± 10.5	150.0 ± 10.0	<0.001
Neck-shaft angle (°)	143.0 ± 7.9	132.1 ± 6.0	<0.001
Femoral neck			
Articulo-trochanteric distance (mm)	21.1 ± 7.9	13.6 ± 8.1	0.001
Femoral neck length ratio[b]	0.929 ± 0.173	0.787 ± 0.281	0.056
Acetabular morphology & subluxation[c]			
Sharp angle (°)	46.7 ± 4.8	44.9 ± 5.5	0.030
Acetabular roof angle (°)	17.1 ± 7.4	16.3 ± 8.0	0.408
LCEA (°)	23.3 ± 6.1	23.9 ± 8.0	0.717
Medial joint space width ratio[b]	1.408 ± 0.518	1.396 ± 0.489	0.507
CHDD[b] (%)	9.2 ± 5.5	6.2 ± 5.1	0.003

†Wilcoxon signed rank test
[a]The values are given as the mean and the standard deviation
[b]Unilateral cases only ($N = 14$)
[c]Two hips which underwent pelvic osteotomy concurrent with hemi-epiphysiodesis were excluded

Table 3 Preoperative and postoperative data of the contralateral hips

$N = 14$	Preoperative status[a]	Latest follow-up[a]	P value[†]
Proximal femur			
Hilgenreiner-epiphyseal angle (°)	22.4 ± 5.9	23.0 ± 5.4	0.802
Head-shaft angle (°)	154.3 ± 5.4	152.7 ± 6.9	0.221
Neck-shaft angle (°)	138.8 ± 6.3	133.0 ± 5.3	0.005
Femoral neck			
Articulo-trochanteric distance (mm)	18.4 ± 3.4	18.9 ± 4.8	0.777
Femoral neck length ratio	Not applicable	Not applicable	
Acetabular morphology & subluxation			
Sharp angle (°)	48.7 ± 3.8	44.7 ± 5.5	0.002
Acetabular roof angle (°)	12.6 ± 4.9	7.4 ± 7.3	0.002
LCEA (°)	24.7 ± 5.6	31.6 ± 5.7	0.002
Medial joint space width ratio	Not applicable	Not applicable	
CHDD (%)	Not applicable	Not applicable	

†Wilcoxon signed rank test
[a]The values are given as the mean and the standard deviation

the index operation but that of the contralateral side did not ($p < 0.001$ and $p = 0.221$, respectively). The NSA significantly decreased on both sides after the index operation, but the amount of change was not significantly different between the two sides ($p = 0.285$). At the latest follow-up, the means of both HSA and NSA became close to zero degrees.

The mean ATD of the operated side was 3.2 ± 5.5 mm longer than that of the contralateral side preoperatively which significantly decreased during follow-up ($p = 0.001$). Meanwhile, the ATD of the contralateral side changed little. As a result, the mean ATD of the operated side was 5.6 ± 9.1 mm shorter than that of the contralateral side at the latest follow-up. Femoral neck length ratio also decreased in 11 hips (79%) ($p = 0.056$).

Regarding acetabular morphology and subluxation, the Sharp angle significantly decreased on both sides, but the amount of change between them was not significantly different ($p = 0.401$) (Tables 2 and 3). Over the follow-up period, Acetabular roof angle and LCEA improved significantly on the contralateral side from normal growth of the acetabulum, while those of the operated side did not show significant changes. MJS width ratio did not change significantly. The mean CHDD improved after the index operation but remained over 6% at the latest follow-up (Table 2).

The screws were changed into longer ones, in five of the hips during the follow-up period postoperatively at 21.8 ± 4.7 months (range, 14 to 29 months), because the

Table 4 Differences of radiologic parameters between the operated and contralateral sides

N = 14	Preoperative status[a]	Latest follow-up[a]	P value†
Proximal femur			
Difference of HEA[b] (°)	16.9 ± 15.1	2.4 ± 12.4	0.008
Difference of HSA[c] (°)	15.5 ± 11.2	−2.5 ± 13.0	0.001
Difference of NSA[c] (°)	5.5 ± 5.6	0.9 ± 6.6	0.056
Femoral neck			
Difference of ATD[c] (mm)	3.2 ± 5.5	−5.6 ± 9.1	0.001
Difference of femoral neck length ratio	Not applicable	Not applicable	
Acetabular morphology & subluxation[d]			
Difference of Sharp angle[c] (°)	−1.9 ± 6.2	0.33 ± 7.7	0.187
Difference of acetabular roof angle[c] (°)	3.3 ± 6.1	8.3 ± 9.3	0.011
Difference of LCEA[b] (°)	2.1 ± 7.8	8.1 ± 9.1	0.009
Difference of CHDD (%)	Not applicable	Not applicable	

†Wilcoxon signed rank test
[a]The values are given as the mean and the standard deviation
[b]These values were calculated by subtracting the values of the operated hips from the values of the contralateral hips
[c]These values were calculated by subtracting the values of the contralateral hips from the values of the operated hips
[d]Two hips which underwent pelvic osteotomy concurrent with hemi-epiphysiodesis were excluded

proximal femora outgrew the screws. Patient's age at the index operation was 6.1 ± 1.6 years (4.3 to 7.7). The HEA increased until the revision surgery by 13.1° ± 5.7° (4.9° to 19.1°) and increased until the latest follow-up by 10.1° ± 5.8° (2.8° to 16.6°) over the mean period of 34 ± 25 months (2 to 60).

Screws were removed in 11 of 18 hips at the mean age of 10.9 ± 2.0 years (8.0 to 14.5). Six of the 11 hips underwent removal of the screw before skeletal maturity at the mean age of 9.6 ± 1.4 years (8.0 to 11.3) and were followed for more than 6 months after screw removal. In these six hips, HEA and HSA did not significantly change from the time of screw removal to the latest follow-up over the mean period of 24.5 ± 12.4 months (6 to 42).

The mean length of the operated legs was 12.6 ± 6.2 mm (0 to 22) longer than that of the contralateral legs preoperatively and 3.2 ± 8.8 mm (−11.6 to 19.7) longer at the latest follow-up. The mean growth of the operated legs significantly diminished compared to that of the contralateral legs over the follow-up period (p = 0.006).

There were no complications associated with screw hemi-epiphysiodesis such as penetration of the articular

surface by the screw, chondrolysis, proximal femoral fracture, irritation symptom at the screw insertion site, or infection.

Discussion

In this study, we reported the outcome of percutaneous medial hemi-epiphysiodesis using a transphyseal screw to correct caput valgum associated with DDH. We quantified caput valgum deformity using HEA and HSA, which were significantly different between the operated and contralateral sides before the index operation. These parameters on the operated hips became similar to those on the contralateral normal hips at the latest follow-up. We tried to evaluate the change of 'fovea valga' over the follow-up period, but could not complete this evaluation because the fovea capitis could not be delineated in many cases; probably due to the altered anatomy of the hip with type 2 osteonecrosis. Our data concur with those of Torode et al., which reported increase of proximal femoral physeal orientation and HSA [13] and McGillion et al. showed improvement of the HEA [17]. Along with the previous studies, taken collectively, our data support the efficacy of screw hemi-epiphysiodesis for caput valgum associated with DDH although previous studies and out data could not prove that this intervention improves the long-term prognosis regarding prevention of osteoarthritis.

In our study, preoperative HSA on the operated side was significantly larger than that of the contralateral side, but NSA was not. This means that the caput valgum deformity was not necessarily associated with coxa valga. After screw hemi-epiphysiodesis, HSA of the operated side decreased much more than that of the contralateral side. However, the decrease of NSA was not significantly different between sides. This result was not concordant to previous animal studies reporting a significant decrease of NSA by screw medial hemi-epiphysiodesis [14–16]. This discrepancy might arise from anatomical differences between animals and humans, or from differences in the measurement methods for NSA. There are several different definitions of NSA [30] and in our study, NSA was measured based upon femur neck orientation [14]. Our data suggest that screw medial hemi-epiphysiodesis corrects mainly caput valgum rather than coxa valga.

In the present study, the ATD of the operated side was longer than that of the contralateral side preoperatively as a result of caput valgum deformity, which became shorter than that of the contralateral side at the latest follow-up. Moreover, femoral neck length ratio also decreased over the follow-up period. This finding concurs with that of the animal study by McCarthy et al. [16] and implies that screw medial hemi-epiphysiodesis cannot prevent shortening of the femoral neck and that it remains a coxa brevis deformity even after the correction of the caput valgum.

In our study, the changes of the Sharp angle on the operated and contralateral sides were similar regardless of screw placement, which was close to the natural course of unoperated cases of caput valgum in a previous study [9]. Furthermore, acetabular roof angle and LCEA did not exhibit a significant improvement on the operated side although it is reported to improve along with normal growth of acetabulum [31, 32]. MJS width ratio also changed very little, and the CHDD remained over 6% in predicting poor acetabular development even after the index operation [29]. Based on these results, screw medial hemi-epiphysiodesis did not make significant impacts on acetabular morphology and femoral head coverage. Lack of significant differences might be because screw placement was performed at relatively older ages when only limited acetabular remodeling potential remained [32].

We could correct HEA by up to 35° even in hips with negative values of HEA preoperatively (Fig. 2). However, this does not imply that every caput valgum deformity can be corrected with screw hemi-epiphysiodesis. For the hips with an established lateral bony bridge or the hips close to skeletal maturity, screw medial hemi-epiphysiodesis would have only an effect preventing the progression of caput valgum, but not correcting the deformity. In such cases, additional procedures need to be considered for significant preexisting caput valgum.

Chang et al. reported that a bony bar formed across the epiphyseal plate along the screw tract in 5 of 8 pigs' hips and a fibrous band formed in another three specimens [14]. In another animal study, the hip which underwent screw hemi-epiphysiodesis showed severe histological changes with epiphyseal plate closure over half the section [15]. In accordance with previous results, caput valgum did not recur in the hips that underwent screw removal before skeletal maturity even without a visible bony bar on plain radiographs. These findings suggest the permanent effect of screw hemi-epiphysiodesis, even after removal of the screw.

Screw medial hemi-epiphysiodesis in addition to pre-existing lateral growth disturbance is expected to suppress the longitudinal growth of the femur. Although important determinants of skeletal growth such as gender and age were diverse, LLD which existed preoperatively decreased by 2.4 mm/year over the follow-up period, which was similar to the normal growth rate of the proximal femur [33]. Even though shortening of the leg makes the ipsilateral hip in a position of relative abduction to the pelvis which is favorable condition for the hip with DDH, the decision on screw hemi-epiphysiodesis should be made cautiously in young patients.

There were no complications associated with screw hemi-epiphysiodesis in our study. Other studies with cerebral palsy patients [18] or with DDH patients [13] also reported no complications. Since the height of the inferomedial part of the epiphysis is low due to caput valgum deformity, screw placement can sometimes be tricky. Therefore, we usually performed an intraoperative arthrogram and checked the position of the screw tip in various positions of the hip to avoid penetration of the articular cartilage.

This study had several limitations. Firstly, because it was a retrospective case series, age at screw placement and follow-up period were variable, which might lead to bias in assessing the effect of a transphyseal screw. And our cases did not compare with an untreated group of hips with caput valgum which can serve as a control group. Secondly, ~40% of patients did not reach skeletal maturity (7 of 18). Next, although radiographs were taken with the pelvis in acceptable positions and the hip in patella facing forward, the shape of the proximal femoral physis varied by femoral rotation, which may affect measurements of some of the radiologic parameters. And a femoral head which is a three-dimensional organ was evaluated two-dimensionally only using X-ray. Lastly,

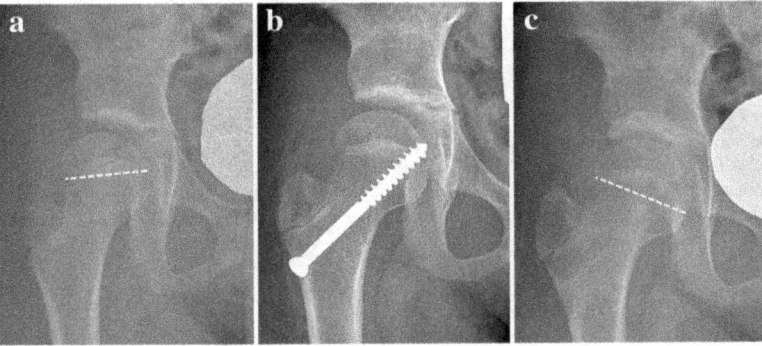

Fig. 2 a A 8.2-year-old female patient was treated for developmental dysplasia of the hip by open reduction at age 2.0 years, showing caput valgum with Hilgenreiner-epiphyseal angle (HEA) -9°. **b** Medial screw hemi-epiphysiodesis changed the HEA to 5° in 1 year. **c** At age 10.9 years, the HEA remained at 25°

although it was the largest study to date investigating screw medial hemi-epiphysiodesis, the sample size was relatively small for powerful statistical analysis [13, 17, 18].

Conclusions

Percutaneous medial hemi-epiphysiodesis using a transphyseal screw can correct caput valgum associated with DDH effectively and safely. However, this procedure does not correct coxa brevis deformity and does not appear to make a significant impact on acetabular morphology and subluxation.

Abbreviations
AP: Anteroposterior; ATD: Articulo-trochanteric distance; CHDD: Center-head distance discrepancy; CI: Confidence interval; DDH: Developmental dysplasia of the hip; HEA: Hilgenreiner-epiphyseal angle; HSA: Head-shaft angle; LCEA: Lateral center-edge angle; LLD: Leg-length-discrepancy; MJS: Medial joint space; NSA: Neck-shaft angle

Acknowledgements
Not applicable.

Funding
No funding was obtained for this study.

Authors' contributions
CHS and TJC drafted the manuscript. CHS, WKH, and DJL performed data collection and data analysis. WJY, IHC, and TJC conceived of the study, participated in the design of the study, performed data interpretation, and participated in coordination. All authors read and approved the final manuscript.

Competing interests
The authors declare that they have no competing interests.

References
1. Brougham DI, Broughton NS, Cole WG, Menelaus MB. Avascular necrosis following closed reduction of congenital dislocation of the hip. Review of influencing factors and long-term follow-up. J Bone Joint Surg Br. 1990; 72(4):557–62.
2. Morcuende JA, Meyer MD, Dolan LA, Weinstein SL. Long-term outcome after open reduction through an anteromedial approach for congenital dislocation of the hip. J Bone Joint Surg Am. 1997;79(6):810–7.
3. Roposch A, Stohr KK, Dobson M. The effect of the femoral head ossific nucleus in the treatment of developmental dysplasia of the hip. A meta-analysis. J Bone Joint Surg Am. 2009;91(4):911–8.
4. Shin CH, Yoo WJ, Park MS, Kim JH, Choi IH, Cho TJ. Acetabular remodeling and role of osteotomy after closed reduction of developmental dysplasia of the hip. J Bone Joint Surg Am. 2016;98(11):952–7.
5. Malvitz TA, Weinstein SL. Closed reduction for congenital dysplasia of the hip. Functional and radiographic results after an average of thirty years. J Bone Joint Surg Am. 1994;76(12):1777–92.
6. Kalamchi A, MacEwen GD. Avascular necrosis following treatment of congenital dislocation of the hip. J Bone Joint Surg Am. 1980;62(6):876–88.
7. Siffert RS. Patterns of deformity of the developing hip. Clin Orthop Relat Res. 1981;160:14–29.
8. Kim HW, Morcuende JA, Dolan LA, Weinstein SL. Acetabular development in developmental dysplasia of the hip complicated by lateral growth disturbance of the capital femoral epiphysis. J Bone Joint Surg Am. 2000; 82-A(12):1692–700.
9. Joo SY, Oh CW, Grissom L, Kumar SJ, MacEwen GD. Three-dimensional computerized tomographic analysis of the deformity of lateral growth disturbance of proximal femoral physis. J Pediatr Orthop. 2009;29(6):540–6.
10. Oh CW, Joo SY, Kumar SJ, Macewen GD. A radiological classification of lateral growth arrest of the proximal femoral physis after treatment for developmental dysplasia of the hip. J Pediatr Orthop. 2009;29(4):331–5.
11. Roposch A, Ridout D, Protopapa E, Nicolaou N, Gelfer Y. Osteonecrosis complicating developmental dysplasia of the hip compromises subsequent acetabular remodeling. Clin Orthop Relat Res. 2013;471(7):2318–26.
12. Cerezal L, Kassarjian A, Canga A, Dobado MC, Montero JA, Llopis E, Rolon A, Perez-Carro L. Anatomy, biomechanics, imaging, and management of ligamentum teres injuries. Radiographics. 2010;30(6):1637–51.
13. Torode IP, Young JL. Caput valgum associated with developmental dysplasia of the hip: management by transphyseal screw fixation. J Child Orthop. 2015;9(5):371–9.
14. Chang CH, Chi CH, Lee ZL. Progressive coxa vara by eccentric growth tethering in immature pigs. J Pediatr Orthop B. 2006;15(4):302–6.
15. d'Heurle A, McCarthy J, Klimaski D, Stringer K. Proximal femoral growth modification: effect of screw, plate, and drill on asymmetric growth of the hip. J Pediatr Orthop. 2016.
16. McCarthy JJ, Noonan KJ, Nemke B, Markel M. Guided growth of the proximal femur: a pilot study in the lamb model. J Pediatr Orthop. 2010; 30(7):690–4.
17. McGillion S, Clarke NM. Lateral growth arrest of the proximal femoral physis: a new technique for serial radiological observation. J Child Orthop. 2011; 5(3):201–7.
18. Lee WC, Kao HK, Yang WE, Ho PC, Chang CH. Guided growth of the proximal femur for hip displacement in children with cerebral palsy. J Pediatr Orthop. 2016;36(5):511–5.
19. Boniforti FG, Fujii G, Angliss RD, Benson MK. The reliability of measurements of pelvic radiographs in infants. J Bone Joint Surg Br. 1997; 79(4):570–5.
20. Tonnis D. Normal values of the hip joint for the evaluation of X-rays in children and adults. Clin Orthop Relat Res. 1976;119:39–47.
21. Weinstein JN, Kuo KN, Millar EA. Congenital coxa vara. A retrospective review. J Pediatr Orthop. 1984;4(1):70–7.
22. Foroohar A, McCarthy JJ, Yucha D, Clarke S, Brey J. Head-shaft angle measurement in children with cerebral palsy. J Pediatr Orthop. 2009;29(3):248–50.
23. Edgren W. Coxa plana. A clinical and radiological investigation with particular reference to the importance of the metaphyseal changes for the final shape of the proximal part of the femur. Acta Orthop Scand Suppl. 1965;Suppl 84:1–129.
24. de Farias TH, Borges VQ, de Souza ES, Miki N, Abdala F. Radiographic study on the anatomical characteristics of the proximal femur in Brazilian adults. Rev Bras Ortop. 2015;50(1):16–21.
25. Sharp I. Acetabular dysplasia. Bone Joint J. 1961;43(2):268–72.
26. Tönnis D. Congenital dysplasia and dislocation of the hip in children and adults: Springer Science & Business Media. Berlin: Springer Verlag; 1987.
27. Wiberg G. Studies on dysplastic acetabula and congenital subluxation of the hip joint: with special reference to the complication of osteoarthritis. Acta Chir Scand. 1939;83(58):53–68.
28. Yoo W, Choi I, Cho T-J, Chung C, Shin Y-W, Shin S. Shelf acetabuloplasty for children with Perthes' disease and reducible subluxation of the hip. Bone Joint J. 2009;91(10):1383–7.
29. Chen IH, Kuo KN, Lubicky JP. Prognosticating factors in acetabular development following reduction of developmental dysplasia of the hip. J Pediatr Orthop. 1994;14(1):3–8.
30. Boese CK, Dargel J, Oppermann J, Eysel P, Scheyerer MJ, Bredow J, Lechler P. The femoral neck-shaft angle on plain radiographs: a systematic review. Skelet Radiol. 2016;45(1):19–28.
31. Shi YY, Liu TJ, Zhao Q, Zhang LJ, Ji SJ, Wang EB. The normal centre-edge angle of Wiberg in the Chinese population: a population-based cross-sectional study. J Bone Joint Surg Br. 2010;92(8):1144–7.
32. Harris NH. Acetabular growth potential in congenital dislocation of the hip and some factors upon which it may depend. Clin Orthop Relat Res. 1976; 119:99–106.
33. Menelaus MB. Correction of leg length discrepancy by epiphysial arrest. J Bone Joint Surg Br. 1966;48(2):336–9.

19

Preoperative prone position exercises: a simple and novel method to improve tolerance to kyphoplasty for treatment of single level osteoporotic vertebral compression fractures

Guangzhou Li[1,2], Hao Liu[2*], Qing Wang[1*] and Dejun Zhong[1]

Abstract

Background: The proper choice of anesthesia for kyphoplasty remains controversy. There are only a few clinical studies specially focusing on and giving detailed information about this treatment under local anesthesia with or without conscious sedation. To evaluate the effect of preoperative prone position exercises on patient tolerance to percutaneous kyphoplasty under local anesthesia.

Methods: Eighty-three patients with single level osteoporotic vertebral compression fractures were nonrandomly assigned to undergo percutaneous kyphoplasty under local anesthesia with preoperative prone position exercises or without. The number of procedure with or without a pause, need for intravenous sedation, and patient satisfactory were recorded and analyzed. Clinical outcomes were assessed using the visual analog scale and the Oswestry Disability Index. The follow-up time was 6 months.

Results: The baseline characteristics of both groups were comparable. The number of procedure without a pause in the exercises group was more than the control group (30/42 patients and 10/41 patients, respectively, $P < 0.001$), and fewer patients required intravenous sedation in the exercises group (7/42 and 28/41, respectively, $P < 0.001$). Patients in the exercises group were more satisfied compared to the control group (41/42 and 32/41, respectively, $P < 0.01$). There were no significant differences between the two groups with regard to improvement in pain and functional scores at all postoperative intervals.

Conclusions: Prone position exercises may improve patient tolerance and satisfaction and reduce the need for intravenous sedation for those with single level vertebral compression fracture undergoing kyphoplasty under local anesthesia. We expect large sample size and multi-center randomized controlled trial studies to be conducted.

Keywords: Kyphoplasty, Prone position, Exercises, Osteoporotic vertebral compression fractures

* Correspondence: pro_liuhao@163.com; jzwk2010@163.com
The abstract of this study was presented as an oral speech at the Global Spine Congress and World Forum for Spine Research 2016 that took place in Dubai at the Grand Hyatt Dubai Convention Centre and published in Global Spine J 2016; 06-GO216 DOI: 10.1055/s- 0036- 1582873.
[2]Department of orthopedics, Sichuan University West China Hospital, Sichuan Province, Chengdu, China
[1]Department of Spine Surgery, the Affiliated Hospital of South-west Medical University, No.25 Taiping St, Luzhou, Sichuan 646000, China

Background

Kyphoplasty (KP), developed from vertebroplasty (VP), is a minimally invasive procedure for the treatment of several vertebal diseases [1–3]. Osteoporotic vertebral compression fractures (OVCF) is the mostly common pathologic condition treated. Compared with VP, KP has a better effect on reducing kyphosis and restoring the height of the vertebral body [4, 5]. However, KP is technically more demanding and complex, and patients undergoing such procedure are generally older and may have numerous illnesses simultaneously, which may especially impair the ability to lie in a prone position for a long time during this procedure, resulting in abandoning the surgery and increasing the risk of anesthesia-related complications [6, 7]. Many authors performed this treatment with patients under general anesthesia [8, 9]. The proper choice of anesthesia for kyphoplasty remains controversy. On the other hand, a few clinical studies reported KP under local anesthesia without detailed information [4, 10].

Ideally, KP should be performed with the patient under local anesthesia with or without conscious sedation. This study was undertaken to evaluate the effect of preoperative prone position exercises (PPE) on patient tolerance to KP under local anesthesia and to determine if such exercises would improve postoperative clinical outcome.

Methods

Study design

Between February 2010 and December 2012, 83 patients with single level painful OVCF not more than 4 weeks old were enrolled in the study. Patients with previous surgery of the spine, psychological diseases, or neurologic deficits, were excluded from participation. This study was approved by Affiliated Hospital of South-west Medical University review board. In our department, two senior spinal surgeons (Q.W. and D.Z.) performed KP in two treatment groups, respectively. One surgeon (Q.W.) preferred that all patients should do PPE, whereas the other one (D.Z.) did not recommend it to patients. So, patients were assigned to undergo KP with PPE or without depending on the surgeon they were referred. Consequently, 42 patients were included in the PPE group (exercises group), and 41 patients in the without PPE group (control group).

A comprehensive assessment of the patients' general condition was performed after admission. On the day before operation, the purpose and procedures involved in the study were fully explained to the patients, and informed consent was obtained before data collection. The PPE was essentially a tolerance test. In the exercises group, with the participators lying in the prone position, one or two soft pillow was placed under their chest. The patients were placed in prone position for 40 to 60 min,

depending on tolerance of oneself, and an investigator recorded the duration and if there was any discomfort. Patients did prone exercises twice. If someone who could not maintain the prone position for 40 min, we placed him/her prone for 20–30 min. In the control group, patients did not do PPE, and no any other exercises given.

Surgical procedures

Surgical procedure was performed under local anesthesia with the patient positioned prone on a radiolucent table with his/her spine extended by chest and pelvic bolsters. C-arm fluoroscopy was used throughout the procedure.

In addition to local anesthesia using 10 ml of 1% lidocaine, if the patient complained inadequate anesthesia during surgical procedure, he or she would be sedated using intravenous fentanyl 0.5 μg/kg and intravenous propofol 0.5 mg.kg^{-1}, and the depth of sedation was monitored by anesthetists to make sure the patient in a safe condition.

With fluoroscopy visualization, transpedicular (in the lumbar vertebrae) or extrapedicular (in the thoracic vertebrae) puncture was performed unilaterally. After reaching the posterior margin of the vertebral body, the bone needle was exchanged for a working cannula. A Balloon with radio-opaque media was inserted into the fractured vertebral body to restore the damaged vertebral body until adequate height restoration and kyphosis correction were obtained or when the inflation pressure reached 220 psi. Then, the balloon was deflated and withdrawn, and the resultant intravertebral cavity was filled with polymethylmethacrylate (PMMA) cement. Monitoring was continued on the ward for 8 h after the operation.

Outcome assessment

Clinical data were prospectively collected and analyzed by one independent observer. On the first postoperative day (the day after the operation), patients were asked whether they were satisfied with such treatment and whether they would undergo the procedure again. The number of interventions that had to be discontinued and the patients who received intravenous sedation were recorded and analyzed.

Pain was evaluated using a visual analogue scale (VAS: 0 = no pain at all, 10 = worst pain imaginable) before and after operation (the first postoperative day), continuing postoperatively at 3 and 6 months. The functional outcome was assessed using the Oswestry Disability Index (ODI) preoperatively and postoperatively at 3 and 6 months.

Statistical analysis

For quantitative variables (the VAS and ODI scores), the groups were compared preoperatively and postoperatively using a paired student's t-test, and the comparisons between the two groups were made by student's t-test. For qualitative variables, the comparisons were made by Chi-square or Fischer's exact test where appropriate. Analyses were performed using SPSS statistical software (Version 13.0, SPSS Inc., Chicago, IL). For all comparisons, a P value < 0.05 was considered significant.

Results

The baseline characteristics of both groups were comparable (Table 1). After 6 months, no patient was lost to follow-up and was excluded from the study. Before operation, one patient with severe thoracic kyphotic deformity just did PPE for 25 min each time, and the others 41 tolerated PPE well without discomfort.

All operations were performed with patients under local anesthesia with or without conscious sedation. No complications related to procedures, anesthesia and sedation occurred, which was confirmed by anesthetists' recorded. No statistically significant difference was observed when the mean duration of operations was compared between the groups (43.8 ± 12.2 min for the exercises group and 47.3 ± 13.7 min for the control group, respectively).

The number of procedure without a pause in the exercises group was more than the control group (30/42 patients and 10/41 patients, respectively, $P < 0.001$), and fewer patients required intravenous sedation in the exercises group (7/42 and 28/41, respectively, $P < 0.001$). More patients in the exercises group were more satisfied compared to the control group ($P < 0.01$, Table 2).

The score of VAS decreased significantly in both groups (Table 3). In the exercises group, the mean pain score decreased from 7.8 ± 1.1 (range, 5–9) before operation to 2.4 ± 1.0 (range, 1–4) on the first postoperative day ($P < 0.001$) and to 2.3 ± 0.7 (range, 1–3) at 6 months after operation ($P < 0.001$); In the control group, VAS score improved from 7.6 ± 1.0 (range, 6–9) preoperatively to 2.4 ± 1.0 (range, 1–4) on the first postoperative day ($P < 0.001$) and to 2.4 ± 0.8 (range, 1–4) at 6 months postoperatively ($P < 0.001$). The ODI score had a similar trend. The mean ODI score decreased from 60.5 ± 6.4 (range, 48–72) preoperatively to 30.6 ± 4.9 (range, 22–42) ($P < 0.001$) and 30.0 ± 4.6 (range, 22–42) ($P < 0.001$) at 3 and 6 months, respectively, in the exercises group; The ODI score improved from 61.1 ± 5.4 (range, 48–72) preoperatively to 29.9 ± 4.1 (range, 24–41) ($P < 0.001$) and 30.1 ± 4.5 (range, 24–42) ($P < 0.001$) at 3 and 6 months, respectively, in the control group. There were no significant differences between the two groups with regard to improvement in pain and functional scores at all postoperative intervals.

Discussion

As the ageing of the population of all over the world, the incidence of OVCF is likely to increase rapidly and provides a great challenge to health care workers and patients [11, 12]. KP has been proven to be an effective minimally invasive procedure for the treatment of OVCF [2–5]. However, KP usually is performed with the patient under general anesthesia [8, 9, 13–15]. This do cause a therapeutic dilemma that patients undergoing such procedure are generally older and may have numerous illnesses which may pose a higher risk for general anesthesia than the minimally invasive procedure per se [6, 7]. Ideally, KP is performed with the patient under local anesthesia. There are only a few clinical studies specially focusing on and giving detailed information about KP under local anesthesia with or without conscious sedation [4, 7, 10, 16, 17]. To the best of our knowledge, there is no report about preparing patients with PPE to study the effect on patient tolerance under local anesthesia and the clinical outcome in the literature so far.

The present study demonstrates that through PPE patients tolerated operation better, with fewer requiring intravenous sedation, and patients were more satisfied with such procedure. The reason why PPE improves patient tolerance under local anesthesia might be: In addition to poor physical function caused by the vertebral fracture and numerous illnesses simultaneously, psychosocial factors, including lack of confidence, low mood, anxiety, distress, may also play a key role in impairing the ability of patients with OVCF to lie in a prone position for a long time. Through the process of PPE, we built up patients' physical adaptation to prone position and patients' confidence, and thus improved patients' psychological and physical tolerance to KP. During PPE, a kind of comprehensive intervention measures

Table 1 Characteristics of the study population

	Exercises group	Control group
No.patients	42	41
Patient age(y)(range)	71.4 ± 8.5(56–92)	70.51 ± 7.8(56–84)
Sex[No.(%)]		
Male	11 (26.2)	13 (31.7)
Female	31 (73.8)	28 (68.3)
Distribution of the fractured vertebrae [No.(%)]		
Thoracic(T6-T10)	8 (19.0)	9 (22.0)
Thoracolumbar(T11-L2)	30 (71.4)	27 (65.9)
Lumbar(L3-L5)	4 (9.5)	5 (12.2)
Chronic obstructive pulmonary disease	13	11
Coronary heart disease	8	9
Diabetes	7	7
Hypertension	17	16
Thoracic kyphosis deformity	11	12

Table 2 Comparison of procedure-related data and patient satisfaction using Chi- square or Fischer's exact test

	Exercises group (n = 42)	Control group (n = 41)	P value
Procedure without a pause (yes/no)	30/12	10/31	P < 0.001
Need for intravenous sedation(yes/no)	7/35	28/13	P < 0.001
Patient willing to repeat(yes/no)	41/1	32/9	P < 0.01

was implemented for preoperative preparation, including physical training, psychological support, and patient education. This reminds us that a combination of preoperative management, including physiotherapy, psychological support and patient education should be taken for such patients before operation.

Although the causes of pain in OVCF are multifactorial, it is known that this is due mainly to micromovement of the vertebral fracture [18]. Effective and rapid relief from pain and satisfactory clinical outcomes can be obtained after elimination of the microfractures, vertebral stabilization, and the chemical neurolytic and thermal neurolytic effect of the PMMA [5, 19]. All these could explain that although PPE improved patient tolerance and satisfaction, there were no statistically significant differences in pain alleviation and functional improvement between the two groups postoperatively. Due to various reasons, some authors still supported assisted sedation for KP or VP [7, 17, 20]. However, considering that patients with OVCF are generally older and may have numerous illnesses, reducing the use of additional sedation or general anesthesia means more safety and less potential risks for patients undergoing KP or VP treatment. Although our PPE did not improvement patients' pain and functional scores compared with patients in the control group, it still might provide potential value to health care workers and patients.

PPE brings some advantages as follows: Firstly, it spares the use of additional intravenous sedation or general anesthesia with its potential complications [21, 22]. Secondly, it may help patients resume their daily activities early after operation. Thirdly, although we did not compare the cost of between the two groups, exercises group appears to be more cost-effective since

Table 3 Comparison of preoperative and postoperative mean VAS scores

	Preoperation	The first postoperative day	3 months after operation	6 months after operation
Exercises group	7.8 ± 1.1	2.4 ± 1.0*	2.4 ± 0.9*	2.3 ± 0.7*
Control group	7.6 ± 1.0	2.4 ± 1.0*	2.5 ± 1.0*	2.4 ± 0.8*

Abbreviations: *VAS* visual analogue scale (VAS: 0 = no pain at all, 10 = worst pain imaginable)

potential adverse events related to intravenous sedation would be reduced.

Our study has a few limitations that should be mentioned. First, all patients in our study were with single level OVCF. For 2 or more than 2 levels OVCFs, the duration time of KP would be too long to use local anesthesia without intravenous sedation, and sometimes we initially recommended general anesthesia for them. So we did not enroll patients with 2 or more OVCF in the current study. Second, we did not randomize the patients between the groups because such randomization might cause ethical concerns. In our study, patients were allocated to different groups depending on the surgeons they were referred. So, any significant selection bias should have been fairly well mitigated. Third, the follow-up was 6 months. With no statistically significant differences in pain alleviation and functional improvement between the two groups during the 6-month follow-up, we did not expect that a long-term follow-up would bring significant differences. In addition, additional morbidities and mortality related to this elderly population may prohibit long-term follow-up. Other limitations of our study include the small sample size and non-multicenter study.

Conclusions

Considering the limitation of the current study by its small number of patients and nonrandomized comparative design, we carefully suggest that PPE may improve patient tolerance and satisfaction and reduce the need for intravenous sedation for those with single level vertebral compression fracture undergoing KP under local anesthesia. However, to confirm and validate the results of our study, large sample size and multi-center randomized controlled trial studies should be conducted.

Abbreviations
KP: Kyphoplasty; ODI: Oswestry Disability Index; OVCF: Osteoporotic vertebral compression fractures; PMMA: Polymethylmethacrylate; PPE: Prone position exercises; VAS: Visual analogue scale; VP: Vertebroplasty

Acknowledgments
The abstract of this study was presented as an oral speech at the Global Spine Congress and World Forum for Spine Research 2016 that took place in Dubai at the Grand Hyatt Dubai Convention Centre and published in Global Spine J 2016; 06-GO216 DOI: 10.1055/s- 0036- 1582873.
This article did not receive any form of pharmaceutical or industry support. We would like to express our sincere gratitude to our hospital colleagues, nurses, physical therapists, and patients who participated in the study.

Funding
No any funding was received to support the study.

Authors' contributions
GL worked through the whole study from designing the study, acquisition of data, analysis and interpretation of data, and drafting the manuscript. HL

made substantial contributions to conception to this paper and contributed in critically revising the manuscript. QW contributed in designing the study and revising the manuscript, and the author performed half of operation for our cases. DZ was in charge of performing the operations and revising the manuscript for important intellectual content. All authors reviewed and approved the final version of the manuscript.

Competing interests
The authors declare that they have no competing interests.

References
1. Voggenreiter G. Balloon kyphoplasty is effective in deformity correction of osteoporotic vertebral compression fractures. Spine. 2005;30:2806–12.
2. Serra L, Kermani FM, Panagiotopoulos K, et al. Vertebroplasty in the treat- ment of osteoporotic vertebral fractures: results and functional outcome in a series of 175 consecutive patients. Minim Invasive Neurosurg. 2007;50:12–7.
3. Taylor RS, Fritzell P, Taylor RJ. Balloon kyphoplasty in the management of vertebral compression fractures: an updated systematic review and meta-analysis. Eur. Spine J. 2007;16:1085–100.
4. CW Y, Hsieh MK, Chen LH, Niu CC, TS F, Lai PL, et al. Percutaneous balloon kyphoplasty for the treatment of vertebral compression fractures. BMC Surg. 2014;14(1):1–6.
5. Dong RB, Chen L, Tang TS, et al. Pain reduction following vertebroplasty and kyphoplasty. Int Orthop. 2013;37:83–7.
6. Lieberman IH, Dudeney S, Reinhardt MK, Bell G. Initial outcome and efficacy of "kyphoplasty" in the treatment of painful osteoporotic vertebral compression fractures. Spine. 2001;26:1631–8.
7. Mohr M, Pilich D, Kirsch M, et al. Percutaneous balloon kyphoplasty with the patient under intravenous analgesia and sedation: a feasibility study. Am J Neuroradiol. 2011;32(4):649–53.
8. Berlemann U, Franz T, Orler R, et al. Kyphoplasty for treatment of osteopo- rotic vertebral fractures: a prospective non-randomized study. Eur. Spine J. 2004;13:496–501.
9. Li X, Yang H, Tang T, et al. Comparison of kyphoplasty and vertebroplasty for treatment of painful osteoporotic vertebral compressionfractures: twelve-month follow-up in a prospective nonrandomized comparative study. J Spinal Disord Tech. 2012;25(3):142–9.
10. Shim J, Lee K, Kim H, et al. Outcome of balloon kyphoplasty for the treatment of osteoporotic vertebral compression fracture in patients with rheumatoid arthritis. BMC Musculoskeletal Disorders. 2016;17(1):365. Published online 2016 Aug 24. https://doi.org/10.1186/s12891-016-1215-4.
11. Riggs BL, Melton LJ 3rd. The worldwide problem of osteoporosis: Insights afforded by epidemiology. Bone.1995; 17(5Suppl): 505–11.
12. Lyles KW, Gold DT, Shipp KM, Pieper CF, Martinez S, Mulhausen PL. Association of osteoporotic vertebral compression fractures with impaired functional status. Am J Med. 1993;94(6):595–601.
13. Kobayashi K, Shimoyama K, Nakamura K, et al. Percutaneous vertebroplasty immediately relieves pain of osteoporotic vertebral compression fractures and prevents prolonged immobilization of patients. Eur Radiol. 2005;15:360–7.
14. Heini PF, Orler R. Kyphoplasty for treatment of osteoporotic vertebral fractures. Eur. Spine J. 2004;13:184–92.
15. Luginbuhl M. Percutaneous vertebroplasty, kyphoplasty and lordoplasty: implications for the anesthesiologist. Curr Opin Anaesthesiol. 2008;21:504–13.
16. Cagli S, Isik HS, Zıleli M. Vertebroplasty and kyphoplasty under local anesthesia: review of 91 patients. Turk Neurosurg. 2010;20(4):464–9.
17. Guglielmino A, Sorbello M, Barbagallo G, et al. Osteoporotic vertebral compression fracture pain (back pain): our experience with balloon kyphoplasty. Minerva Anestesiol. 2007;73(1–2):77–100.
18. Barr JD, Barr MS, Lemley TJ, McCann RM. Percutaneous vertebroplasty for pain relief and spinal stabilization. Spine. 2000;25:923–8.
19. Shah RV. Sacral kyphoplasty for the treatment of painful sacral insufficiency fractures and metastases. Spine J. 2012;12:113–20.
20. Venmans A, Klazen CA, Lohle PN, van Rooij WJ. Percutaneous vertebroplasty and procedural pain. Am J Neuroradiol. 2010;31(5):830–1.
21. Weill A, Chiras J, Simon JM, Rose M, Sola-Martinez T, Enkaoua E. Spinal metastases: indications for and results of percutaneous injection of acrylic surgicalcement. Radiology. 1996;199(1):241–7.
22. Sesay M, Dousset V, Liguoro D, et al. Intraosseous lidocaine provides effective analgesia for percutaneous vertebroplasty of osteoporotic fractures. Can J Anaesth. 2002;49(2):137–43.

20

Acceptability of a digital health intervention alongside physiotherapy to support patients following anterior cruciate ligament reconstruction

Emma Dunphy[1,2*] , Fiona L. Hamilton[1], Irena Spasić[3] and Kate Button[4,5]

Abstract

Background: Physiotherapy rehabilitation following surgical reconstruction to the Anterior Cruciate Ligament (ACL) can take up to 12 months to complete. Given the lengthy rehabilitation process, a blended intervention can be used to compliment face-to-face physiotherapy with a digital exercise intervention. In this study, we used TRAK, a web–based tool that has been developed to support knee rehabilitation, which provides individually tailored exercise programs with videos, instructions and progress logs for each exercise, relevant health information and a contact option that allows a patient to email a physiotherapist for additional support. The aim of this study was to evaluate the acceptability of TRAK–based blended intervention in post ACL reconstruction rehabilitation.

Methods: A qualitative research design using semi-structured interviews was used on a convenience sample of participants following an ACL reconstruction, and their treating physiotherapists, in a London NHS hospital. Participants were asked to use TRAK alongside face-to-face physiotherapy for 16 weeks. Interviews were carried out, audio recorded, transcribed verbatim and coded by two researchers independently. Data were analyzed using thematic analysis.

Results: Of the 25 individuals that were approached to be part of the study, 24 consented, comprising 8 females and 16 males, mean age 30 years. 17 individuals used TRAK for 16 weeks and were available for interview. Four physiotherapists were also interviewed. The six main themes identified from patients were: the experience of TRAK rehabilitation, personal characteristics for engagement, strengths and weaknesses of the intervention, TRAK in the future and attitudes to digital healthcare. The main themes from the physiotherapist interviews were: potential benefits, availability of resources and service organization to support use of TRAK.

Conclusions: TRAK was found to be an acceptable method of delivering ACL rehabilitation alongside face-to-face physiotherapy. Patients reported that TRAK, specifically the videos, increased their confidence and motivation with their rehabilitation. They identified ways in which TRAK could be developed in the future to meet technological expectations and further support rehabilitation. For Physiotherapists time and availability of computers affected acceptability. Organization of care to support integration of digital exercise interventions such as TRAK into a blended approach to rehabilitation is required.

Keywords: Anterior cruciate ligament, Physiotherapy, Surgery, Rehabilitation, E-health, Internet

* Correspondence: emma.dunphy@ucl.ac.uk
[1]E-Health Unit, Research Department of Primary Care and Population Health, Upper Third Floor UCL Medical School (Royal Free Campus), Rowland Hill Street, NW3 2PF, London, UK
[2]Homerton University Hospital NHS Trust, Homerton Row E96SR, London, UK
Full list of author information is available at the end of the article

Background

Anterior cruciate ligament (ACL) injury represents a significant burden of serious knee injuries. An American study estimates that 100,000 ACL reconstructions are performed per year [1]. A UK based study estimates that in a 'catchment area of 400,000 population, accident and emergency departments can expect to see two acute ACL injuries per week [2]. There is a significant commitment to rehabilitation required for patients who wish to return to an active, athletic life [3–5].

There are many protocols for ACL rehabilitation available and evidence for both physical and psychological recovery continues to inform best practice in optimizing function [5–10]. Still, a high percentage of individuals never return to their pre-injury level of function [3, 6, 11–14]. Potential reasons for this are loss of confidence and self-efficacy [6, 11, 15] combined with poor engagement with the rehabilitation process [16], which is known to be lengthy in nature, often requiring commitment for a year or more [14]. Patients struggle with motivation, compliance and a clear understanding of what is recommended at each stage of their recovery [5, 16]. Patient knowledge and engagement are key to successful rehabilitation [17]. There is evidence to suggest that digital tools can support engagement with healthcare [18–22]. Patients can use the Internet to gain access to correct information and utilize digital tools such as progress logs and personalized prompts in order to be informed, motivated and encouraged [21, 23, 24]. One such tool is TRAK, a digital intervention developed to support self-management of knee conditions [24, 25]. TRAK, provides a platform for individually tailored exercise programs with videos, detailed instructions and progress logs for individual exercises, a health information section, and a contact option that allows a patient to email a physiotherapist for additional support. TRAK has recently been modified with specific content for ACL rehabilitation based on the best available evidence [4, 5, 9, 10, 16, 26]. The ACL-specific version of TRAK includes over 200 new exercise videos, mostly to support advanced stages of physiotherapy including return to sport activities. These exercises (see Fig. 1 for an example), target modifiable factors such as strength, neuromuscular control, motor learning, sport specific skills and fatigue resistance, and are specifically tailored to an ACL population of patients, who tend to be younger and more active, and therefore have higher expectations regarding knee function [27]. ACL-related health information focuses on managing expectations given a lengthy recovery process by providing detailed information, milestones and common problems associated with each stage of rehabilitation.

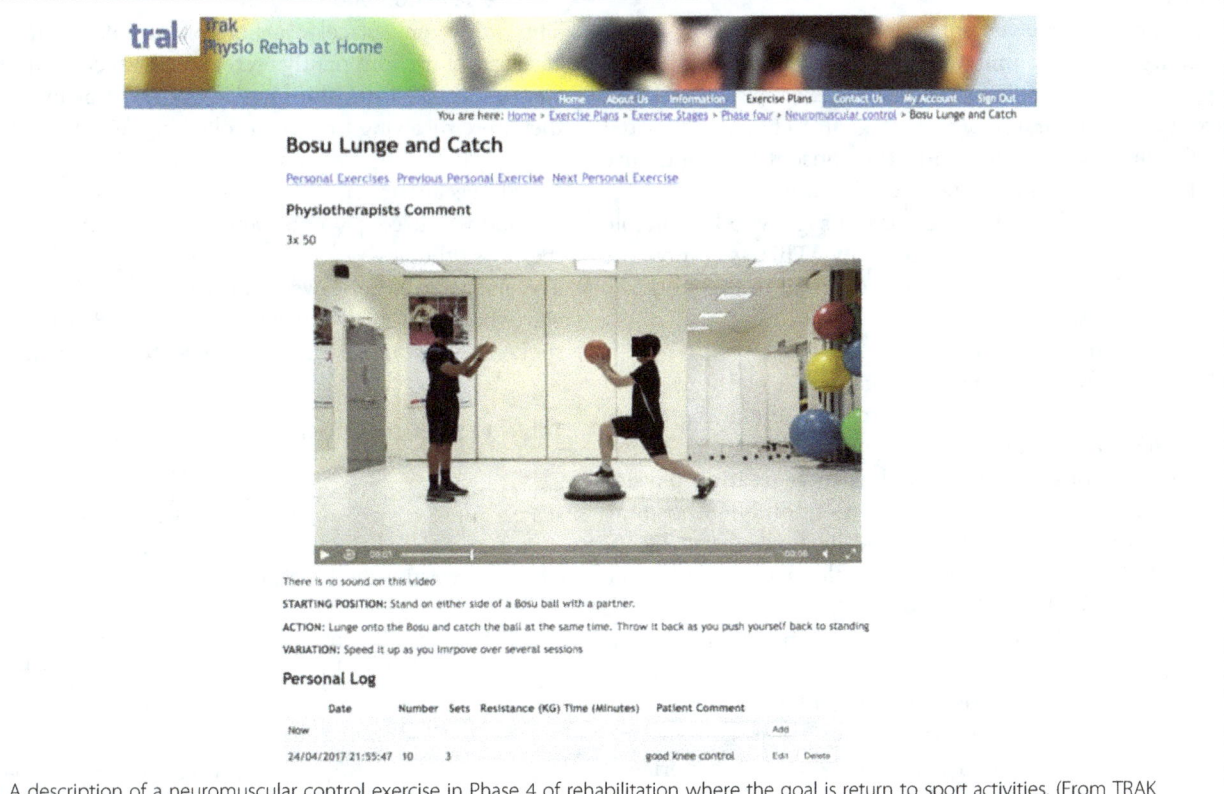

Fig. 1 A description of a neuromuscular control exercise in Phase 4 of rehabilitation where the goal is return to sport activities. (From TRAK website with permission)

As part of the development and testing of digital interventions, we need to understand the relationship between individuals' initial reactions to newly developed online interventions, the intention to use it and their actual use [28]. The usability study conducted for the initial version of TRAK, which was implemented originally as a Facebook app, suggested that a digital exercise intervention would facilitate communication, provide information, help recall information, improve understanding, enable exercise progression, and support self-management in general [24]. These finding were subsequently confirmed when a new version of TRAK re–implemented as web–based app (which is also the version discussed in this study) was integrated into routine healthcare and evaluated for its impact on the patient, clinician and organization [25, 29]. The aim of the current study, however, was to evaluate the acceptability of TRAK to a specific patient population – those following ACL reconstruction, whose rehabilitation on average takes 12 months to complete and, therefore, may struggle with long–term engagement. In addition to patients themselves, we also evaluated the acceptability of TRAK to physiotherapists. These findings will be used to inform more effective integration of TRAK into a blended exercise intervention, which should capture patients' needs over an extended duration of recovery pathway.

Methods
Patient public involvement
Patients and the public were involved in the early development of this study by suggesting exercise content appropriate to their rehabilitation goals. They participated in the filming of videos and gave consent for public use of these videos. They informed the study methodology by suggesting that a trial period of usage who be suitable to assess the website acceptability. This was not the group of patients who were the recruited to the study.

Study design
This research was done with qualitative methods using semi-structured interviews to ascertain the acceptability of TRAK to a population receiving rehabilitation following ACL reconstruction as well as their treating physiotherapists, who were based at one London NHS hospital. Five physiotherapists were trained on how to use TRAK and integrate it into patient care alongside face-to-face physiotherapy. They then used TRAK for four months with a group of patients who were at varying stages following ACL reconstruction. After four months semi-structured interviews were conducted by lead researcher ED, at a location convenient to both types of participants. The interviews focused on the overall experience of ACL rehabilitation and in particular experience of using TRAK. In relation to the latter, we examined the

influence of contextual factors related to acceptability of new digital tools including performance expectancy, effort expectancy, social influence, facilitating conditions, self-efficacy, anxiety and behavioral intentions [28].

Standard ACL rehabilitation pathway
All patients who undergo ACL reconstruction are invited to follow a standard ACL rehabilitation pathway, which has been designed around published evidence and is delivered in a group format. [5, 7–10, 16, 26, 30]. This pathway consists of four rehabilitation stages (Table 1.). Progression through the stages is based on pre-set functional criteria. Treatment is delivered within a group environment. Individual consultations are provided for within that structure. Exercise prescription is individually tailored and in line with American College of Sports Medicine guidance [31].

There is a significant variety in patients' individual experiences and goals. TRAK rehabilitation is designed so that it can reflect any individual's pathway within these stages. It is designed to facilitate improved engagement, confidence, motivation and self-efficacy away from the class. The personalized exercise plans with videos, exercise log, information and remote e-mail support for any questions or concerns are in addition to the standard care ACL program.

Sample selection and recruitment
This study took place in a London hospital with an NHS caseload of predominantly recreational athletes. All patients were recruited from the physiotherapy department, where they were receiving treatment following ACL reconstructive surgery. Between two and four new ACL patients are referred weekly from orthopedics. A convenience sample method was used: patients were recruited from all stages of the physiotherapy post-operative ACL pathway (see Fig. 2). The inclusion criteria were: all patients on the ACL pathway who could freely consent, were over 18 years old, who spoke English fluently and had access to a smartphone. The

Table 1 Stages of ACL rehabilitation in standard care

Stage 1, 0–6 weeks approximately, depending on milestones achieved: focuses on restoration of active range of motion, muscle activation, gait and the management of swelling, pain and wound healing.

Stage 2, 6 weeks to 3 months approximately, depending on milestones achieved: weekly classes which initiate strength training and neuromuscular control.

Stage 3, from 3 months approximately, depending on milestones achieved: strength gains are consolidated and motor control is challenged with increasing dynamic activity. Some participants will complete care and return to sport in this stage where goals do not include cutting and pivoting activities such football, hockey, dancing etc.

Stage 4, from 6 months approximately, depending on milestones achieved: advanced sports specific skills and movement patterns are trained toward patient goals.

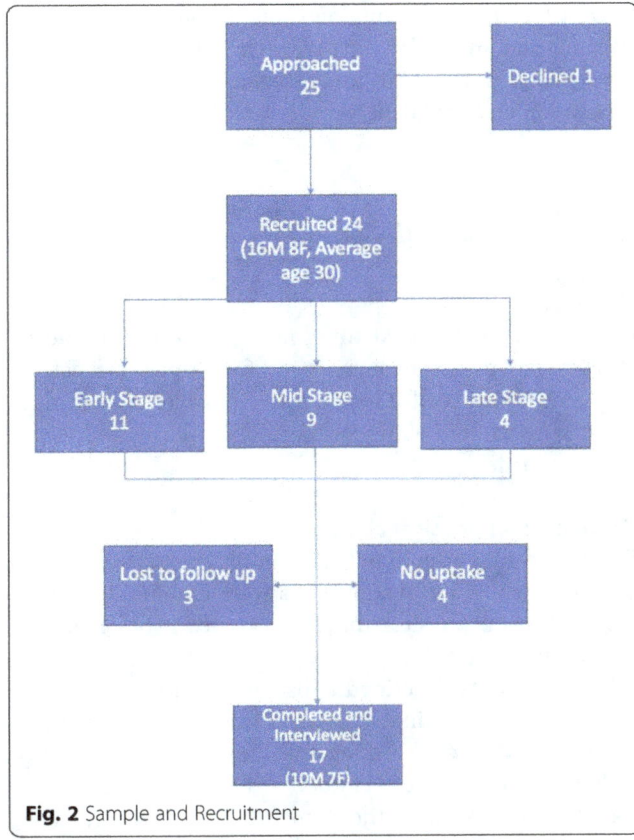

Fig. 2 Sample and Recruitment

exclusion criteria were: patients with multi-ligament reconstruction, revision ACL surgery or fractures, or patients with a poor command of English. Twenty-five patients were asked to take part in the study. One patient declined participation because of time concerns. A sample of 24 patients was recruited. Four patients withdrew from the study due to time constraints. Seventeen patients completed the study and were interviewed. Following provision of an information leaflet and obtaining written informed consent, participants were trained on how to use TRAK by their treating physiotherapist who provided them with a personalized exercise plan. This was delivered in a one-to-one session and patients were offered informal user guidance as needed.

The Principal Investigator (PI) was one of 5 treating physiotherapists in the ACL group from Band 5, 6 and 7 level of experience. Thirteen participants knew the PI before being recruited but were unaware of any role or motivation in the study. Physiotherapist training on how to use TRAK as part of the standard care took place over a 30 min period in a group session led by the lead researcher. The TRAK exercise programs were maintained and updated by all physiotherapists involved in the group.

Data collection
Semi-structured interviews took place at a convenient time and place for the participants, at the hospital, over

the phone and in two cases at an agreed, appropriate public place. All physiotherapists were interviewed in the physiotherapy department. All interviews were digitally audio recorded and transcribed verbatim by the lead researcher. All interviews were participant and PI only.

The interview questions were guided by topics that arose in previous related studies and from ongoing informed discussion within the research team [20, 24, 25]. The topic guide was minimally refined throughout the process to responds to emerging data.

Data analysis
Data from the interviews were analyzed using pragmatic thematic analysis to inform factors that relate to acceptability of new digital tools like TRAK. This sees the data itself rather than the theory driving the process. The themes emerging from the interviews are grouped stringently so all the interview data relating to a particular theme are recorded. Data are weighted and reported secondary to frequency of occurrence or explanatory value [32]. The data were analyzed and coded by the principal investigator and separately coded by another team member. Saturation of data was agreed upon. A dialectic process followed until agreement was reached. Data are presented in the results as a descriptive narrative to reflect the patient and physiotherapist experience [32].

Results
Ten male and seven female patients with an average age of 30 were interviewed. Four Physiotherapists were also interviewed. The patient and physiotherapists interviews have been reported separately to illustrate with clarity how using TRAK alongside face-to-face physiotherapy was experienced by patients and physiotherapists. Key quotes from the interviews are included to express the specific words of the participants. The results show how and why users accept or do not accept TRAK. They explore in particular, performance and effort expectancy, social conditions and environment, self-efficacy, anxiety and behavioral intentions relating to the combination of TRAK with standard care [28].

Patient interviews
Theme 1 – Experiences of the blended approach of standard ACL rehabilitation with TRAK
Using TRAK blended with standard physiotherapy enhanced the patient experience for most participants. The blended combination of their face-to-face care and the use of the website to support self-management gave patients access to the resources they needed at all times.

P13: There are certain things that I couldn't remember from week to week but it was good to be able to go back and look at it again.

P8: Oh definitely, I couldn't imagine it (rehab) without it. It is such a lot of work … it's been 6 months since my surgery. You have to put in so much work. You need that support to keep.

P10: I mean…I do refer to internet anyway because of the accessibility issue. It's so easy. So I think there are positives for that reason alone. It's so easy to get to. If there is detailed information on there, I want to use it. I think it's a good thing.

Patients found that the group structure was a positive experience. They discussed the learning environment and the support they felt from one another. They also described replacing something of the loss of their usual activities while they rehabilitated.

P2: I wasn't sure how it would be to be part of a class but I really like it. I know it helps with volume control but actually it's really nice to be around other people who have gone through the same thing and see the different stages before and ahead and how far you have come. How people are doing. And … I also think it's a pretty good job of providing one to one during those classes too.

P9: One thing I really like was to come here and see the guys who had the same injury I had and you ask them, hey mate, what happened to you and they say football. Me too!

P6: Motivation and comparing yourself. It's important to review other people and their training and it tells you a lot about what you should be doing. Why are you so good at that and why are you doing that so much better than what I do? You know it drives you. I had a very joyful moment of three times ten at 80 kg and others from my level couldn't do it. I felt proud.

Eight patients mentioned that they felt lucky to have been in an area where ACL injury and surgery are commonplace and so an evidence-based rehabilitation group is provided with high levels of support. Their perception was that NHS care was varied and they felt lucky to be in this particular hospital.

P14: I felt very lucky to have happened to live in the right area.

P5: I think it's really good because I have heard that other hospitals …doesn't have a programme that is as good as yours and physios that look after you.

P6: I feel like I am one of those who won the postcode lottery.

P7: I think it has been pretty brilliant, the support I have received in comparison to other people I know who have gone to other hospitals.

Theme 2 - Personal characteristics and rehabilitation engagement

Patients broadly seemed to find the ACL rehabilitation experience exceeded their expectations, but the commitment to rehabilitation was undoubtedly a burden for many patients and marked their lives in a significant way. Key concepts that recurred for patients were, commitment, motivation and confidence in physical ability.

Commitment
P7: There is a lot to do …you have work and your life and then this rehab is a whole other thing.

Motivation
P2: I think the toughest thing now is to keep the motivation to go to the gym three or four times a week. … you need to think of it as a lifestyle change, to keep fit…. Just trying to fit it with work and commuting and everything is hard.

Confidence in physical ability
P7: I felt like I couldn't do (things) and was letting people down. A lot of those jobs were hinging on me being able to do physical things. … so yes it has really affected me quite a lot.

Many patients described a loss of function and participation after ACL injury. There was a sense of being changed and often a feeling that the extent of their loss of function was not understood.

P6: I tried skiing without my ACL, I tried and tried but it felt awful. The more I thought about it, I needed the surgery. It would have ended up being injured more if I continued on that knee.

P9: I was in pain… I had 1 or 2 times …where I took a step and my knee just collapsed.

Some people reflected on how their pre-existing personality traits affected the way they engaged with both traditional physiotherapy and TRAK. Those who were disposed to improve self-care with the use of technology did so, whereas those who saw themselves as being differently motivated or skilled, engaged differently.

P14: In terms of tracking on the website I haven't done it that well and I have been trying to work out why … and I am not very good at being consistent with my methods in anything in life and it includes that.

P1: I am lazy with the internet and it's easier to watch a video and just do it but I'll not report or log.

Theme 3 – Attitudes to the internet and healthcare
As there are so many websites providing healthcare advice and services, patients expressed concern about knowing with confidence what information is 'safe' when it comes to digital resources. They worried about self-diagnosis, poor exercise technique and inappropriate advice exercise apps or websites where their personal injury and abilities were not fully understood and taken into account. Patients were very clear that they go online for information despite the risks and that they feel the

NHS should be providing them with approved digital rehabilitation tools and information sources.

P5: it's overwhelming too. You might think there is something wrong with you and you might do the wrong thing. You need to check with a real professional.

P14: Even if you think of putting that on YouTube with every other videos people will all go to the one that is NHS approved. Obviously that's the one people would pick.

P6: If I don't know how to do an exercise or something and I will go on YouTube or whatever but you get a varied standard and some may be downright dangerous. It is not good, for obvious reasons. So I think opt have a site that I know my physios or the hospital I am with, the NHS, has approved that these are the good stuff to do or links to the right stuff. That is kind of important.

Theme 4 – Benefits of using TRAK for rehabilitation

The patient participants gave positive patient feedback on the key functions of TRAK. They felt that all the key functions (video-based personal plans, information, exercise logs and email support) impacted directly on their knowledge, motivation and confidence, but to differing degrees.

Patients felt that they went to the videos to inform their technique and give them confidence that they were doing the exercises correctly. They also reported that the videos reminded them of what exercises they should be doing.

P10: You can't rate it highly enough really. It's somewhere to go and check on what you're supposed to be doing and make sure to do it right.

There was a mixed response to the exercise log, it was popular as a method to monitor progress but it was reported to be somewhat user-unfriendly and did not provide an option of a general progress report.

P6: It really makes me because I think, oh god I haven't filled anything in to my log this week and it looks so bad. It really drags me to the gym, I look at it and think, I have to do something. I have to do something ... even when I feel yuk.

P8: Again at the beginning I was inputting few things but it was adding half an hour onto my gym session. Trying to get a connection and all that.

The information section was popular immediately post-operatively and at phase-to-phase transitional points. Several patients suggested that the information was too wordy and would be improved by presenting it in video format and linking it with the exercise phases, i.e. a more seamless transition between the personal plans and information.

P6: In the beginning when you have more issues and you are fresh out of surgery and a bit ahhhhh. Then it's very useful.

The 'contact us' section was not as popular as expected. Patients reported that they wanted the face-to-face reassurance when they had concerns. This identified a challenge for new technology to find effective ways of reassuring patients through a digital medium.

P10: I thought before I started using it that I would use the contact us more but didn't because I waited until the session and asked my questions there. Maybe I didn't come into such huge problems where I had to contact you urgently.

Some individuals emphasized the importance of TRAK to support rehabilitation when they were unable to attend physiotherapy due to work commitments or because of personal circumstances.

P14: I think the videos are like a revolution! It's amazing ...but it's not like what you see on YouTube because you trust it. ... it doesn't exist anywhere else as far as I can see.

P3: There are lots of exercises that people can do. And if it's too easy for you, you can move up different stages. Some harder ones and some easier ones... I think it gives you a focus and a way to approach it. It's like a weekly target to do it and not think of the long road.

It also acted as a motivator to comply with their rehabilitation:

P6: Well TRAK works very well for me. Firstly, it makes me go to the gym. It really makes me because I think, oh god I haven't filled anything in to my log this week and it looks so bad. I love the videos; I look at them every time before I do my exercise. Because I am paranoid about bad technique and sometimes so paranoid about it that I stay away from doing things.

Theme 5 – Limitations of TRAK for rehabilitation

Patients were asked about their user experience of TRAK as a tool to support self-management. The answers were broadly divided into extrinsic and intrinsic factors. Patients discussed extrinsic problems they experienced, which could have been addressed by better physiotherapist management of the personal plans or e-mail links.

P4: in terms of communication. Right from the off, I write a couple of messages in the contact us section and I never received anything back. It kind of killed the point of the website for me... to a degree.

P10: I refer back to the paper in the class sometimes as that is more up to date than my plan....

Other extrinsic factors such as access to and the speed of Internet connection also affected usability. Without exception, every patient mentioned this as a limitation.

P15: The problem is the internet connection, in the gym it's impossible to navigate between pages so I just gave up. Some apps you can use offline, that is what is needed.

P8: Again at the beginning I was inputting few things but it was adding half an hour onto my gym session. Trying to get a connection and all that.

Intrinsic factors referred to the website function itself. Patients discussed functional limitations of TRAK in comparison to other apps they were exposed to through the commercial market.

P9: (I used it) out of commitment (to the study). If it was more designy (sic) or there was an app easy to use then definitely.... If it was done like the Nike one, you can bet there would have been so many downloads.... There is nothing on there to say 'come on'. Like the Nike app, if you run there is this voice saying 'great job, you did 5 K today'.

P14: I found it difficult, well, clunky to add it add the bottom of every page. To put that in each time. It's the kind of ins and out of the techy stuff ... it wasn't smooth.

Theme 6 – TRAK in the future: How to increase the impact on positive behaviors

Patients saw the use of TRAK blended together with face-to-face physiotherapy as the future of ACL rehabilitation. They agreed universally that a digital exercise intervention was needed and they used their own experience with new technology to provide more information about their user needs. They would like to see the usability of existing functions improved, e.g. the ways of providing health-related information (educational videos alongside written information), easier identification of exercises (thumbnails alongside their descriptions), easier logging of exercise progression (slider scales and speech notes as an alternative to text input). New functionality that TRAK could benefit from mainly focused on personalization aspects such as prompts and cues that could be set individually, summary of overall progress, web chat, etc. The majority of patients felt that the web site needed to be converted into an app accessible on handheld devices such as tablets and smartphones and in particular with functions that are accessible offline.

P4: I would very much like to stress that it should be an app. It's just that it would really help because it is really tricky on the phone. It's hard in the gym I want to look at the examples really quick and remind myself ... an app would be better. You can use it offline.

P9: I want it to prompt me, I want it to give me a weekly record, I want it to shout at me through the phone that I need to be doing my single leg squats today, that kind of thing. Something that comes up saying 'don't forget this, do this today'.

They requested further prompts to emphasize exercises they may be missing, prompt a help link, a chat log that you could refer back to, a dashboard of completed sessions and milestones that can generate a weekly report, a set of different workouts that the can be automatically generated such as A, B & C, per week, a body

map to show where they should feel the exercises, further links to relevant resources such as evidence or sport-specific information and pop ups that remind them where they are relative to milestones.

P6: I wish I could reflect all the exercise that I am doing. Even stuff that's not on TRAK, so I can keep a complete record of my exercise and progress. Drills, squats that aren't on TRAK. Sounds banal but there is a pride in showing all that I have done to myself and the physio. It's what I do to get better.

P7: the kind of comparison I have is when I was going to do a half marathon and I used this app and it told me every day. Go and run this far, now do a strength and conditioning class and now go do some yoga.

Patients were very clear that they did not think TRAK was a replacement for physiotherapy, but should be used to complement face-to-face treatment in a 'blended approach'. They were very keen to explain that it was an aid to their self-care when they were not in physiotherapy. Interestingly several patients who were in the middle stage of their rehabilitation did say that when they became too busy at times they were happy to manage through the website and attend physiotherapy less often.

P16: I would like to have both but I wouldn't have it instead.

Physiotherapist interviews

Physiotherapist discussed the benefit of having a website to enhance their patients' self-management during rehabilitation. Physiotherapists explained that they want to improve their patients' confidence, quality of exercise technique and compliance with exercise as the evidence suggests this would ensure better outcomes. The website provides a more evolved way of influencing these factors than traditional exercise handouts. They also noted that digital health options do not interest all patients and that patients' self-selection is key to acceptability of digital interventions.

Theme 1 - Benefits to physiotherapists

Physiotherapists expressed enthusiasm for TRAK on behalf of themselves and their patients, however they also seemed to acknowledge that not all patients would be suitable for this digital tool.

PHY1: We are giving back that locus of control to the patient .... You pick a patient who is appropriate for it. I mean there are so many patients who you may have say 6 appointments with, the middle three might just be exercise progressions. Some patients would be more than happy with email review... well, you could save the patient time too.

PHY4: Anyone that wants. Self-selecting group and definitely. I am refusing to be ageist because I have 80-year-old patients who email me and who are very engaged with technology. Equally I have 30 years olds that don't care or don't get it.

Rotational physiotherapists particularly felt that they used the website to educate themselves. That it was a go to summary of the education for each stage and a library of exercise ideas that they could use to help patients.

PHY3: As a junior physio I found it really useful in terms of information and a quick go to resource for reviewing milestones and do's and don'ts…. I quite relied on it and it fed me information. Especially band 5 physios who come into a trust new and it's a great learning tool to help you.

PHY1: If we had much more digital contact with patients I would be very happy with that. We could be emailing patients and caring a lot remotely. Simple progressions and checking on exercises could save contact time, patients' own time and money I guess.

Theme 2 - Suggestions to improve the usability of TRAK for physiotherapists

Of particular concern to physiotherapists was the time it took to build personal exercise programs and maintain them as patients progressed. Practical suggestions that recurred in interviews included the use of tablets in class to update programs quickly, thumbnail images alongside the names of exercises so they could quickly see what each one was without having to click on it and load new pages. Another suggestion was an inbuilt spelling checker, as one dyslexic physiotherapist felt they were slow in adding instructions because this functionality was not available. Physiotherapists would also like to see the exercise section have several 'bolted' key exercises for each stage.

PHY1: It would be good to build a smoother understanding of how we use the TRAK in the sessions. Some patients expect to be updated, some don't and then we don't know… in the sessions, having TRAK open on iPad or something would work. So patients could almost go through it with you as you upgrade it.

One physiotherapist was concerned about the use of patients in the videos because their exercise technique may not be perfect, e.g. a hop that showed inadequate valgus control of the knee. This emphasized the need to upgrade some of the videos. Another physiotherapist was concerned that not enough variations of exercises were available, which meant some exercise videos differed from what the patients were taught in the group.

Importantly, they would like to see a weekly dashboard or a report generated on what the patients have done. This could be printed as a notes record and can be added to paper or digital notes kept in the department instead of duplicating an exercise compliance and progression record.

Physiotherapists discussed the risks associated with TRAK training and management for physiotherapists. They were concerned about delays in picking up patient contacts and felt an emphasis on red flags in the information or red flag pop up reminders might help to identify potentially vulnerable patients.

PHY4: I have a disclaimer about slow contacts on my email and the phone number of the department in case of problems …It needs to have an out of office function or a re-routing function for when therapists are off. The information section, it should have …a clear red flag lists, when to stop and exercise, FAQ's etc. again to reduce anxiety and reassure.

Further suggestions for improvement included providing information on using videos in addition to written material. One physiotherapist suggested that in line with commercial apps, perhaps a celebrity or famous athlete who had a similar injury would be involved in the production of information videos. Patient-experience videos were also suggested as well as voiceover instructions to some of the videos to highlight key guidance on technique. Similar to the patients, the physiotherapists wanted to see prompts and pop ups that engaged patients and directed to different sections of information. They also felt that a group or board should be reviewing the content on an ongoing basis so that the evidence is up to date and exercises or information can be added as appropriate. Opinions were mixed about how much information about physiology or advanced rehabilitation knowledge patients would benefit from. However, it was agreed that links to approved information or research were a good addition.

Discussion

This study found that patients generally accepted a TRAK, a digital self-management support tool that was personalized with their own ACL rehabilitation plan and saw it as a positive addition to be blended with standard care. Physiotherapists likewise engaged well with the website as a support tool for patients and found it helpful to work with patients through this interface. Of the 17 interviewed patients and 4 physiotherapists, all thought that the blended approach of standard care and the website, notwithstanding its ongoing technical improvement, was an improvement on standard care alone. Every interviewed patient thought that the website should be a choice available to all ACL rehabilitated patients on the NHS.

In the interviews, the emergence of social influence, expectations and anxieties regarding TRAK usage reflect the established paradigm for acceptability of new digital technology discussed by Venkatesh et al. [28]. Performance expectancy (the degree to which an individual believes that using the system will help them attain goals), effort expectancy (the degree of ease associated with using the technology), social influence (the degree to which an individual perceives that important others believe they should use) and facilitating conditions (the degree to which an individual believes the organizational and technical infrastructure exist to support use) are considered the key factors in determining acceptability. As well as self-efficacy, anxiety and behavioral intentions.

Social influences in the group were evident where patients described their engagement with one another as an incentive for using the TRAK website. More importantly, individuals reported that interest in TRAK was dependent on the engagement of their physiotherapist. They reported less use if their physiotherapists were slow to respond to e-mails or because personal plans were not updated in a timely manner. This establishes the physiotherapist as the necessary agent behind the blending of standard care with TRAK. Physiotherapists expressed awareness of this and highlighted a number of facilitating conditions that influenced their ability to deliver this. Clinical time was the main challenge for TRAK management, but they felt that through use of better hardware such as tablet devices and improved organization of TRAK data, they could improve efficiency and maintenance of personalized programs.

Performance and effort expectancy of TRAK found a gap in functionality between this prototype and participants' experience of commercial health apps such as 'the Nike App'. In particular, they wished to see TRAK as an app with offline functions. Physiotherapists wanted a function for prompts and reminders that could be set by patients depending on patient goals in order to facilitate further engagement, and incentives such as, 'if you achieve these target, you may begin the running program' [33]. Patients and physiotherapists reported that TRAK was easy to use and did not frustrate their effort expectancy, with the exception of maintaining the log, though this was also discussed as having a positive effect on behavior.

The Behavior Change Wheel model outlines the importance of understanding the patients' physical, social and psychological sources of behavior in order to understand developing interventions for changing behavior [34]. This group of patients described their sense of loss, their goals and the burden of a long and physically challenging rehabilitation program. These contextual factors inform their feelings about the target behavior, the rehabilitation program. The patients discussed how the website informed, motivated and improved confidence in carrying out the desired behaviors. Specifically the website functions provided clear plans, videos and instructions as well as persuading them with targeted information and an opportunity to record and monitor

progress [34]. Overall, individuals indicated that TRAK helped them as part of a blended approach to physiotherapy (face-to-face and digital) as opposed to exclusive face-to-face or digital options.

Some patients who participated highlighted that they would not have chosen ordinarily to use a digital health intervention as they were not sure they would like it or it would be beneficial. Interestingly they worried about how their lack of usage would impact on the physiotherapists' opinion of them. They described themselves as 'lazy' and 'sorry' [23]. This raises questions about how organizational changes to incorporate digital tools may affect patients who choose not to use these tools [28, 35]. Morden et al. found that "care must be taken to balance the needs of clinicians and patients whilst avoiding the scenario where patient information becomes a substitute rather than a supplement" [36]. Every patient that was interviewed without exception said that they did not see TRAK as an alternative to their face-to-face physiotherapy appointments but it should be used in a blended approach combining the digital tool with face-to-face. This is an approach taken by Bossen et al. with knee OA [20]. While some patients will continue to prefer standard care, this blended approach facilitates patients who wish to work more independently to do so safely. Some patients did say they would accept TRAK instead of appointments in stage 3 of their rehabilitation where exercise goals were clear and they felt confident to work independently with longer gaps between appointments. This can be explored further in a planned feasibility trial of TRAK for ACL patients [37] . Given the established psychological factors in determining return to function and sport the role of patient confidence in the blended approach is key to its usefulness [15]. As such TRAK is a unique digital tool for ACL reconstructed patients to facilitate the self-care component of their rehabilitation.

Conclusion

Exploring patients' opinions showed an evolved understanding of the potential benefits of a blended approach. TRAK aims to influence patient engagement and behavior change in line with established theory by motivating patients, giving them the capability to perform well and creating opportunities to record development toward well-defined goals. The study results suggest that TRAK, subject to technical improvement, was acceptable to patients in effort and performance expectancy. The value of TRAK was understood by participants to be a personalized reflection of their rehabilitation program with interactive components that aimed to inform, motivate and engage. However, physiotherapists highlighted organizational changes are needed to better integrate its use into standard physiotherapy practice.

Abbreviations
ACL: Anterior Cruciate Ligament; NHS: National Health Service; PI: Principal Investigator; TRAK: Taxonomy for the Rehabilitation of Knee Conditions

Acknowledgements
Emma Dunphy was supported in part by the National Institute for Health Research (NIHR) Collaboration for Leadership in Applied Health Research and Care North Thames at Bart's Health NHS Trust. The views expressed are those of the authors and not necessarily those of the NHS, NIHR, or the Department of Health.

Funding
ED was supported in part by National Institute for Health Research (NIHR) Collaboration for Leadership in Applied Health Research and Care North Thames at Bart's Health NHS Trust.

Authors' contributions
ED was the PI on this study and worked with supervision from KB and FH. KB and IS designed TRAK and ED made content changes to reflect the needs of ACL patients. ED and KB separately analyzed data and prepared the final manuscript for publication. All authors read and approved the final manuscript.

Competing interests
The authors declare that they have no competing interests.

Author details
[1]E-Health Unit, Research Department of Primary Care and Population Health, Upper Third Floor UCL Medical School (Royal Free Campus), Rowland Hill Street, NW3 2PF, London, UK. [2]Homerton University Hospital NHS Trust, Homerton Row E96SR, London, UK. [3]School of Computer Science & Informatics, Cardiff University, Queens Building, 5 The Parade, Cardiff CF24 3AA, UK. [4]School of Healthcare Sciences, Cardiff University, Eastgate House, Newport Road, Cardiff CF24 0AB, UK. [5]Cardiff & Vale University Health Board, Health Park, Cardiff CF14 4XW, UK.

References
1. Bollen S. Advances in the management of anterior cruciate ligament injury. Curr Orthop. 2000;14(5):325–8.
2. Kapoor B, et al. Current practice in the management of anterior cruciate ligament injuries in the United Kingdom. Br J Sports Med. 2004;38(5):542–4.
3. Ardern CL, et al. Fifty-five per cent return to competitive sport following anterior cruciate ligament reconstruction surgery: an updated systematic review and meta-analysis including aspects of physical functioning and contextual factors. Br J Sports Med. 2014:bjsports-2013-093398.
4. Adams D, et al. Current concepts for anterior cruciate ligament reconstruction: a criterion-based rehabilitation progression. J Orthop Sports Phys Ther. 2012;42(7):601–14.
5. Risberg MA, Lewek M, Snyder-Mackler L. A systematic review of evidence for anterior cruciate ligament rehabilitation: how much and what type? Physical Therapy in Sport. 2004;5(3):125–45.
6. Ardern CL, et al. A systematic review of the psychological factors associated with returning to sport following injury. Br J Sports Med. 2013;47(17):1120–6.
7. Herrington L, Myer G, Horsley I. Task based rehabilitation protocol for elite athletes following anterior cruciate ligament reconstruction: a clinical commentary. Physical Therapy in Sport. 2013;14(4):188–98.
8. Risberg MA, Ekeland A. Assessment of functional tests after anterior cruciate ligament surgery. J Orthop Sports Phys Ther. 1994;19(4):212–7.
9. Risberg MA, et al. Design and implementation of a neuromuscular training program following anterior cruciate ligament reconstruction. J Orthop Sports Phys Ther. 2001;31(11):620–31.
10. EltzEn I, et al. A progressive 5-week exercise therapy program leads to significant improvement in knee function early after anterior cruciate ligament injury. J Orthop Sports Physic Ther. 2010;40(11):705–21.
11. Ardern CL, et al. The impact of psychological readiness to return to sport and recreational activities after anterior cruciate ligament reconstruction. Br J Sports Med. 2014;48(22):1613–9.
12. Ardern CL, et al. Return-to-sport outcomes at 2 to 7 years after anterior cruciate ligament reconstruction surgery. Am J Sports Med. 2012;40(1):41–8.
13. Ardern CL, et al. Return to sport following anterior cruciate ligament reconstruction surgery: a systematic review and meta-analysis of the state of play. Br J Sports Med. 2011:bjsports76364.
14. Ardern CL, et al. Return to the preinjury level of competitive sport after anterior cruciate ligament reconstruction surgery two-thirds of patients have not returned by 12 months after surgery. Am J Sports Med. 2011;39(3):538–43.
15. Ardern CL, et al. Psychological responses matter in returning to preinjury level of sport after anterior cruciate ligament reconstruction surgery. Am J Sports Med. 2013;41(7):1549–58.
16. Lynch AD, et al. Consensus criteria for defining 'successful outcome'after ACL injury and reconstruction: a Delaware-Oslo ACL cohort investigation. Br J Sports Med. 2013:bjsports-2013-092299.
17. Croft P, Porcheret M, Peat G. Managing osteoarthritis in primary care: the GP as public health physician and surgical gatekeeper. Br J Gen Pract. 2011;61.
18. Grindem H, et al. Online registration of monthly sports participation after anterior cruciate ligament injury: a reliability and validity study. Br J Sports Med. 2013:bjsports-2012-092075.
19. van Mechelen DM, Van Mechelen W, Verhagen EA. Sports injury prevention in your pocket?! Prevention apps assessed against the available scientific evidence: a review. Br J Sports Med. 2014;48(11):878–82.
20. Bossen D, et al. Effectiveness of a web-based physical activity intervention in patients with knee and/or hip osteoarthritis: randomized controlled trial. J Med Internet Res. 2013;15(11):e257.
21. Alkhaldi G, et al. The effectiveness of prompts to promote engagement with digital interventions: a systematic review. J Med Internet Res. 2016;18(1)
22. Semple JL, et al. Using a mobile app for monitoring post-operative quality of recovery of patients at home: a feasibility study. JMIR mHealth and uHealth. 2015;3(1):e18.
23. Moore GC, Benbasat I. Development of an instrument to measure the perceptions of adopting an information technology innovation. Inf Syst Res. 1991;2(3):192–222.
24. Spasić I, et al. TRAK app suite: a web-based intervention for delivering standard care for the rehabilitation of knee conditions. JMIR research protocols. 2015;4(4)
25. Button K, et al. TRAK ontology: defining standard care for the rehabilitation of knee conditions. J Biomed Inform. 2013;46(4):615–25.
26. Risberg MA, et al. Neuromuscular training versus strength training during first 6 months after anterior cruciate ligament reconstruction: a randomized clinical trial. Phys Ther. 2007;87(6):737–50.
27. Magnussen RA, et al. Cross-cultural comparison of patients undergoing ACL reconstruction in the United States and Norway. Knee Surgery Sports Traumatology Arthroscopy. 2010;18(1):98.
28. Venkatesh V, et al. User acceptance of information technology: toward a unified view. MIS Q. 2003:425–78.
29. Button KSI. Implementation of the TRAK intervention to enable e-rehab for knee conditions: a web-based intervention suite to support self-management in. Rehabilitation. 2017.
30. Myer GD, et al. Rehabilitation after anterior cruciate ligament reconstruction: criteria-based progression through the return-to-sport phase. J Orthop Sports Phys Ther. 2006;36(6):385–402.
31. Garber CE, et al. American College of Sports Medicine position stand. Quantity and quality of exercise for developing and maintaining cardiorespiratory, musculoskeletal, and neuromotor fitness in apparently healthy adults: guidance for prescribing exercise. Med Sci Sports Exerc. 2011;43(7):1334–59.
32. Pope C, Ziebland S, Mays N. Analysing qualitative data. Br Med J. 2000; 320(7227):114.
33. Knight E, et al. Public health guidelines for physical activity: is there an app for that? A review of android and apple app stores. JMIR mHealth and uHealth. 2015;3(2):e43.
34. Michie S, van Stralen MM, West R. The behaviour change wheel: a new method for characterising and designing behaviour change interventions. Implement Sci. 2011;6(1):42.
35. Bossen D, et al. Adherence to a web-based physical activity intervention for patients with knee and/or hip osteoarthritis: a mixed method study. J Med Internet Res. 2013;15(10):e223.

21

Musculoskeletal extremity pain in Danish school children – how often and for how long? The CHAMPS study-DK

Signe Fuglkjær[1][*][iD], Jan Hartvigsen[1,2], Niels Wedderkopp[3,4], Eleanor Boyle[1,5], Eva Jespersen[1,6], Tina Junge[1,7], Lisbeth Runge Larsen[8] and Lise Hestbæk[1,2]

Abstract

Background: Musculoskeletal pain is common in childhood and adolescence, and may be long-lasting and recurrent. Musculoskeletal problems tend to follow adolescents into adulthood, and therefore it is important to design better prevention strategies and early effective treatment. To this end, we need in-depth knowledge about the epidemiology of musculoskeletal extremity problems in this age group, and therefore, the aim of this study was to determine the prevalence, frequency and course of musculoskeletal pain in the upper and lower extremities in a cohort of Danish school children aged 8–14 years at baseline.

Methods: This was a prospective 3-year school-based cohort study, with information about musculoskeletal pain collected in two ways. Parents answered weekly mobile phone text messages about the presence or absence of musculoskeletal pain in their children, and a clinical consultation was performed in a subset of the children.

Results: We found that approximately half the children had lower extremity pain every study year. This pain lasted on average for 8 weeks out of a study year, and the children had on average two and a half episodes per study year. Approximately one quarter of the children had upper extremity pain every study year that lasted on average 3 weeks during a study year, with one and a half episodes being the average. In general, there were more non-traumatic pain episodes compared with traumatic episodes in the lower extremities, whereas the opposite was true in the upper extremities. The most common anatomical pain sites were 'knee' and 'ankle/ft'.

Conclusion: Lower extremity pain among children and adolescents is common, recurrent and most often of non-traumatic origin. Upper extremity pain is less common, with fewer and shorter episodes, and usually with a traumatic onset. Girls more frequently reported upper extremity pain, whereas there was no sex-related difference in the lower extremities. The most frequently reported locations were 'knee' and 'ankle/ft'.

Keywords: Adolescent health, Epidemiology, Cohort, Leg, Arm, Limb, Injury, Complaint, Prevalence

* Correspondence: sfuglkjaer@health.sdu.dk
[1]Department of Sports Science and Clinical Biomechanics, Faculty of Health Sciences, University of Southern Denmark, Campusvej 55, 5230 Odense M, Denmark
Full list of author information is available at the end of the article

Background

Musculoskeletal (MSK) pain is common in childhood and adolescence [1–3], and may be long-lasting and recurrent [4–6]. MSK pain in the lower extremities occurs both in children [3, 7] and in adolescents [1], with ankle and foot problems being more common in children [7, 8], and knee problems being more common during adolescence [1]. Importantly, one study found that half the Danish adolescents aged 12–15 years with knee pain also reported knee pain when asked 1 year later [9]. Similarly, in another study, one third of the Finnish children with lower extremity (LE) pain reported its presence one and/or 4 years later [4]. MSK problems tend to follow adolescents into adulthood [10, 11], and therefore, it is important to design better prevention strategies and early effective treatment. To this end, we need in-depth knowledge about the epidemiology of MSK extremity problems in children and adolescents, including frequency and course.

Traditionally, data on MSK health in children and adolescents have been obtained from clinical assessments in emergency departments or in primary care physicians' practices. This type of research provides valid information about patterns of care-seeking, mainly for traumatic problems such as fractures and distortions [12, 13]. However, such studies rarely provide information about non-traumatic problems, which have been shown to be more common compared to traumatic problems in these age groups [3, 14]. Knowledge about MSK problems in the general population, including non-traumatic problems, has traditionally been collected via questionnaires completed by children or their parents. However depending on recall period, questionnaire data may suffer from recall bias, especially for minor problems [15, 16], and therefore short recall periods are needed to collect reliable estimates [17]. Mobile phone text messages at short time-intervals is one practical and user-friendly method to reduce recall bias [18, 19], and thus, may be a more valid way to track information about MSK problems in children. In addition, this method makes it possible to estimate occurrence by prevalence rather than incidence, which has been suggested to be the most appropriate way to describe non-traumatic MSK problems, because of the long-lasting and recurrent nature of these complaints [20]. Therefore, we set out to determine the frequency and course of upper extremity (UE) and LE pain in 8–14-year-olds. Specifically, we wanted to describe the following four areas using information about their MSK pain reported by their parents via weekly mobile phone text messages, as well as data obtained in a clinical examination for a subset of this cohort:

1) MSK pain as reported by the parents

   The sex-specific prevalence of any type of UE or LE pain
   The frequency and duration of UE or LE pain episodes

2) Pain distribution as reported from the clinical examination

   The prevalence of pain in specific anatomical sites
   The distribution of 1) pain episodes in girls versus boys and 2) traumatic versus non-traumatic episodes including a comparison of traumatic versus non-traumatic episodes in relation to frequency

Methods

Setting

This was a prospective three-year school-based cohort study nested within the Childhood Health, Activity and Motor Performance School Study (CHAMPS Study-DK). It started in 2008, and in August 2011, additional funding made it possible to prolong the study until June 2014. It was a dynamic cohort study, thus children could enter or leave the study at any time during the study period. The main purpose of the CHAMPS Study-DK was to evaluate the effectiveness of extra physical education on children's general health. Schools were divided into two groups: intervention schools received six lessons of physical education per week, whereas control schools only received two lessons. The intervention was performed from 2008 to 2012. With regard to MSK pain, data was obtained over the complete study period (2008 to 2014). The CHAMPS Study-DK is described in detail elsewhere [21]. Data on incidence and prevalence of MSK extremity injuries from 2008 to 2011 have been reported previously [7, 14]. The current study includes data from 2011 to 2014, and the prevalence and course of spinal pain in the children has been reported previously [22].

Study population

In August 2011, all pupils attending the third to seventh grade in 13 out of 17 public primary schools in the municipality of Svendborg, Denmark, were invited to participate in the study. Svendborg is a Danish municipality with 58,000 inhabitants and is comparable to the rest of Denmark in terms of age, sex and income, but has a slightly higher unemployment rate (5.3% versus 4.5%) [23]. In Svendborg, 84% of children attend public schools. The children and adolescents in the study were from families that represented all levels of socio-economic status.

Data collection

Musculoskeletal pain as reported by the parents

Every Sunday, parents received three mobile phone text message questions (SMS questions); one about presence or absence of MSK pain in their child and two about the child's sports participation. For this study, only the data in response to the question about MSK pain were used. The exact wording of the question was as follows: "Has [name of child] had any pain during the past week in: 1-Neck or back; 2-Shoulder, arm or hand; 3-Hip, leg or foot; or 4-No pain, and no further instructions were given regarding pain registration. It was possible to report pain in more than one area. If parents did not reply they received up to two reminders at intervals of 48 h. The SMS questions were sent out every week except for 6 weeks during the summer holidays (July and August) and 1 week during the Christmas holidays.

If parents texted a '1', '2' and/or '3' for the MSK pain question, they were telephoned within 5 days by a member of the clinical team, consisting of licenced and experienced physiotherapists and chiropractors. A standardized interview was performed about the nature of their child's pain, including information about duration of pain and mode of onset. If the pain seemed to be of MSK origin, a clinical examination was scheduled at the child's school within 2 weeks from the date parents received the SMS question. On the other hand, if the pain was perceived to be non-MSK in nature or had disappeared, no further action was taken. To assemble comprehensive information on all MSK problems, information obtained from the telephone interview or the clinical examination about children being examined or treated elsewhere (e.g. emergency department) was collected concurrently. Relevant information from medical records was registered for analyses without a clinical examination performed by a member of the clinical team.

Pain distribution as reported from the clinical examination

A member of the clinical team performed the clinical examination, and parents were informed about the result of the examination by telephone or letter. If deemed necessary, the child was referred to a medical specialist for further examination.

Based on the clinical examination, the UE and LE pain were categorized into one of the following anatomical sites: 'shoulder', 'upper arm', 'elbow', 'lower arm', 'wrist/hand/fingers', 'hip/groin', 'thigh', 'knee', 'lower leg', 'ankle/ft', 'unspecific upper extremity' and 'unspecific lower extremity'. If a child had several MSK problems at different anatomical sites within the same extremity, the clinician defined the primary pain site based on the child's report of impact, and this was used for analyses. Further, for the analyses in the current study, we classified all

examined anatomical episodes as either traumatic or non-traumatic using information from the clinical examination. A traumatic episode was defined as an injury resulting from a specific identifiable event, whereas a non-traumatic episode was not related to an identifiable event [24].

Variables

Descriptive variables, which included age and sex, and outcome variables, are listed below:

MSK pain as reported by the parents

    UE pain the last week (Y/N)
    LE pain the last week (Y/N)

Pain distribution as reported from the clinical examination

    Anatomical pain site
       Shoulder
       Upper Arm
       Elbow
       Lower Arm
       Wrist/Hand/Fingers
       Hip/groin
       Thigh
       Knee
       Lower leg
       Ankle/Foot
       Unspecific Upper Extremity
       Unspecific Lower Extremity

Anatomical pain sites were divided according to causation

    Traumatic episodes
    Non-traumatic episodes

Data analysis

STATA 15.0 (StataCorp, College Station, Texas, USA) was used for the analyses. UE and LE pain were reported separately, and the significance level was set at 0.05. To avoid breaks in data continuity due to the summer holidays, we chose to report by study year rather than for 3 full calendar years. Therefore, study year 1 represents the period from August 2011 to June 2012 (44 weeks), study year 2 was the period from August 2012 to June 2013 (47 weeks); and study year 3 covers August 2013 to June 2014 (46 weeks).

To obtain a satisfactory observation period, the child had to participate at the start and at the end of a study year, to be included in the analyses. More specifically, children should be included in the study for at least a full study year minus 1 week, e.g. 43 weeks in study year 1. Within this period, missing answers were allowed; however, parents had to respond in at least 85% of the weeks within a study year, or the child would be excluded due to low SMS compliance.

Chi-squared or unpaired t-tests were performed to determine whether there were any differences in demographics between the children who were included in the analysis and those who were not, either due to declining participation in the project, low SMS-compliance, or dropping out of the study.

Research has shown that MSK pain varies between the sexes [1, 25]. Therefore, we calculated sex-specific *prevalence rates* with 95% confidence intervals of UE pain and LE pain for each study year. Trend in prevalence rates with age was assessed using generalized estimating equations.

The *total number of pain weeks* was calculated as the sum of weeks where pain was reported for each study year. They were categorized based on the distribution of data, and results were expressed in numbers, proportions and means with 95% confidence intervals, and medians with interquartile ranges. An episode was deemed to have started when pain was reported in an area from which no pain had been reported in the previous week. Similarly, an episode was deemed to have ended when pain was not reported in the area for at least 1 week. To assess the robustness of this definition, we repeated the analysis using a 4-week 'no-pain-in-the-area' gap instead of the 1-week gap. In the 4-week definition, at least 4 weeks of no pain was needed before a subsequent episode was categorized as a *new* episode.

The *number of episodes* per child was calculated as the sum of episodes for each child during a study year.

For each episode, we calculated the *length of an episode* by summing the number of weeks where pain was reported. Number of episodes and length of episodes were categorized based on the distribution of data, and results were expressed in numbers, proportions and means with 95% confidence intervals, and medians with interquartile ranges.

We formulated the following decision rules to account for missing SMS answers. If four or fewer consecutive SMS answers were missing, they were imputed with the same value as the previous week's SMS answer, provided it was the same as for the week after the missing SMS answers. Otherwise, we defined the end of that episode as occurring at the week prior to the missing SMS answers. If the number of consecutive missing SMS answer weeks was greater than four, we also defined the end of the episode as occurring at the week prior to the missing SMS answer.

We performed a sensitivity analysis to estimate the impact of these decision rules by treating missing answers in two extreme ways to determine the range within which the correct value would lie: first, we imputed the missing answers to be the same as the last SMS answer, regardless of the value of the next report. This would potentially inflate episode lengths and diminish the number of episodes. Second, we imputed the SMS answer 'no pain' for all weeks with missing answers, which would do the opposite.

Prevalence rates of pain from each anatomical site based on the clinical examination were calculated with 95% confidence intervals for each study year in the same way as above. Likewise, trend in prevalence rates with age was assessed using generalized estimating equations. To identify possible differences between boys and girls, and between traumatic and non-traumatic episodes regarding anatomical pain sites, results for all 3 study years were used, and the boy:girl ratios and the traumatic:non-traumatic ratios were calculated. Finally, the mean number of episodes per child was calculated for traumatic and non-traumatic pain episodes and a potential difference was tested using a mixed effect regression model, reported by a *p* value.

Results
Study sample
During the entire study period, 1917 children were invited to participate in the CHAMPS-Study DK, and 1465 (76%) were enrolled. During the study period, 296 children dropped out (Fig. 1).

The average weekly response rate for all three study years was 96.4%. After excluding children with low SMS compliance, the final sample consisted of 982 children in study year 1; 1100 children in study year 2; and 1033 children in study year 3. In total, 401, 448 and 359 children received a clinical examination the three study years respectively (Fig. 2). In study year 1, 70 (7.1%) children had an anatomical pain site registered in UEs, and 361 (36.8%) children in the LEs. In study year 2, there were 108 (9.8%) and 392 (35.6%) children with pain in UEs and LEs, respectively, and for study year 3, the numbers were 91 (8.8%) and 312 (30.1%).

The children were 8–14 years of age at baseline in 2011, and mean age increased from 10.7 (SD 1.4) years in study year 1 to 11.6 (SD 1.4) years in study year 2, and 12.5 (SD 1.4) years in study year 3. During all 3 study years, 52% of the children were girls.

We found no significant differences between the children who either declined participation, had low SMS compliance or dropped out, when compared to the study sample in relation to sex, but the dropouts

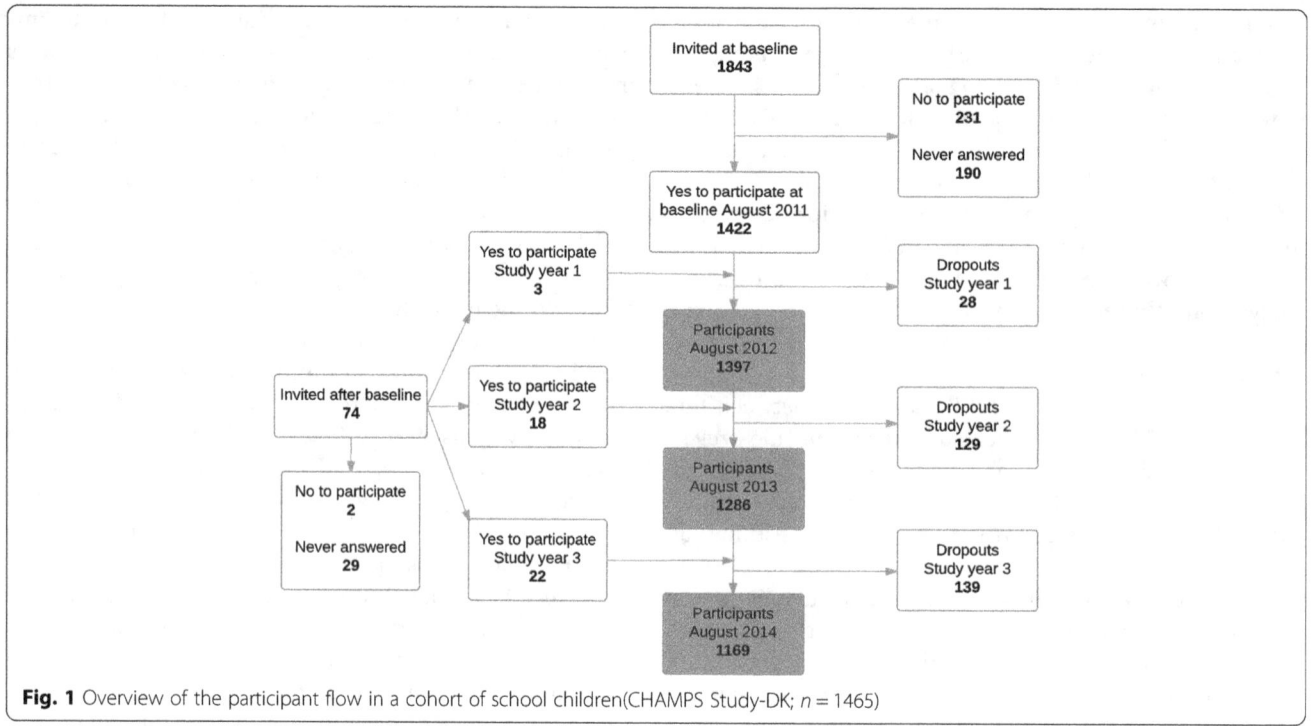

Fig. 1 Overview of the participant flow in a cohort of school children(CHAMPS Study-DK; *n* = 1465)

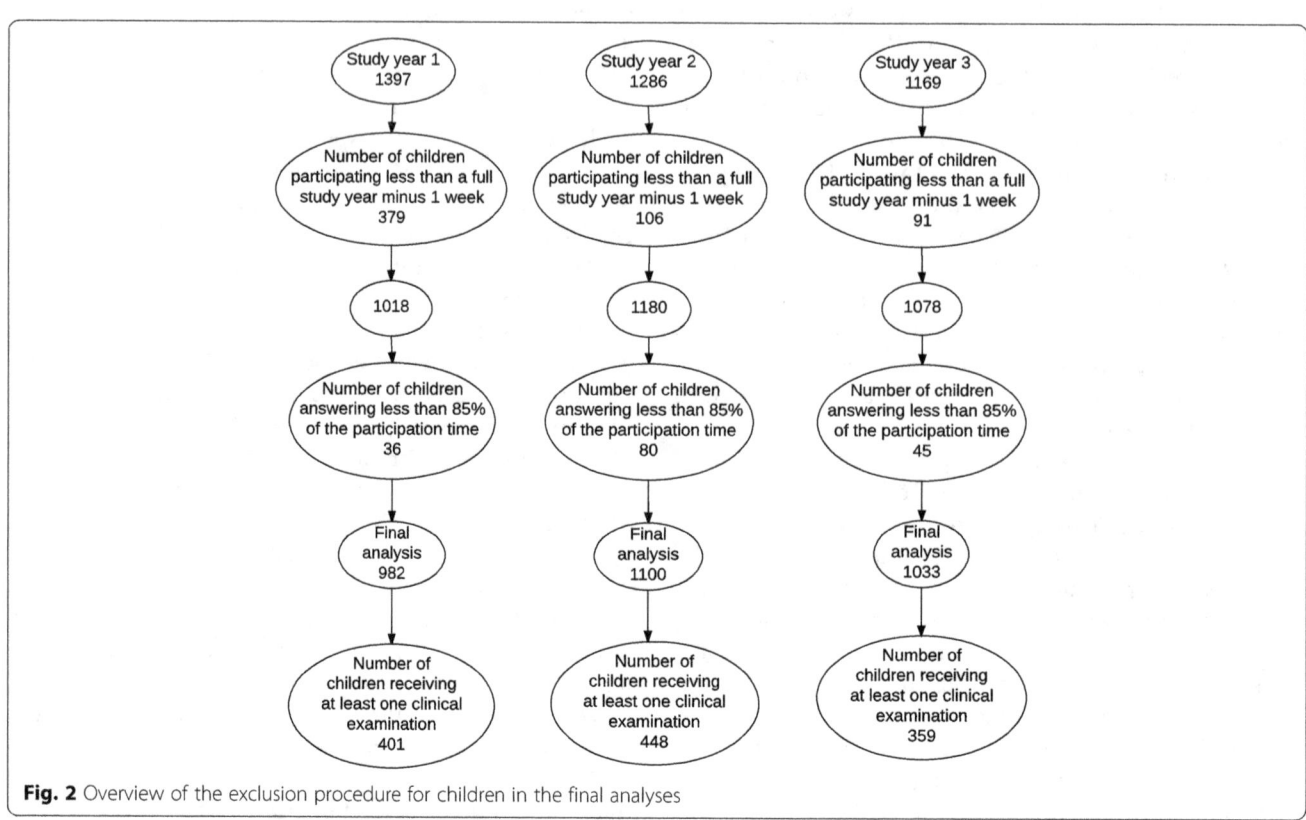

Fig. 2 Overview of the exclusion procedure for children in the final analyses

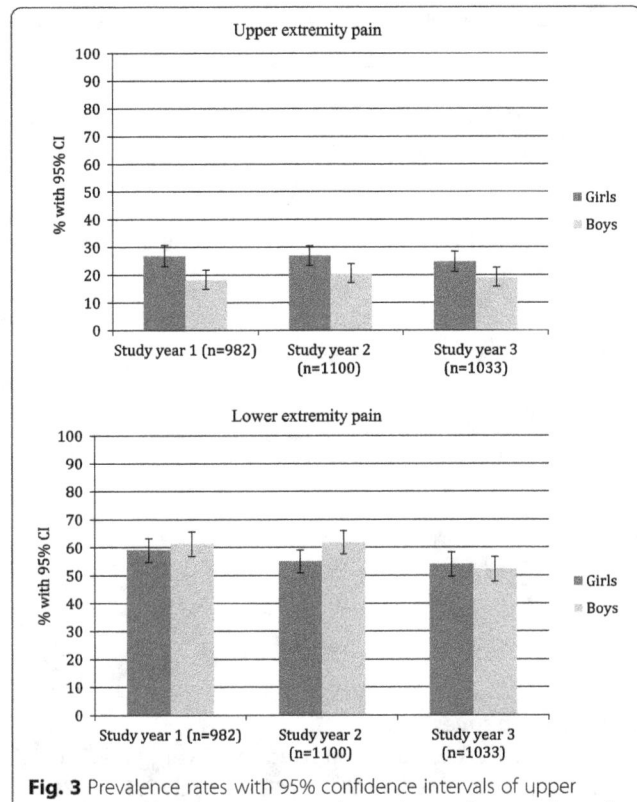

Fig. 3 Prevalence rates with 95% confidence intervals of upper extremity and lower extremity pain by study year, from a cohort of Danish school children. CI: confidence intervals

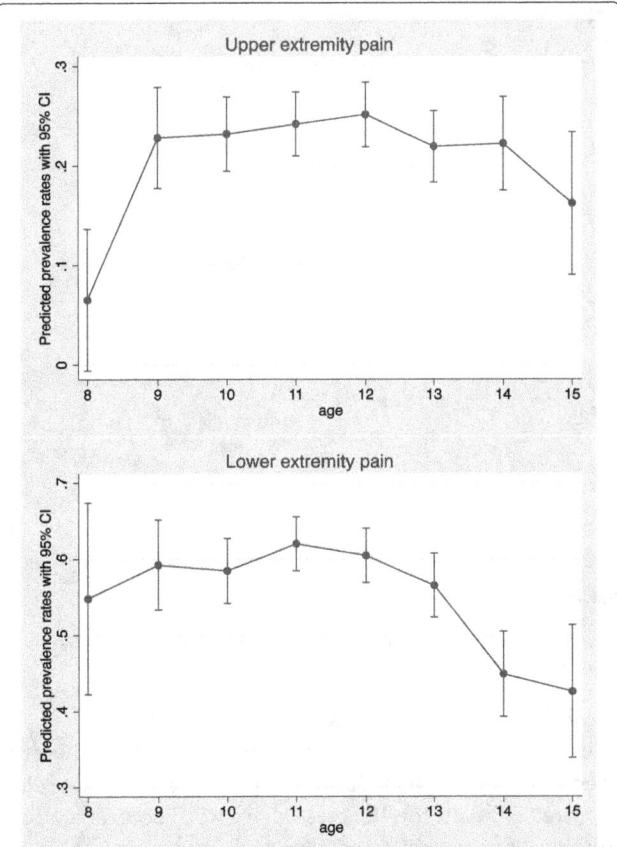

Fig. 4 Predicted prevalence rates with 95% confidence intervals of upper and lower extremity pain by age, from a cohort of Danish school children. CI: confidence intervals

were on average older compared to children who remained in the study (12.5 years of age versus 10.6 years of age, $p < 0.001$).

1) Musculoskeletal pain as reported by the parents

Upper extremity
Sex-specific and age-specific prevalence rates by study year
Approximately a quarter of the girls and a fifth of the boys reported pain in the UEs, with no change with age (Figs. 3 and 4).

Total number of pain weeks
On average, the children who reported UE pain reported its presence close to 3 weeks in study year 1, and this increased to more than 4 weeks in study year 3 (Table 1). In study year 1, 48% of the children reporting UE pain, reported its presence for only 1 week; and in study year 3 this decreased to 40%. Approximately 7% reported pain for 8 weeks or more in study year 1, increasing to 15% in study year 3.

Number of episodes
Children with UE pain reported on average 1.5 (95% CI 1.3–1.6), 1.6 (95% CI 1.5–1.8) and 1.6 (95% CI 1.4–1.7) episodes per year, for the 3 study years

respectively. The median number of episodes was 1 (25%–75%: 1–2), for all 3 study years. Approximately two-thirds of the children with reported UE pain, reported one episode of UE pain per study year, and few children reported more than four episodes per study year (Fig. 5).

Length of episodes
The total number of UE pain episodes per study year was 325, 427 and 354, respectively. On average, an episode of UE pain lasted for 2 weeks in study year 1, increasing to almost 3 weeks in study year 3. More than half the episodes lasted for just 1 week, and only a few episodes lasted for more than 12 weeks (Table 2).

Lower extremity
Prevalence by study year
Approximately half the children reported LE pain, with no difference between the sexes (Fig. 3). The risk of reporting LE pain decreased with age, odds ratio 0.91 (p value = 0.001). More specifically, there was a statistically significant decrease in prevalence rate from the age of 11 to 15 years (Fig. 4).

Table 1 Proportion of children who experienced upper extremity pain expressed by number of pain weeks, from a cohort of Danish school children

Number of pain weeks	Study year 1 (44 weeks)		Study year 2 (47 weeks)		Study year 3 (46 weeks)	
	n	% (95% CI)	n	% (95% CI)	n	% (95% CI)
1	108	48.7 (41.9–55.4)	116	44.3 (38.2–50.5)	91	40.1 (33.7–46.8)
2	36	16.2 (11.6–21.)	47	17.9 (13.5–23.1)	28	12.3 (8.4–17.3)
3	22	9.9 (6.3–14.6)	29	11.1 (7.5–15.5)	32	14.1 (9.8–19.3)
4	13	5.9 (3.2–9.8)	21	8.0 (5.0–12.0)	22	9.7 (6.2–14.3)
5	11	5.0 (2.5–8.7)	6	2.3 (0.8–4.9)	8	3.5 (1.5–6.8)
6	8	3.6 (1.6–7.0)	6	2.3 (0.8–3.9)	8	3.5 (1.5–6.8)
7	9	4.1 (1.9–7.6)	9	3.4 (1.6–6.4)	4	1.8 (0.5–4.5)
8–43	15	6.8 (3.8–10.9)	28	10.7 (7.2–15.1)	34	15.0 (10.6–20.3)
Total[a]	222	100.0	262	100.0	227	100.0
Median (25%–75%)[b]		2 (1–4)		2 (1–4)		2 (1–4)
Mean (95% CI)[b]		2.9 (2.5–3.3)		3.4 (2.9–3.9)		4.4 (3.6–5.2)

children without reported pain are not included
CI Confidence intervals
[a]number of participants reporting upper extremity pain during 1 study year
[b]number of weeks

Total number of pain weeks

During all 3 study years, approximately 20% of the children reporting LE pain did so for 1 week, and another 20% reported LE pain for 12 weeks or more. The average total number of pain weeks was 8 for each study year (Table 3).

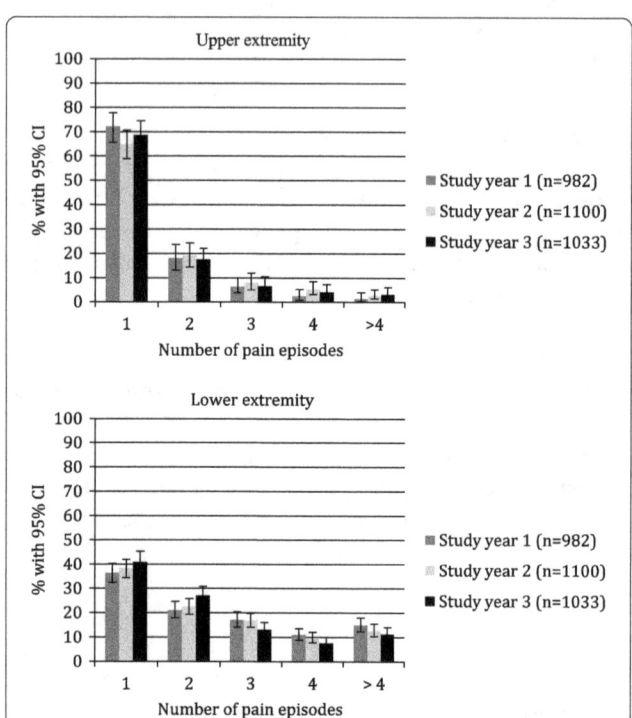

Fig. 5 Proportions of children who experienced 1 to more than 4 episodes of upper and lower extremity pain, in a cohort of Danish school children. Children with no reported pain episodes are not included. CI: confidence intervals

Number of episodes

Children with LE pain reported on average 2.7 (95% CI 2.5–2.9), 2.5 (95% CI 2.4–2.7) and 2.4 (95% CI 2.2–2.5) episodes per study year, for the 3 years respectively. Approximately one-third of the children reported one episode per study year, and one-third reported three episodes or more per study year (Fig. 5).

Length of episodes

The total number of LE pain episodes was 1587, 1603 and 1220, for the 3 study years respectively. An episode of LE pain lasted on average 3 weeks in study year 1, increasing to 3.5 weeks in study year 3. Approximately half the episodes lasted for 1 week in all 3 study years. In study year 1, 3% of the episodes lasted more than 12 weeks, and in study year 3, it was 6% (Table 2).

Pain distribution as reported from the clinical examination

Prevalence of anatomical pain sites by study year

The subset of the cohort with registration of an anatomical pain site consisted approximately of one-third of the children with reported UE pain, and close to two-thirds of those with reported LE pain. In total, 1729 anatomical pain sites were registered during the three study years.

The two most frequent pain sites were 'knee' and 'ankle/ft'. 'Knee' was registered in approximately 15% of the children each study year. 'Ankle/ft' was registered in 19% of the children in study year 1, decreasing to 10% in study year 3. The least frequent pain sites were upper and lower arm, with prevalence rates of less than 1% (Fig. 6). The risk of reporting 'ankle/ft' decreased with

Table 2 Proportion of episodes according to length of episodes of upper and lower extremity pain, from a cohort of Danish school-children

	Length of episodes	Study year 1 (44 weeks)		Study year 2 (47 weeks)		Study year 3 (46 weeks)	
Upper extremity		n	% (95% CI)	N	% (95% CI)	N	% (95% CI)
	1 week	197	60.6 (55.1–65.9)	283	66.3 (61.6–70.6)	180	50.9 (45.5–56.2)
	2–3 weeks	86	26.5 (21.7–31.6)	86	20.1 (16.4–24.3)	107	30.2 (25.5–35.3)
	4–11 weeks	40	12.3 (8.9–16.4)	55	12.9 (9.9–16.4)	55	15.5 (11.9–19.7)
	≥ 12 weeks	2	0.6 (0.1–2.2)	3	0.7 (0.1–2.0)	12	3.4 (1.8–5.8)
	Total[a]	325	100.0	427	100.00	354	100.0
	Median						
	(25%–75%)		1 (1–2)		1 (1–2)		1 (1–3)
	Mean (95% CI)		2.0 (1.8–2.2)		2.1 (1.9–2.3)		2.8 (2.4–3.1)
Lower extremity	1 week	814	51.3 (48.8–53.8)	816	50.9 (48.4–53.4)	615	48.0 (45.3–50.8)
	2–3 weeks	403	25.4 (23.3–27.6)	407	25.4 (23.3–27.6)	337	26.3 (23.9–28.8)
	4–11 weeks	316	19.9 (18.0–22.0)	297	18.5 (16.7–20.5)	247	19.3 (17.2–21.6)
	≥ 12 weeks	54	3.4 (2.6–4.4)	83	5.2 (4.1–6.4)	81	6.3 (5.1–7.8)
	Total[a]	1587	100.0	1603	100.0	1220	100.0
	Median						
	(25%–75%)		1 (1–3)		1 (1–3)		2 (1–4)
	Mean (95% CI)		3.0 (2.8–3.2)		3.3 (3.1–3.5)		3.6 (3.4–3.9)

children without reported pain are not included
CI Confidence interval[a]number of pain episodes during 1 study year

Table 3 Proportion of children who experienced lower extremity pain by number of pain weeks reported for each study year, from a cohort of Danish school children

Number of pain weeks	Study year 1 (44 weeks)		Study year 2 (47 weeks)		Study year 3 (46 weeks)	
	n	% (95% CI)	n	% (95% CI)	n	% (95% CI)
1	118	20.0 (16.8–23.5)	140	21.8 (18.2–25.2)	120	21.9 (18.5–25.6)
2	83	14.1 (11.4–17.1)	77	12.0 (9.6–14.8)	77	14.0 (11.2–17.2)
3	57	9.7 (7.4–12.3)	74	11.5 (9.2–14.3)	48	8.7 (6.5–11.4)
4	40	6.8 (4.9–9.1)	58	9.1 (6.9–11.5)	41	7.5 (5.4–10.0)
5	38	6.4 (4.6–8.7)	28	4.4 (2.9–6.3)	29	5.3 (3.6–7.5)
6	25	4.2 (2.8–6.2)	20	3.1 (1.9–4.8)	29	5.3 (3.6–7.5)
7	30	5.1 (3.5–7.2)	27	4.2 (2.8–6.1)	17	3.1 (1.81–4.9)
8	16	2.7 (1.6–4.4)	22	3.4 (2.2–5.2)	21	3.8 (2.4–5.8)
9	17	2.9 (1.7–4.6)	19	3.0 (1.8–4.6)	16	2.9 (1.7–4.7)
10	14	2.4 (1.3–3.9)	13	2.0 (1.1–3.4)	15	2.7 (1.5–4.5)
11	17	2.9 (1.7–4.6)	12	1.9 (1.0–3.2)	9	1.6 (0.8–3.1)
12	12	2.0 (1.1–3.5)	14	2.2 (1.2–3.6)	9	1.6 (0.8–3.1)
13–45	123	20.9 (17.6–24.4)	137	21.4 (18.3–24.8)	118	21.5 (18.1–25.2)
Total[a]	590	100.0	641	100.0	549	100.00
Median						
(25%–75%)[b]		4 (2–11)		4 (2–11)		4 (2–10)
Mean (95% CI)[b]		8.3 (7.5–9.1)		8.3 (7.5–9.1)		8.7 (7.8–9.6)

children without reported pain are not included
CI Confidence intervals
[a]number of participants reporting lower extremity pain during 1 study year
[b]number of weeks

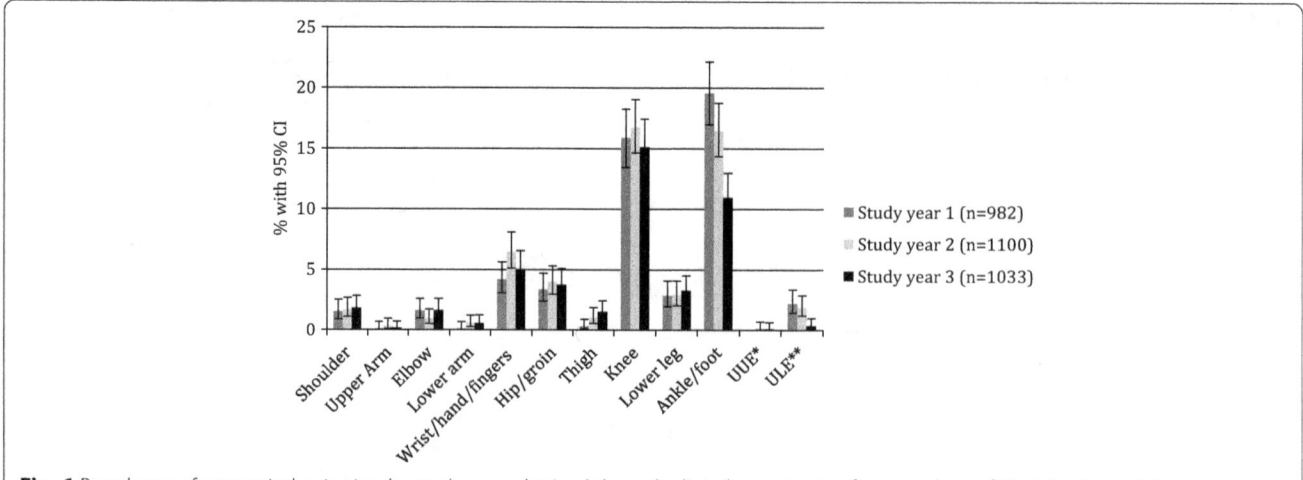

Fig. 6 Prevalence of anatomical pain sites by study year, obtained through clinical examination from a cohort of Danish school children. *unspecific upper extremity, **unspecific lower extremity

age, odds ratio 0.82 (*p* value <0.001). More specifically, there was a statistically significant decrease in prevalence rate from the age of 10 to 14 years.

Distribution by sex

In general, more pain sites were registered in girls than boys, noticeably 'unspecific lower extremities' 2.3 times, 'shoulder' 2.1 times and 'wrist/hand/fingers' 1.6 times more. Only 'thigh' pain was more frequent in boys, with 2.2 times more pain episodes than in girls.

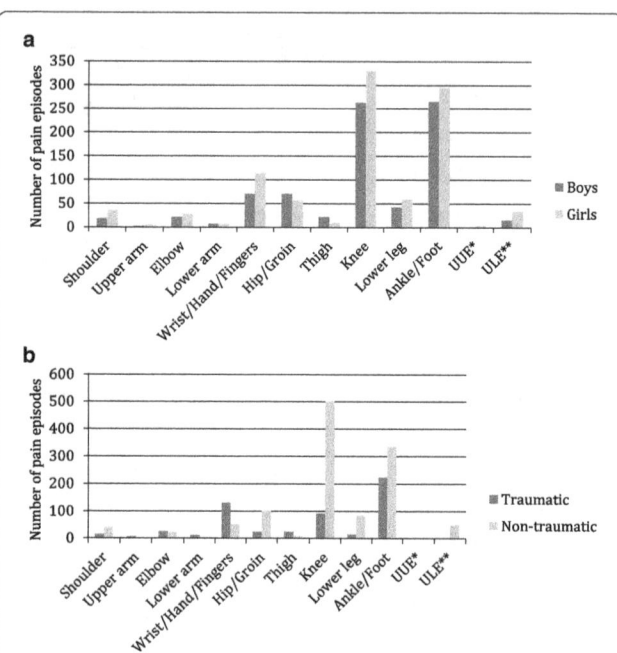

Fig. 7 Total number of pain episodes over three study years by **a)** sex and **b)** causation, in a subset of a cohort of Danish school children. The total number of pain episodes was 1729, distributed in 777 children. * unspecific upper extremity ** unspecific lower extremity

In 'ankle/ft', 'hip/groin', 'lower arm' and 'elbow', there was an equal distribution between boys and girls (Fig. 7a).

Distribution by complaint type

In general, for the UEs, there were more traumatic than non-traumatic episodes. For 'wrist/hand/fingers', 'upper arm' and 'lower arm', there were 2.5 to 6.0 times more traumatic episodes compared with non-traumatic episodes, whereas there was an equal distribution between traumatic and non-traumatic episodes in the 'elbow'. The opposite pattern was found in 'shoulder', with 2.7 times more non-traumatic episodes compared with traumatic. Conversely, in the LEs, non-traumatic episodes were more common than traumatic episodes. In 'knee', 'hip/groin' and 'lower leg' 4.0 to 6.1 times more episodes were categorized as non-traumatic, and in 'ankle/ft' there were approximately 1.5 times more non-traumatic episodes. The opposite pattern was found in 'thigh' with 3.0 times more episodes categorized as traumatic (Fig. 7b). The prevalence rates of non-traumatic 'ankle/ft' episodes decreased significantly from 13% (95% CI 11.0–15.3) in study year 1 to 6% (95% CI 4.6–7.6) in study year 3.

Comparison of traumatic versus non-traumatic pain episodes by number and length of episodes

On average, children with non-traumatic episodes reported more episodes compared with children with traumatic episodes, 1.8 (95% CI 1.7–1.9) versus 1.5 (95% CI 1.4–1.5) (*p* value <0.001).

Definition of a new episode (sensitivity analysis)

We compared the definition of an episode used in the analyses (a new episode was deemed to have started when pain was reported in an area from which no pain was reported the previous week) to a four-week 'no-pain-in-the-area' gap. As expected, the mean number of episodes decreased whereas the mean length of episodes increased, when 4 weeks of 'no pain' were needed before a subsequent episode was considered to be a new episode. Importantly, analyses showed the same pattern of MSK pain with more LE pain and more LE episodes compared with UE episodes. The length of episodes increased on average with 70% in LE, and 40% in UE when a four-week-gap of 'no pain' was needed, indicating LE episodes were more recurrent compared with UE episodes (Additional file 1).

Missing data

For UEs, both when missing data were imputed as the same as the last answer and as no pain, we found similar results. For LEs, analyses resulted in fewer and longer episodes when missing data were imputed as the same as the last SMS answer. Furthermore, we found shorter pain periods in two out of three situations, when missing data were imputed as 'no pain' (Additional file 2).

Discussion

In a three-year study of Danish school children aged 8–14 years at baseline, we found that approximately half the children had LE pain, and one-quarter of the children reported UE pain every study year. The children with LE pain had on average more and longer pain episodes compared with the children with UE pain. The two most common anatomical pain sites for the subset of the children, who were examined, were 'knee' and 'ankle/ft'.

Previous studies have also found LE pain to be more common than UE pain [25–28], but to our knowledge, this is the first study to closely follow MSK problems in this age group over a longer period of time. Although the exact location and type of problem is unknown, the number of episodes of LE pain demonstrates that more than half of the affected children have recurrent problems in the LE. This confirms results from two other cohort studies [4, 9]. Our finding of 'knee' and 'ankle/ft' as the most common pain sites is also in line with previous findings [1, 8]. In the years leading up to this study, information about MSK pain was collected from the same cohort, where 'ankle/ft' injuries were found to be the most common, followed by 'knee' injuries [7]. We found a significant decrease in the prevalence rate of 'ankle/ft' problems with age, especially in non-traumatic pain episodes. This may be because of a reduction in growth-related symptoms, or potentially a decreased amount of physical activity in adolescence.

Methodological considerations

There was not a large attrition bias, but the dropouts were slightly older than the children who remained in the study, which potentially could result in an underestimation of pain, since MSK pain seems to increase during adolescence [26, 29, 30].

There might be some limitations with regard to the SMS answers. Parents answered SMS questions continuously every week for more than 5 years, and therefore some response fatigue could be anticipated. Nevertheless, the response rate was high, although we do not know if some parents reported 'no pain' to avoid a subsequent phone call, again resulting in an underestimation of the reporting of pain. Furthermore, the breaks in data continuity were also a limitation, as we do not know how the holidays influence the prevalence of MSK pain.

Parent reporting is often used as a proxy measure for children reporting their pain themselves. To determine concordance between parent reporting and the children's actual pain, 685 children, aged 8 to 14 years, were questioned about presence, location and severity of MSK pain. When compared with the SMS answers, poor parent-child concordance was found [31]. Interestingly, the child often reported pain that was not reported by their parents, whereas the opposite was rarely the case. Thus, we probably have lower estimates of pain in this study, compared with child-reported data. A better concordance was seen for pain of greater intensity, which could indicate that parents did not report minor pain. This is in line with another study showing that minor complaints were more likely to be under-reported by parents [16], whereas better concordance was found when children were more severely ill [32].

Another limitation may be an unknown change in the parent/child relationship with age. We expect this potential bias to be limited, because of the children's relatively young age. If such a bias was present, it was most likely to be independent of location, i.e. the effect would be the same for all pain sites. It might be that non-traumatic episodes are easier to hide, potentially resulting in a higher traumatic/non-traumatic ratio with age, if the child became less communicative.

Major strengths include the large population-based cohort, and the high response rate of the text messages. Furthermore, our results appear robust because imputing missing data and sensitivity analyses did not change our results. We believe that the combination of these parental pain reports, and the information from clinical examinations, provides a comprehensive overview of MSK problems in this age group, but more research in other settings of general and clinical populations is needed.

Conclusion

Lower extremity pain among children and adolescents is common, recurrent and most often of non-traumatic origin. Upper extremity pain is less common, with fewer and shorter episodes, and usually with a traumatic onset. Girls more frequently reported upper extremity pain, whereas there was no sex-related difference in the lower extremities. The most frequently reported locations were 'knee' and 'ankle/ft'. These findings should encourage a stronger focus on prevention and early effective treatment of lower extremity pain in children and adolescents.

Abbreviations

CHAMPS Study-DK: Childhood Health, Activity and Motor Performance School Study; LE: Lower extremity; MSK: Musculoskeletal; SMS answer: Mobile phone text message answer; SMS question: Mobile phone text message question; UE: Upper extremity

Acknowledgements

We acknowledge the participants and their parents, the participating schools and 'Sport & Uddannelse Svendborg Kommune'. Finally we would like to thank all members of the CHAMPS Study-DK, and Suzanne Capell for assisting with proof reading.

Funding

The authors gratefully acknowledge the following organisations for funding individual researchers and for funding the CHAMPS Study Denmark part II: the Nordea Foundation, the TRYG Foundation, the IMK Foundation, the Region of Southern Denmark, the University of Southern Denmark, the University College Lillebaelt's Department of Physiotherapy, the Danish Chiropractic Research Foundation, the Svendborg Project, the Municipality of Svendborg, as well as the Nordic Institute of Chiropractic and Clinical Biomechanics. No funding bodies were involved in the analysis of data, interpretation of the data or publication decisions.

Authors' contributions

NW was responsible for the concept and design of the CHAMPS Study-DK. SF, EJ, TJ and LRL participated in the collection of data. LH, JH and SF conceived the idea for the present study. EB prepared the data for the statistical analyses, and SF conducted those with assistance from EB. SF, LH and JH participated in the interpretation of the results and for the first draft of the manuscript. All authors revised the manuscript critically for intellectual content and approved the final version. All authors agree to be accountable for all aspects of the work in ensuring that questions related to the accuracy or integrity of any part of the work are appropriate investigated and resolved.

Competing interests

LH is a member of the Editorial Board of BMC Musculoskeletal Disorders. The authors declare that they have no competing interests.

Author details

[1]Department of Sports Science and Clinical Biomechanics, Faculty of Health Sciences, University of Southern Denmark, Campusvej 55, 5230 Odense M, Denmark. [2]Nordic Institute of Chiropractic and Clinical Biomechanics, Campusvej 55, 5230 Odense M, Denmark. [3]Institute of Regional Health Services Research, University of Southern Denmark, Winsloewparken 193, 5000 Odense C, Denmark. [4]Sports Medicine Clinic, Orthopaedic Department, Hospital Lillebaelt, Østre Hougvej 55, 5500 Middelfart, Denmark. [5]Dalla Lana School of Public Health, University of Toronto, 155 College St, Toronto, ON M5T 3M7, Canada. [6]Department of Rehabilitation, Odense University Hospital, Odense, Denmark and National Centre of Rehabilitation and Palliation, University of Southern Denmark, Odense, Denmark. [7]Health Sciences Research Centre, University College Lillebaelt, Niels Bohrs Allé 1, 5230 Odense M, Denmark. [8]Research and Innovation Center for Human Movement and Learning, Inter-Faculty Educational Resources, University College Lillebælt, Niels Bohrs Alle 1, 5230 Odense M, Denmark.

References

1. Rathleff MS, Roos EM, Olesen JL, Rasmussen S. High prevalence of daily and multi-site pain–a cross-sectional population-based study among 3000 Danish adolescents. BMC Pediatr. 2013;13:191.
2. Jeffries LJ, Milanese SF, Grimmer-Somers KA. Epidemiology of adolescent spinal pain - a systematic overview of the research literature. Spine. 2007; 32(23):2630–7.
3. El-Metwally A, Salminen JJ, Auvinen A, Kautiainen H, Mikkelsson M. Risk factors for traumatic and non-traumatic lower limb pain among preadolescents: a population-based study of Finnish schoolchildren. BMC Musculoskelet Disord. 2006;7:3.
4. El-Metwally A, Salminen JJ, Auvinen A, Kautiainen H, Mikkelsson M. Lower limb pain in a preadolescent population: prognosis and risk factors for chronicity–a prospective 1- and 4-year follow-up study. Pediatrics. 2005; 116(3):673–81.
5. Aartun E, Hartvigsen J, Wedderkopp N, Hestbaek L. Spinal pain in adolescents: prevalence, incidence, and course: a school-based two-year prospective cohort study in 1,300 Danes aged 11-13. BMC Musculoskelet Disord. 2014;15:187.
6. Jones MA, Stratton G, Reilly T, Unnithan VB. A school-based survey of recurrent non-specific low-back pain prevalence and consequences in children. Health Educ Res. 2004;19(3):284–9.
7. Jespersen E, Rexen CT, Franz C, Moller NC, Froberg K, Wedderkopp N. Musculoskeletal extremity injuries in a cohort of schoolchildren aged 6-12: a 2.5-year prospective study. Scand J Med Sci Sports. 2015;25(2):251–8.
8. Verhagen E, Collard D, Paw MC, van Mechelen W. A prospective cohort study on physical activity and sports-related injuries in 10-12-year-old children. Br J Sports Med. 2009;43(13):1031–5.
9. Rathleff CR, Olesen JL, Roos EM, Rasmussen S, Rathleff MS. Half of 12-15-year-olds with knee pain still have pain after one year. Dan Med J. 2013; 60(11):A4725.
10. Hestbaek L, Leboeuf-Yde C, Kyvik KO, Manniche C. The course of low back pain from adolescence to adulthood: eight-year follow-up of 9600 twins. Spine (Phila Pa 1976). 2006;31(4):468–72.
11. Jones GT, Silman AJ, Power C, Macfarlane GJ. Are common symptoms in childhood associated with chronic widespread body pain in adulthood? Results from the 1958 British birth cohort study. Arthritis Rheum. 2007;56(5):1669–75.
12. Clark EM. The epidemiology of fractures in otherwise healthy children. Current osteoporosis reports. 2014;12(3):272–8.
13. Waterman BR, Owens BD, Davey S, Zacchilli MA, Belmont PJ Jr. The epidemiology of ankle sprains in the United States. J Bone Joint Surg Am. 2010;92(13):2279–84.
14. Jespersen E, Holst R, Franz C, Rexen CT, Klakk H, Wedderkopp N. Overuse and traumatic extremity injuries in schoolchildren surveyed with weekly text messages over 2.5 years. Scand J Med Sci Sports. 2014;24(5):807–13.
15. Moshiro C, Heuch I, Astrom AN, Setel P, Kvale G. Effect of recall on estimation of non-fatal injury rates: a community based study in Tanzania. Inj Prev. 2005;11(1):48–52.
16. Sundblad GM, Saartok T, Engstrom LM. Child-parent agreement on reports of disease, injury and pain. BMC Public Health. 2006;6:276.
17. Harel Y, Overpeck MD, Jones DH, Scheidt PC, Bijur PE, Trumble AC, Anderson J. The effects of recall on estimating annual nonfatal injury rates for children and adolescents. Am J Public Health. 1994;84(4):599–605.
18. Axen I, Bodin L, Bergstrom G, Halasz L, Lange F, Lovgren PW, Rosenbaum A, Leboeuf-Yde C, Jensen I. The use of weekly text messaging over 6 months was a feasible method for monitoring the clinical course of low back pain in patients seeking chiropractic care. J Clin Epidemiol. 2012;65(4):454–61.

19. Johansen B, Wedderkopp N. Comparison between data obtained through real-time data capture by SMS and a retrospective telephone interview. Chiropr Osteopat. 2010;18:10.
20. Bahr R. No injuries, but plenty of pain? On the methodology for recording overuse symptoms in sports. Br J Sports Med. 2009;43(13):966–72.
21. Wedderkopp N, Jespersen E, Franz C, Klakk H, Heidemann M, Christiansen C, Moller NC. Leboeuf-Yde C: study protocol. **The childhood health, activity, and motor performance school study Denmark (the CHAMPS-study DK)**. BMC Pediatr. 2012;12:128.
22. Dissing KB, Hestbaek L, Hartvigsen J, Williams C, Kamper S, Boyle E, Wedderkopp N. Spinal pain in Danish school children - how often and how long? **The CHAMPS Study-DK**. *BMC Musculoskelet Disord*. 2017;18(1):67.
23. **Statistics Denmark** [http://www.statistikbanken.dk].
24. Fuller CW, Ekstrand J, Junge A, Andersen TE, Bahr R, Dvorak J, Hagglund M, McCrory P, Meeuwisse WH. Consensus statement on injury definitions and data collection procedures in studies of football (soccer) injuries. Br J Sports Med. 2006;40(3):193–201.
25. Hoftun GB, Romundstad PR, Zwart JA, Rygg M. Chronic idiopathic pain in adolescence–high prevalence and disability: the young HUNT study 2008. Pain. 2011;152(10):2259–66.
26. Krul M, van der Wouden JC, Schellevis FG, van Suijlekom-Smit LW, Koes BW. Musculoskeletal problems in overweight and obese children. Ann Fam Med. 2009;7(4):352–6.
27. Hulsegge G, van Oostrom SH, Picavet HS, Twisk JW, Postma DS, Kerkhof M, Smit HA, Wijga AH. Musculoskeletal complaints among 11-year-old children and associated factors: the PIAMA birth cohort study. Am J Epidemiol. 2011; 174(8):877–84.
28. Mikkelsson M, Salminen JJ, Kautiainen H. Non-specific musculoskeletal pain in preadolescents. Prevalence and 1-year persistence. Pain. 1997;73(1):29–35.
29. Bot SD, van der Waal JM, Terwee CB, van der Windt DA, Schellevis FG, Bouter LM, Dekker J. Incidence and prevalence of complaints of the neck and upper extremity in general practice. Ann Rheum Dis. 2005;64(1):118–23.
30. Bishop JL, Northstone K, Emmett PM, Golding J. Parental accounts of the prevalence, causes and treatments of limb pain in children aged 5 to 13 years: a longitudinal cohort study. Arch Dis Child. 2012;97(1):52–3.
31. Kamper SJ, Dissing KB, Hestbaek L. Whose pain is it anyway? Comparability of pain reports from children and their parents. Chiropr Man Therap. 2016;24:24.
32. Mock C, Acheampong F, Adjei S, Koepsell T. The effect of recall on estimation of incidence rates for injury in Ghana. Int J Epidemiol. 1999;28(4):750–5.

22

The relationship between preoperative American Society of Anesthesiologists Physical Status Classification scores and functional recovery following hip-fracture surgery

Li-Huan Chen[1,2], Jersey Liang[3,4], Min-Chi Chen[5], Chi-Chuan Wu[6], Huey-Shinn Cheng[7], Hsiu-Ho Wang[1] and Yea-Ing Lotus Shyu[6,8,9,10*]

Abstract

Background: Little is known about the relationship of the American Society of Anesthesiologists Physical Status Classification scores (ASA scores) on patient outcomes following hip fracture surgery in Asian countries. Therefore, this study explored the association of patients' preoperative ASA scores on trajectories of recovery in physical functioning and health outcomes during the first year following postoperative discharge for older adults with hip-fracture surgery in Taiwan.

Methods: The data for this study was generated from three prior studies. Participants (N = 226) were older hip-fracture patients from an observational study (n = 86) and two clinical trials (n = 61 and n = 79). Participants were recruited from the trauma wards of one medical center in northern Taiwan and data was collected prior to discharge and at 1, 3, 6, and 12 months after hospital discharge. Participants were grouped as ASA class 1–2 (50.5%; ASA Class 1, n = 7; ASA Class 2, n = 107) and ASA class 3 (49.5%, n = 112). Measures for mortality, service utilization, activities of daily living (ADL), measured by the Chinese Barthel Index, and health related quality of life, measured by Medical Outcomes Study Short Form-36, were assessed for the two groups. Generalized estimating equations (GEE) were used to analyze the changes over time for the two groups.

Results: During the first year following hip-fracture surgery, ASA class 1–2 participants had significantly fewer rehospitalizations (6%, p = .02) and better scores for mental health (mean = 70.29, standard deviation = 19.03) at 6- and 12-months following discharge than those classified as ASA 3. In addition, recovery of walking ability (70%, p = .001) and general health (adjusted mean = 58.31, p = .003) was also significantly better than ASA 3 participants.

Conclusions: There was a significant association of hip-fracture patients classified as ASA 1–2 with better recovery and service utilization during the first year following surgery. Interventions for hip fractured patients with high ASA scores should be developed to improve recovery and quality of life.

Keywords: American Society of Anesthesiologists scores, Asa, Health-related quality of life, Hip-fractured adults, Mortality, Physical function recovery, Service utilization

* Correspondence: yeaing@mail.cgu.edu.tw
[6]Department of Orthopedic Surgery, Chang Gung Memorial Hospital, Linkou, 5 Fu-Hsing Street, Guishan District, Taoyuan 33305, Taiwan
[8]School of Nursing, College of Medicine, and Healthy Aging Research Center, Chang Gung University, 259 Wenhua 1st Road, Guishan District, Taoyuan 33302, Taiwan
Full list of author information is available at the end of the article

Background

The worldwide incidence of hip fracture in 2000 was 1.6 million and is expected to rise dramatically as of 2050 to approximately 6.3 million, due to the ongoing aging of the world's population [1]; an estimated 50% of those hip fractures are expected to occur in Asian populations [2]. Hip fracture affects the life expectancy and mortality of persons aged 65 years and older [3]. The mortality rate for elderly patients with hip fracture has been estimated to be between 21.5% to 27.3% within 1 year of fracture [3, 4]. In a previous study the 1-year mortality rate of elderly Taiwanese persons with hip fracture was found to be 15.5%, with only 56.1% recovering their previous performance of activities of daily living (ADL) and 37.9% recovering their instrumental ADL (IADL) 1 year following hip fracture [5].

One widely used measure of preoperative function is the American Society of Anesthesiologists Physical Status Classification (ASA class), which has been found to predict patient outcomes after hip fracture. For example, patients with an ASA class of 1 or 2 (healthy or with mild systemic illness, respectively) were more likely to be living at home 1 year after hip fracture [6, 7]. Similarly, 1-year mortality following surgery for hip fracture was almost 9-times higher for patients with an ASA class of 3 or 4 (severe systemic illness) than patients with an ASA class 1 or 2 [8]. In addition, higher ASA grades were associated with poorer 30-day outcomes, which included higher mortality, number of comorbidities, and number of inpatient readmissions [9, 10]. Higher ASA scores have also been associated with greater pain, less distance walked and poorer movement [11].

Currently, there is little knowledge regarding the correlation between preoperative ASA classes of hip fracture for persons in Asian countries and patient outcomes. Although the ASA score has been correlated with several factors regarding patient outcomes [2, 12] no studies have explored the association between ASA scores and the trajectory of recovery or longitudinal changes in health outcomes following hip fracture surgery in Taiwan [13]. Therefore, the aim of the present study was to determine the association, if any, of the preoperative ASA classes of a sample of older hip fracture patients in Taiwan on recovery trajectories as measured by physical functioning and health outcomes over the course of the first year following hospital discharge. We hypothesized that during the first year after surgical treatment for hip fracture, older patients with severe preoperative systemic disease (ASA score 3 and 4) would have higher mortality as well as increased service utilization, emergency room visits, and institutionalization. In addition, we hypothesized these patients would have poorer recovery in walking ability, performance of ADLs, and health-related quality of life than those with mild systemic disease (ASA grade 1 and 2) or healthy patients.

Methods

Data source and participants

This was a secondary analysis of data from three previously published studies of 285 participants recruited from the trauma wards of a medical center in northern Taiwan. We excluded 59 of the participants due to incomplete data relevant to this study. The hip-fracture participants for this analysis ($N = 226$) were from an observational study ($n = 86$ [13]), and control groups were non-interventional participants from two clinical trials ($n = 61$ [14] and $n = 79$ [15]). The Chang Gung Memorial Hospital Research Ethics Board approved these studies (NHRI-EX92-9023PL: CMRP819, 89–25, and 94-422c) and written informed consent was obtained for each participant. Data for these three studies were collected at baseline (prior to hospital discharge) and at 1-, 3-, 6-, and 12-month post-discharge. For all three studies, the inclusion criteria for hip-fracture patients were as follows: 1) age ≥ 60 years, 2) hospitalization resulting from a hip fracture that was subsequently treated with internal fixation or arthroplasty, 3) a place of residence located in northern Taiwan, and 4) a lack of any severe cognitive impairment as determined by a physician or by a score of ≥10 on the Chinese Mini-Mental State Examination (CMMSE) [16]. Because data was collected from self-report measures, patients found to have severe cognitive impairment were excluded if they were unable to complete the measures.

Measures

ASA score

An anesthesiologist, aware of the study, assessed participants' ASA scores, which was determined by the participant's medical history. In Taiwan, ASA scores are divided into six classes: a completely healthy patient is given a class 1 ASA score; a patient with mild systemic disease is considered class 2; a patient with a severe but not incapacitating systemic disease is class 3 ASA; a patient with an incapacitating disease that is also life-threatening is class 4 ASA; and a moribund patient not expected to live for 24 h with or without surgery is class 5. A class 5 ASA score is also taken to indicate a need for emergency surgery. A class 6 ASA score is provided to patients classified as brain-dead and eligible to be designated as organ donors. The validity of using ASA scores to indicate a patient's long-term mortality and complications following total hip arthroplasty [6, 17] and hip-fracture surgery [8] has been well established. ASA scores are routinely used in Taiwan to assess for anesthesia and surgery risk.

Activities of daily living (ADL)

The Chinese Barthel Index (CBI) was used to measure each patient's ability to perform ADL. The CBI exhibits satisfactory reliability and validity when used as an assessment tool for assessing Taiwanese older adults with hip fracture [18]. Specifically, the CBI is used to measure the level of dependency of a patient with regard to each of the following activities: bathing, grooming, dressing, eating, using the toilet, transferring, climbing stairs, and bowel/bladder control. CBI scores range from 0 (indicating complete dependence on assistance from others in performing all of the ADL) to 100 (indicating complete independence from others in performing all of the ADL).

Recovery of walking ability

The recovery of each patient's walking ability was evaluated using the item of the CBI that assesses independence in walking; a comparison was made between the patient's postoperative walking ability score and his or her score prior to the fracture, with said pre-facture walking ability being assessed retrospectively according to the patient's recall at the time of admission. If the patient's postoperative walking ability score was the same as or greater than his or her walking ability before the fracture, it was coded as 1, whereas it was coded as 0 if it was more limited than his or pre-fracture walking ability [5, 19].

Health-related quality of life (HRQoL)

The Taiwan version of the Medical Outcomes Study Short-Form 36 (SF-36) [15, 19, 20] was used in order to assess each patient's HRQoL. The SF-36 includes a total of 36 items used to assess a variety of health-related domains: bodily pain (BP), physical functioning (PF), vitality (VT), the role of disability due to physical health problems (RP), and general perceptions of health. Among elderly hip-fracture patients who are independent before their hip fracture, approximately half become partially or wholly dependent on others after the fracture in terms of social functioning (SF), self-care ability [5], general mental health, and role disability due to emotional problems (RE). The total score for each of these relevant sub-scales range from 0 to 100, with better health outcomes being indicated by higher scores.

Procedures

The Committee on Human Research at the hospital approved all three studies, all of which were conducted using the same research procedure. Specifically, research assistants identified possible study participants subsequent to each patient's surgery but before each patient was discharged from the hospital. After a potential participant was identified, a research assistant then invited him or her to participate in the given study. Patients who agreed to take part in the study then signed a written informed consent, after which they were assessed at five different time points: prior to hospital discharge, and at 1, 3, 6, and 12 months after discharge. Relevant covariate data, such as demographic data and data on cognitive functioning, were collected from the patients prior to hospital discharge.

Covariates

In the analysis for predictors of outcome variables, we controlled for covariates of time, gender, age, type of surgery (internal fixation or arthroplasty), pre-fracture performance of ADLs, and data set membership (study of origin). Pre-fracture ADL performance was measured by patients' self-reported CBI score. To control for possible significant differences among the three data sets, they were identified as covariates by including two dummy variables in the regression analysis of generalized estimating equations (GEE).

Statistical analysis Data analysis was performed using Statistical Analysis Software [21]. The overall participant sample consisted of patients with ASA scores from 1 to 3. Participants were sub-divided into two groups: healthy or mild systemic disease (class 1–2) and severe systemic disease (class 3) [8]. For demographic variables such as gender, educational background, mortality, institutionalization and emergency room visits, Chi-square tests compared the differences between the two groups. Student's t-test, two-tailed, compared the differences in continuous variables between the two groups. GEE analysis determined whether patients could be expected to recover pre-fracture abilities for ADL, walking, and HRQoL in the first 12 months after hospital discharge. GEE can account for possible correlations in repeated measures over time and can explore the differences at different time points. In longitudinal studies, GEE analysis is especially useful for data belonging to participants who die or are lost to follow up; analysis can be applied to attrition without using imputation [22]. Therefore, data for participants with at least one observation were included in the analysis, if participants died or were lost to follow up during the year post-discharge. The participants with at least one observation were analyzed by the GEE approach, which included a total of 114 participants in the ASA 1–2 group, and 112 participants in the ASA 3 group. The number of participants remaining at each time point for each group are listed in Table 2. Time, gender, age, type of surgery, pre-fracture ADL performance data set membership was controlled for as a covariate in the GEE analysis [21]. Level of significance was set at $p < .05$ [23].

Results
Participant characteristics

Participants consisted of patients with ASA scores from 1 to 3. Comparison of hip-fractured older adults classified as ASA 1–2 and ASA 3 showed no significant differences in demographics, with the exception of age (Table 1). Significant differences for only two clinical characteristics were seen for participants classified as ASA 3: number of comorbidities ($p = .024$) and the presence of heart disease ($p = .04$) (Table 1).

Table 1 Demographic and clinical characteristics for all hip-fractured participants, and differences between groups: preoperative ASA scores determined by independent t-test (a) or Chi-squared tests

Variable	Total Participants (n = 226)	Groups		p-Value
		ASA 1–2 (n = 114)	ASA 3 (n = 112)	
Age (years) (mean ± SD)	78.22 ± 7.70	77.06 ± 7.40	79.39 ± 7.85	.023[a]
Gender, n (%)				.14
Male	78 (34.5%)	34 (29.8%)	44 (39.2%)	
Female	148 (65.5%)	80 (70.2%)	68 (60.7%)	
Hospital stay (days) (mean ± SD)	9.96 ± 5.06	10.02 ± 4.91	9.89 ± 5.24	.85
Education, n (%)				.92
None	133 (58.5%)	69 (60.6%)	64 (57.1%)	
Primary	52 (23.0%)	24 (21.1%)	28 (25.0%)	
High School	27 (11.9%)	14 (12.3%)	13 (11.6%)	
College or above	14 (6.2%)	7 (6.1%)	7 (6.2%)	
Fracture classification, n (%)				.73
Femoral neck	113 (50.0%)	57 (50.0%)	56 (50.0%)	
Intertrochanteric	104 (46.0%)	52 (45.6%)	52 (46.4%)	
Subtrochanteric	9 (4.0%)	5 (4.4%)	4 (3.6%)	
Type of surgery, n (%)				.76
Arthroplasty	87 (38.5%)	45 (39.5%)	42 (37.5%)	
Internal fixation	139 (61.5%)	69 (60.5%)	70 (62.5%)	
Number of comorbidities (mean ± SD)	0.90 ± 0.85	0.77 ± 0.86	1.03 ± 0.82	.024[a]
Presence of comorbidity (type), n (%)				
Cardiovascular disease	46 (20.4%)	17 (14.9%)	29 (25.9%)	.04
Hypertension	99 (43.8%)	46 (40.4%)	53 (47.3%)	.29
Diabetes mellitus	58 (25.7%)	25 (21.0%)	33 (29.7%)	.20
Unable to walk independently pre-fracture, n (%)	17 (7.5%)	5 (4.4%)	12 (10.7%)	.07
CBI performance, pre-fracture (mean ± SD)	97.15 ± 6.39	97.72 ± 5.84	96.56 ± 6.88	.174[a]

Abbreviations: *ASA* American Society of Anesthesiologists; *SD* standard deviation; *CBI* Chinese Barthel Index
[a]*P*-value determined by independent t-test, otherwise determined by Chi-square test

Differences in service utilization and mortality

Comparisons of outcomes for participants in the ASA 1–2 and ASA 3 groups at 1-, 3-, 6-, and 12-months following hospital discharge are shown in Table 2, including numbers of remaining participants at each time point for each group. The number of participants readmitted to the hospital at 12 months was significantly greater for those classified as ASA 3 than those classified as ASA 1–2 ($p = .02$). However, there was no significant difference in emergency room visits or mortality rates for these two groups in the first year after discharge (Table 2).

Relationship between ASA score, recovery of physical function, and HRQoL

Outcomes for recovery of walking ability, ADLs, as measured by CBI scores, and scores for subscales of HRQoL were compared for the two groups at the four times post-discharge (Table 2). Participants with ASA 3 had poorer

recovery of walking ability at 1- and 3-months compared with participants classified as ASA 1–2 ($p = .004$ and $p < .001$, respectively). There was no significant difference in CBI scores between groups at any time post-discharge. Differences in some of the subscale scores for HRQoL were significantly lower at various times post-discharge for the ASA 3 group: general health at 1 month ($p = .006$); mental health at 12-months; and role disability/physical at 6-months.

These differences between groups were examined by GEE analysis, controlling for covariates of time, gender, age, type of surgery, and pre-fracture CBI performance data set membership (Table 3). The participants in the group with preoperative ASA 1–2 scores had significantly better scores for walking ability recovery (beta coefficient = 0.38, $p = .001$, Table 3, and Fig. 1) than the ASA 3 group, indicating better walking ability recovery during the first year following discharge. Moreover, the ASA 1–2

Table 2 Comparison of outcomes for participants grouped by preoperative ASA scores following hip-fracture surgery within 1-,3-, 6-and 12-month post-discharge

| Outcome Post-discharge | Participant Group | | p-Value[a] |
	ASA 1–2	ASA 3	
Participants within 1 month, n (% remaining)	114 (100%)	112 (100%)	
Mortality	0 (0.0%)	0 (0.0%)	
Institutionalization	2 (1.8%)	7 (6.3%)	.08
Emergency room visits	7 (6.1%)	9 (8.1%)	.57
Hospital readmissions	6 (5.3%)	13 (11.6%)	.09
Recovery of walking ability	55 (48.2%)	33 (29.5%)	.004
CBI[b] score (mean ± SD)	73.46 ± 19.68	68.57 ± 19.43	.06
HRQOL[c] Subscale Scores (mean ± SD)			
Bodily pain	69.58 ± 24.47	71.96 ± 25.09	.47
General health	62.16 ± 23.41	50.02 ± 25.46	.006
Vitality	57.86 ± 24.55	58.38 ± 24.27	.87
Social functioning	62.61 ± 30.69	61.48 ± 29.82	.78
Role disability/emotional	66.07 ± 44.29	66.97 ± 44.09	.88
Mental health	62.40 ± 22.58	63.09 ± 19.78	.81
Physical functioning	33.93 ± 38.13	28.64 ± 38.43	.30
Role disability/physical	28.57 ± 42.82	22.48 ± 37.88	.26
Participants within 3 months, n (% remaining)	108 (94.7%)	107 (95.5%)	
Mortality	1 (0.9%)	2 (1.8%)	.55
Institutionalization	3 (2.8%)	4 (3.7%)	.71
Emergency room visits	5 (4.6%)	4 (3.7%)	.73
Hospital readmissions	4 (3.7%)	5 (4.6%)	.73
Recovery of walking ability	79 (73.8%)	53 (48.6%)	< .001
CBI[b] score (mean ± SD)	83.19 ± 17.94	80.09 ± 17.52	.20
HRQOL[c] Subscale Scores (mean ± SD)			
Bodily pain	72.10 ± 23.12	75.52 ± 24.89	.31
General health	58.62 ± 24.26	52.56 ± 24.14	.07
Vitality	61.94 ± 21.33	62.43 ± 22.17	.87
Social functioning	59.98 ± 24.60	62.14 ± 28.25	.56
Role disability/emotional	79.17 ± 38.36	81.88 ± 35.78	.60
Mental health	67.25 ± 19.49	65.18 ± 21.44	.47
Physical functioning	31.35 ± 25.35	26.36 ± 26.15	.17
Role disability/physical	20.91 ± 34.33	25.73 ± 38.58	.34
Participants within 6 months, n (% remaining)	102 (89.5%)	97 (86.6%)	
Mortality	2 (1.9%)	4 (3.7%)	.41
Institutionalization	3 (3.0%)	3 (3.1%)	.97
Emergency room visits	9 (8.9%)	10 (10.5%)	.70
Hospital readmissions	7 (6.9%)	11 (11.6%)	.26
Recovery of walking ability	75 (73.5%)	64 (64.6%)	0.17
CBI[b] score (mean ± SD)	85.49 ± 22.37	86.13 ± 17.39	.82
HRQOL[c] Subscale Scores (mean ± SD)			
Bodily pain	78.10 ± 24.69	83.74 ± 22.28	.10
General health	60.11 ± 23.09	57.72 ± 23.87	.49

Table 2 Comparison of outcomes for participants grouped by preoperative ASA scores following hip-fracture surgery within 1-,3-, 6- and 12-month post-discharge *(Continued)*

Outcome Post-discharge	Participant Group		p-Value[a]
	ASA 1–2	ASA 3	
Vitality	63.68 ± 21.38	65.16 ± 21.90	.64
Social functioning	73.08 ± 26.54	75.41 ± 27.60	.56
Role disability/emotional	85.51 ± 32.89	88.30 ± 30.80	.55
Mental health	68.04 ± 20.57	68.09 ± 18.98	.95
Physical functioning	55.75 ± 32.47	57.23 ± 34.75	.76
Role disability/physical	33.60 ± 40.96	47.85 ± 45.54	.03
Participants within 12 months, n (% remaining)	84 (73.7%)	81 (72.3%)	
Mortality	3 (3.1%)	8 (8.1%)	.13
Institutionalization	1 (1.2%)	3 (3.6%)	.31
Emergency room visits	3 (3.6%)	8 (10.0%)	.10
Hospital readmissions	5 (6.0%)	14 (17.3%)	.02
Recovery of walking ability	64 (76.2%)	56 (67.5%)	.21
CBI[b] score (mean ± SD)	85.71 ± 26.94	87.04 ± 19.55	.71
HRQOL[c] Subscale Scores (mean ± SD)			
Bodily pain	70.04 ± 26.46	77.75 ± 25.83	.08
General health	53.77 ± 23.67	50.60 ± 25.24	.45
Vitality	60.59 ± 20.25	59.93 ± 21.91	.85
Social functioning	74.30 ± 27.13	66.37 ± 30.30	.10
Role disability/emotional	91.30 ± 25.98	82.87 ± 37.11	.12
Mental health	70.29 ± 19.03	63.14 ± 22.70	.047
Physical functioning	50.70 ± 29.76	41.99 ± 31.97	.09
Role disability/physical	45.07 ± 43.02	38.19 ± 45.57	.36

[a]p-value determined by student's t-test, two-tailed
[b]CBI (Chinese Barthel Index): higher score indicates greater independence
[c]HRQOL (Health Related Quality of Life); higher score indicates better health outcomes

group had significantly better outcomes for general health (beta coefficient = −4.95, p = .032, Table 3, and Fig. 2) than the ASA 3 group, indicating better overall outcomes in general health during the first year following discharge. However, the ASA 3 group had significantly better scores for coping with bodily pain (beta coefficient = 4.86, p = .028,) than the ASA 1–2 group.

Discussion

To our knowledge, this is the first study to evaluate the relationship between preoperative ASA scores and patient outcomes during one-year following hip-fracture surgery for older adults in Taiwan. ASA classifications were associated with levels of service utilization, mortality, and longitudinal changes in both physical recovery and various aspects of HRQoL.

Our results demonstrated higher preoperative ASA scores correlated with higher hospital readmissions at 6- and 12-months following hospital discharge, which is consistent with previous reports showing higher preoperative ASA scores are associated with more hospital

readmissions [9, 10] and poorer ambulatory recovery [10, 24]. Our findings showed participants with ASA scores of 3 had significantly poorer recovery of walking ability at 1-and 3-months after discharge. However, although post-discharge ADL performance (CBI score) differed at 1-month post-discharge between those classified as ASA 1–2 and ASA 3, there was no difference in long-term outcomes at 1-year, which is consistent with previous findings [8, 25]. However, for the total sample of participants, with no grouping by ASA scores, walking recovery and CBI scores gradually improved over time in the 1 to 12 months after surgery, demonstrating recovery was proportional to time.

Quality of life also gradually improved over time during the first 1- to 6-months following surgery. However, quality of life decreased at 12 months. One explanation may be that physical recovery improved more rapidly during the first 6 months, which has been shown to influence a perception of an improvement in quality of life [5]. However, as the speed of recovery slowed in the latter half of the year following surgery [5], most

Table 3 Association between participants' preoperative ASA score classification and recovery of physical and mental functioning during the first year following hospital discharge for hip-fracture surgery: General Estimating Equation (GEE) analysis

Outcome variable	Time (months post-discharge)								Group		
	1	3[a]		6[a]		12[a]			ASA 1-2[b]		ASA 3
	(%)/Mean	β	(%)/Mean	β	(%)/Mean	β	(%)/Mean		(%)/Mean	β	(%)/Mean
Walking recovery, %[c]	39%	0.97	63%§	1.30	70%§†	1.4	73%§†		70%	0.38	53%#
CBI score, mean[d]	71.91	10.27	82.18§	13.86	85.77§†	1.39	85.85§†		81.24	13	81.62
HRQOL scores, mean[d]											
BP	71.35	2.95	74.31	10.08	81.43§†	2.83	74.18˙		72.89	4.86	77.75#
GH	58.06	−2.47	55.60	0.64	58.71	−7.09	50.98§†˙		58.31	−4.95	53.36#
VT	57.8	3.56	61.37	6.05	63.85§	1.43	59.24˙		59.85	1.43	61.28
SF	62.76	−0.93	61.50	12.06	74.49§†	7.60	70.63§†		67.25	−0.28	66.97
RE	66.88	13.99	80.86§	19.94	86.81§†	18.08	85.68§		79.65	0.82	80.47
MH	62.76	2.95	65.72	4.91	67.67§	2.79	65.55		65.89	−0.93	64.96
PF	32.72	−2.45	30.27	24.22	56.94§†	11.64	44.36§˙		43.05	−3.95	39.10
RP	27.39	−2.46	24.93	13.83	41.23§†	12.14	39.54§†		32.81	0.93	33.74

Abbreviations: *CBI* Chinese Barthel Index, (activities of daily living); HRQOL = health related quality of life; *BP* bodily pain; *GH* general health perception; *VT* vitality; *SF* social functioning; *RE* role disability due to emotional problems; *MH* general mental health; *PF* physical functioning; *RP* role disability due to physical health problems

[a]Time post-discharge compared with 1 month
[b]Participant group ASA 1–2 compared with ASA 3
[c]Percentage was calculated only for categorical outcome variables
[d]Mean = adjusted mean obtained after controlling for time, gender, age, type of surgery, and pre-fracture CBI performance data set membership
#Indicates a significant difference between ASA 1–2 and ASA 3 group, $p < .05$
§Indicates time post-discharge was significantly different compared with 1 month for both ASA 1–2 and ASA 3, $p < .05$
†Indicates a significant difference compared with 3 months for both ASA 1–2 and ASA 3, $p < .05$
˙Indicates a significant difference compared with 6 months for both ASA 1–2 and ASA 3, $p < .05$

dimensions for health-related quality of life had reached a plateau [26]. Hip-fractured patients with ASA scores of 3 also had poorer health outcomes in several subscales for HRQoL at different times post-discharge, as well as the overall trajectories of these subscales, which has not previously been reported. This finding adds new knowledge regarding the relationship of ASA classifications to HRQoL scores.

We found no significant difference in mortality between participants with high or low ASA scores, which is in contrast to previous findings [3, 8]. This might be due to the health and independence of our population. For example, approximately 61.3% of participants in a previous study experienced severe systemic disease (ASA 3 & 4) [10], whereas none of our study participants were classified as having severe (class 4) systemic disease. Therefore, although the mortality rate in our study was higher for the ASA 3 group (12.5%) than the ASA 1–2 group (5.3%), we might need a larger sample to achieve a statistically significant difference.

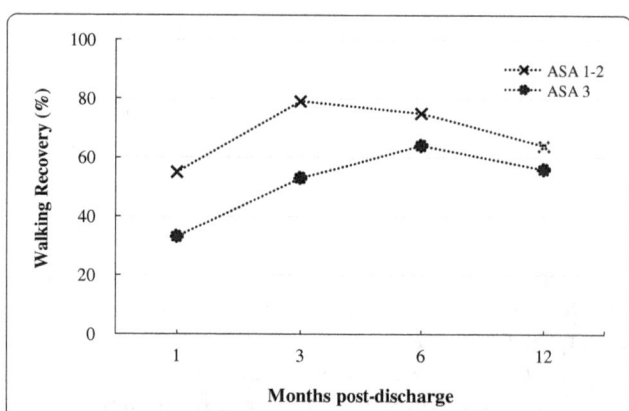

Fig. 1 Trajectory of hip-fracture surgery patients' walking recovery relative to preoperative ASA scores of 1–2 and ASA 3 over time after hospital discharge. (ASA: American Society for Anesthesiologists)

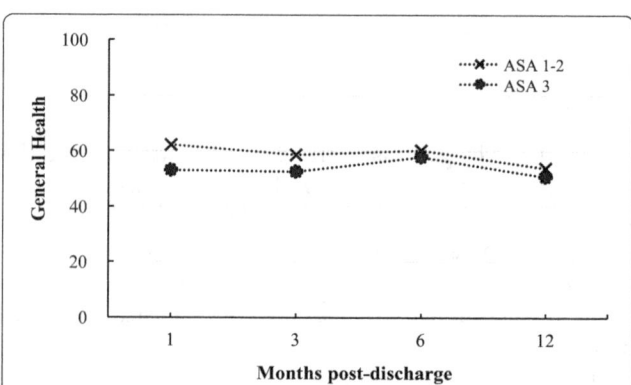

Fig. 2 Trajectory of hip-fracture surgery patients' recovery of general health over time after hospital discharge relative to groups with preoperative ASA scores of 1–2 and ASA 3. (ASA: American Society of Anesthesiologists)

In addition, older patients with high and low preoperative ASA scores [8] have been shown to differ significantly before hip-fracture surgery in the percentages with cardiovascular diseases, diabetes mellitus and walking difficulty. In our study, although greater percentages of participants with higher ASA scores had hypertension, cardiovascular diseases and difficulty in walking before hip-fracture, only cardiovascular disease was statistically significant, which is similar to a previous report showing a correlation between ASA scores and cardiovascular disease [8–10].

The participants in our study were relatively independent before their hip-fracture, with only 6.2% having difficulty walking, whereas 29.2% of participants in a previous study had difficulty walking [8]. However, participants with ASA 3 scores appeared to have significantly better control of coping with bodily pain than the ASA 1–2 group. This finding should be further explored with a larger sample, due to the small variances in independence and health conditions in our sample. Our findings highlight the need to focus on older patients with high preoperative ASA scores during the first year after hospital discharge following hip-fracture surgery, particularly with regards to strategies for preventing hospital readmissions. This should include intervention protocols, which are developed specifically for patients with higher preoperative ASA scores.

Study limitations
The generalizability of the study findings is limited by the use of secondary data as well as the study's utilization of a relatively small convenience sample, the fact that some of the study participants were lost to follow-up, and the lack of participation by patients with severe physical limitations (ASA Class 4). In Taiwan, patients that are Class 4 or higher have an incapacitating disease that is also life-threatening, and thus they seldom receive surgery. Thus, the study findings can only be generalized to that portion of the population of older Taiwanese hip fracture patients who exhibited independence prior to their fractures. Finally, the original studies did not collect information on the specifics of the hip-fracture surgery. Therefore, our secondary analysis did not include data on type of surgical reduction performed for hip-fracture: closed reduction with a sliding hip screw; closed reduction with IM nail; Internal fixation without reduction and with cancellous screws; and open reduction and dynamic condylar screws. The type of surgery may affect outcomes [27, 28] and this was not accounted for in our study. Therefore, we suggest future studies include detailed information regarding the type of surgery performed.

Conclusion
We found higher ASA scores were associated with more hospital readmissions at 1- and 12-months following hospital discharge. In addition, better recovery of walking ability and general health was associated with participants having ASA scores of I-II during the first year following hip-fracture surgery. The present study and its findings could serve as a valuable reference for health care professionals in countries providing care to older adult Chinese/Taiwanese hip-fracture patients.

Abbreviations
ADL: Activities of daily living; ASA class: American Society of Anesthesiologists Physical Status Classification; ASA: American Society of Anesthesiologists; BP: bodily pain; CBI: Chinese Barthel Index; CMMSE: Chinese Mini-Mental State Examination; GEE: generalized estimating equations; HRQoL: Health-related quality of life; IADL: instrumental ADL; MOS SF-36: Medical Outcomes Study Short Form 36; PF: physical functioning; RE: role disability due to emotional problems; RP: role of disability due to physical health problems; SF: social functioning; VT: vitality

Acknowledgments
The authors thank the medical team and patients on the department of Orthopedic Surgery at Chang Gung Memorial hospital for their support in this study.

Funding
This work was supported by grants from the National Health Research Institutes, Taiwan (NHRI-EX92-9023PL), Healthy Aging Research Center, Chang Gung University (EMRPD1G0211), and Chang Gung Medical Foundation (BMRP297, CMRPG8D0743).

Authors' contributions
L. C. developed the original idea and wrote the manuscript. Y. L. S. developed the original idea, supervised the projects, and wrote the manuscript. J. L. and M. C. contributed to data analysis, interpretation, and writing of the results. C. W. and H. C. contributed to data collection and interpretation. H. W. wrote the manuscript. All authors have read and approved the final manuscript.

Competing interests
The authors declare that they have no competing interests.

Author details
[1]Department of Nursing, Yuanpei University of Medical Technology, 306 Yuanpei Street, Hsinchu 30015, Taiwan. [2]Graduate Institute of Clinical Medical Sciences, Chang Gung University, 259 Wenhua 1st Road, Guishan District, Taoyuan 33302, Taiwan. [3]Department of Health Management and Policy, School of Public Health, University of Michigan, 1415 Washington Heights, M3007 SPH II, Ann Arbor, MI 48109, USA. [4]Institute of Gerontology, University of Michigan, 1415 Washington Heights, M3007 SPH II, Ann Arbor, MI 48109, USA. [5]Department of Public Health & Biostatistics Consulting Center, Chang Gung University, 259 Wenhua 1st Road, Guishan District, Taoyuan 33302, Taiwan. [6]Department of Orthopedic Surgery, Chang Gung Memorial Hospital, Linkou, 5 Fu-Hsing Street, Guishan District, Taoyuan 33305, Taiwan. [7]Department of Internal Medicine, Chang Gung Memorial Hospital, Linkou, 5 Fu-Hsing Street, Guishan District, Taoyuan 33305, Taiwan. [8]School of Nursing, College of Medicine, and Healthy Aging Research Center, Chang Gung University, 259 Wenhua 1st Road, Guishan District, Taoyuan 33302, Taiwan.

[9]Department of Nursing, Kaohsiung Chang Gung Memorial Hospital, 123 Dapi Road, Niaosng District, Kaohsiung 83301, Taiwan. [10]Department of Gerontological Care and Management, Chang Gung University of Science and Technology, 261 Wenhua 1st Road, Guishan District, Taoyuan 33303, Taiwan.

References

1. Cooper C, Cole ZA, Holroyd CR, Earl SC, Harvey NC, Dennison EM, Melton LJ, Cummings SR, Kanis JA. Secular trends in the incidence of hip and other osteoporotic fractures. Osteoporos Int. 2011;22(5):1277–88.

2. Dhanwal DK, Dennison EM, Harvey NC, Cooper C. Epidemiology of hip fracture: worldwide geographic variation. Indian J Orthop. 2011;45l(1):15–22.

3. Panula J, Pihlajamaki H, Mattila VM, Jaatinen P, Vahlberg T, Aarnio P, Kivelä SL. Mortality and cause of death in hip fracture patients aged 65 or older: a population-based study. BMC Musculoskeletal Disord. 2011;12:105.

4. Vidal EI, Coeli CM, Pinheiro RS, Camargo KR Jr. Mortality within 1 year after hip record fracture surgical repair in the elderly according to postoperative period: a probabilistic linkage study in Brazil. Osteoporos Int. 2006;17(10): 1569–76.

5. Shyu YIL, Chen MC, Liang J, Wu CC, Su JY. Predictors of functional recovery for hip fractured elders at 12 months following hospital discharge: a prospective study on a Taiwanese sample. Osteoporos Int. 2004;15(6):475–82.

6. Bjorgul K, Novicoff WM, Saleh KJ. American Society of Anesthesiologist Physical Status score may be used as a comorbidity index in hip fracture surgery. J Arthro. 2010;25(Suppl(6)):134–7.

7. Dubljanin-Raspopović E, Marković-Denić L, Marinković J, Nedeljković U, Bumbaširević M. Does early functional outcome predict 1-year mortality in elderly patients with hip fracture? Clin Orthop Relat Res. 2013;471(8):2703–10.

8. Michel JP, Klopfenstein C, Hoffmeyer P, Stern R, Grab B. Hip fracture surgery: is the pre-operative American Society of Anesthesiologists (ASA) score a predictor of functional outcome? Aging Clin Exp Res. 2002;14(5):389–94.

9. Mathew SA, Gane E, Heesch KC, McPhail SM. Risk factors for hospital re-presentation among older adults following fragility fractures: a systematic review and meta-analysis. BMC Med. 2016;14(1):136.

10. Kastanis G, Topalidou A, Alpantaki K, Rosiadis M, Balalis K. Is the ASA score in geriatric hip fractures a predictive factor for complications and readmission? Scientifica. 2016;2016:7096245.

11. Korkmaz MF, Erdem MN, Disli Z, Selcuk EB, Karakaplan M, Gogus A. Outcomes of trochanteric femoral fractures treated with proximal femoral nail: an analysis of 100 consecutive cases. Clin Interv Aging. 2014;9:569–74.

12. Michael A, Eagland K, Doos L. ASA score in hip fracture patients. Eur Geriatr Med. 2012;3(Suppl(1)):s50.

13. Shyu YI, Liang J, Wu CC, Su JY, Cheng HS, Chou SW, Yang CT. A pilot investigation of the short-term effects of an interdisciplinary intervention program on elderly patients with hip fracture in Taiwan. J Am Geriatr Soc. 2005;53(5):811–8.

14. Shyu YI, Liang J, Wu CC, Su JY, Cheng HS, Chou SW, Chen MC, Yang CT. Nterdisciplinary intervention for hip fracture in older Taiwanese: benefits last for 1 year. J Gerontol A Biol Sci Med Sci. 2008;63(1):92–7.

15. Tseng MY, Liang J, Shyu YI, Wu CC, Cheng HS, Chen CY, Yang SF. Effects of interventions on trajectories of health-related quality of life among older patients with hip fracture: a prospective randomized controlled trial. BMC Musculoskelet Disord. 2016;17:114.

16. Yip PK, Shyu YI, Liu SI, Lee JY, Chou CF, Chen RC. An epidemiological survey of dementia among elderly in an urban district of Taipei. Acta Neurol Sinica. 1992;1:347–54.

17. Swanson KC, Valle AG, Salvati EA, Sculco TP, Bottner F. Perioperative morbidity after single-stage bilateral total hip arthroplasty: a matched control study. Clin Orthop Relat Res. 2006;451:140–5.

18. Chen YJ, Dai YT, Yang CT, Wang TJ, Teng YH. A review and proposal on patient classification in long-term care system. Taipei: Department of Health, Republic of China; 1995.

19. Li HJ, Cheng HS, Liang J, Wu CC, Shyu YI. Functional recovery of older people with hip fracture: does malnutrition make a difference? J Adv Nurs. 2013;69(8):1691–703.

20. Shyu YI, Liang J, Tseng MY, Li HJ, Wu CC, Cheng HS, Chou SW, Chen CY, Yang CT. Comprehensive and subacute care interventions improve health-related quality of life for older patients after surgery for hip fracture: a randomised controlled trial. Int J Nurs Stud. 2013;50(8):1013–24.

21. Corp IBM. IBM SPSS statistics for windows, version 20.0. Armonk: IBM Corp; 2011.

22. Twisk J, de Vente W. Attrition in longitudinal studies. How to deal with missing data. J Clin Epidemiol. 2002 Apr;55(4):329–37.

23. Forbes DA. What is a p value and what does it mean? BMJ EBN. 2012;15(2):34.

24. Cho HM, Lee K, Min W, Choi YS, Lee HS, Mun HJ, Shim HY, Lee da G, Yoo MJ. Survival and functional outcomes after hip fracture among nursing home residents. J Korean Med Sci. 2016;31(1):89–97.

25. Richmond J, Aharonoff GB, Zuckerman JD, Koval KJ. Mortality risk after hip fracture. J Orthop Trauma. 2003;17(1):53–6.

26. Shyu YIL, Chen MC, Liang J, Lu JF, Wu CC, Su JY. Changes in quality of life among elderly patients with hip fracture in Taiwan. Osteoporos Int. 2004; 15(2):95–102.

27. Williams DR, Wilson CM. Race, ethnicity, and aging. In handbook of aging and the socail science. 5th ed. San Diego: Academic Press; 2001.

28. Stone R. Asia's looming social challenge: coping with the elder boom. Science. 2010;330(6011):1599.

Locking compression plate distal ulna hook plate fixation versus intramedullary screw fixation for displaced avulsion fifth Metatarsal Base fractures: a comparative retrospective cohort study

Lin Xie[†], Xin Guo[†], Shu-Jun Zhang and Zhen-Hua Fang[*]

Abstract

Background: Intramedullary screw (IMS) fixation was wildly used in fifth metatarsal base fractures (FMBFs) and the results were satisfactory. However, in the comminuted osteoporosis or small displaced avulsion FMBFs, anatomical reduction and stable fixation could not be achieved with IMS. The Locking Compression Plate (LCP) distal ulna hook plate fixation was a novel alternative fixation method. The aim of this retrospective cohort study was to determine if LCP distal ulna hook plate fixation resulted in improved outcomes compared to the traditional IMS fixation in displaced avulsion FMBFs.

Methods: Of 43 patients with displaced avulsion FMBFs, 18 patients were treated with LCP distal ulna hook plate fixation and 25 were treated with IMS fixation. The patients were evaluated clinically and radiographically and followed up to 12 months. The surgery time, time for hospital stay, time for weight-bearing, time for bony union, time for return to daily life, pain relief, functional outcome and complications after treatment with LCP distal ulna hook plate fixation or IMS fixation were compared. The functional outcome was assessed by the AOFAS (American Orthopedic Foot and Ankle Society) mid-foot score at 3, 6, 9, and 12 months after surgery. Meanwhile, pain scores were obtained at 3, 6, 9, and 12 months after surgery.

Results: The two cohorts had similar baseline characteristics. Surgery time was less in LCP distal ulna hook plate fixation cohort compare to IMS fixation cohort ($p < 0.0001$). Time for partial weight-bearing ($p < 0.0001$) and full weight-bearing ($p < 0.0001$) also demonstrated significant improvements in patients with LCP distal ulna hook plate fixation compared to IMS fixation. Patients in the LCP distal ulna hook plate fixation cohort had significantly increased AOFAS at 9 months ($p < 0.0001$) and 12 months ($p < 0.0001$) after surgery compared to the IMS fixation cohort.

Conclusion: In this retrospective cohort study, LCP distal ulna hook plate fixation as an alternative fixation method was better therapy for the displaced avulsion FMBFs compared to IMS fixation. LCP distal ulna hook plate fixation had a short surgery time and improved functional performance.

Keywords: Locking compression plate (LCP), Intramedullary screw (IMS), Fifth Metatarsal Base fractures (FMBFs)

* Correspondence: bone_ghost@hotmail.com
[†]Equal contributors
Department of Orthopedic Surgery, Wuhan Orthopedic Hospital, Wuhan Puai Hospital, Huazhong University of Science and Technology, Hanzheng Street 473#, Wuhan City, Hubei Province 430033, China

Background

The base of fifth metatarsal was defined as the proximal 1.5 cm of the shaft distal to its articular surface. Fifth metatarsal base fractures (FMBFs) were the most common type of the fifth metatarsal fractures [1]. The fracture typically occurred when an adduction force was applied to the forefoot with the ankle plantarflexed. The base was usually divided anatomically into three zones [2] (its tuberosity, meta-diaphyseal junction and proximal shaft). Fractures in zone 1 were the most familiar ones which comprised about 93% of all the proximal fifth metatarsal fractures [1]. In our study, displaced avulsion FMBFs were defined as the displaced fractures in zone 1 [3, 4] (Fig. 1).

Most un-displaced avulsion FMBFs can be treated with conservative treatment [3, 5]. Non-weight-bearing with cast immobilization has been the main treatment of this injury [5, 6]. However, this injury often was a source of lost work productivity and associated with nonunion rates of 7% to 28% [2]. Fractures displaced more than 2 mm frequently required surgical treatment to achieve anatomic reduction of the articular surface, early weight-bearing and restoration of peroneus longus and brevis tendons [2]. Surgery treatment of displaced avulsion FMBFs was challenging because of its subcutaneous location, comminuted fracture, its attachment of peroneus longus and brevis muscles and its weight-bearing function [3, 7]. Intramedullary screw (IMS) fixation was wildly used in FMBFs [7–9] (Fig. 2). Previous studies showed that the screw was larger in both diameter and length the better [10]. However, the comminuted or small displaced avulsion FMBFs were difficulty to treat with large IMS and function outcomes following IMS remained unsatisfactory because of late weight-bearing [11]. Meanwhile, the IMS was associated with many complications, including lateral gapping, distraction of the fracture site and mal-reduction of the fractures [10, 12].

The Locking Compression Plate (LCP) distal ulna hook plate fixation was a novel alternative fixation method [13, 14] (Fig. 2). In addition, case series with LCP distal ulna hook plate fixation had shown improved clinical outcomes [14]. The purpose of this retrospective cohort study was to determine if LCP distal ulna hook plate fixation resulted in improved outcomes compared to the IMS fixation.

Methods

Patient eligibility

From July 2013 to July 2016, 42 patients (43 cases) with displaced avulsion Fifth Metatarsal Base Fractures were treated surgically and evaluated retrospectively. Ethical approval and informed consent from every single patient was obtained. Eligible patients were included in our study when they met the following criteria: (1) diagnosed with displaced (more than 2 mm) avulsion FMBFs; (2) over 18 years of age and in full possession of their mental faculties; (3) 4 days or less after injury; and (4) be treated with LCP distal ulna hook plate fixation (Fig. 3) or IMS (Fig. 4) and be follow-up until 12 months.

Patients with the following condition were excluded: (1) soft tissue injury: open fracture type Gustilo-

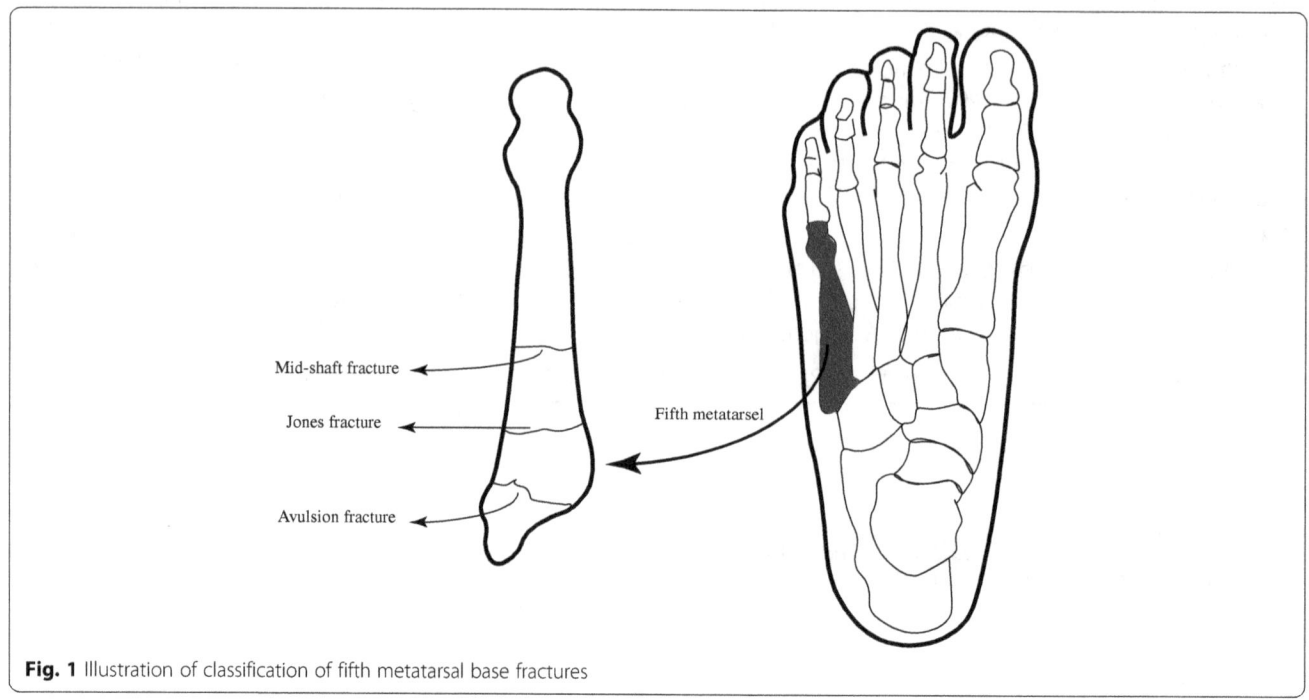

Fig. 1 Illustration of classification of fifth metatarsal base fractures

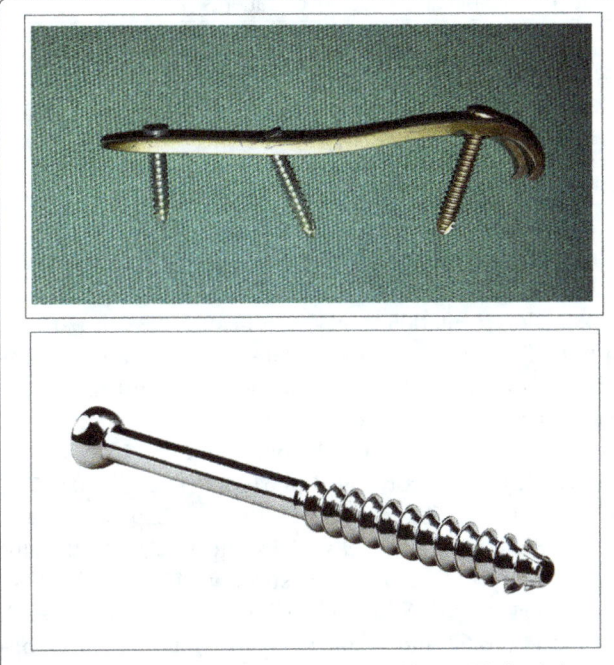

Fig. 2 Photograph of Locking Compression Plate (LCP) distal ulna hook plate and Intramedullary Screw

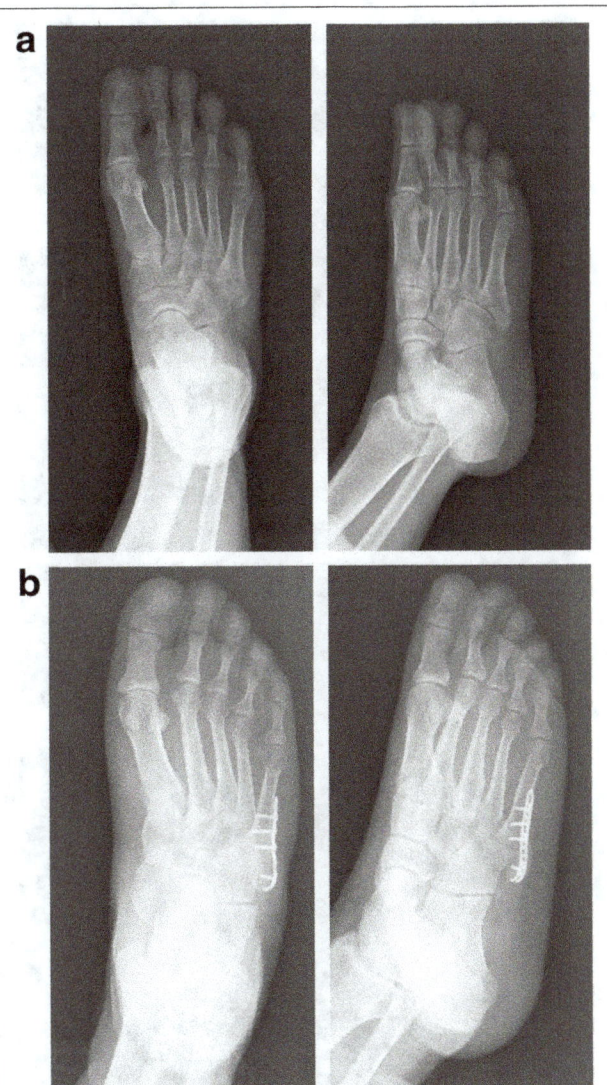

Fig. 3 Pre- (**a**) and postoperative (**b**) radiographs of a fifth metatarsal base fracture that was treated surgically using the Locking Compression Plate (LCP) distal ulna hook plate fixation

anderson Type II or higher; (2) pathological fracture or re-fracture; (3) additional zone 2 and 3 fractures; and (4) bilateral fracture.

Surgical treatment and rehabilitation protocol

All patients were surgically treated by a single, senior surgeon (ZHF) with the goals of anatomic reduction of the articular surface, achieve stable fixation and re-built the attachment of peroneus longus and brevis tendons. A lateral approach was used for direct visualization of the fractures as previously described. Patients in both cohorts were subject to the same postoperative rehabilitation protocol, which included no weight-bearing with short leg cast for 3 weeks. Radiographs were taken only on initial presentation to the clinic and in those patients with a great deal of pain clinically at the fracture site at the 6-week stage. Fracture union was defined radio graphically by bridging bone on at least 3 of 4 cortices.

Clinical and function outcome assessments

The baseline characteristics including age, male, and smoking were collected. Patient-reported weight-beating time, pain relief, and clinical functional outcomes were prospectively collected at predetermined intervals of 3,6,9, and 12 months postoperatively. Subjective clinical outcomes were measured using the American Ortho-pedic Foot and Ankle Society Score (AOFAS). It was one of the most widely used clinician-reporting tools for foot and ankle conditions. Developed in 1994, AOFAS is

a clinician-based score that measures outcomes on four different anatomic regions of the foot: The ankle-hindfoot, midfoot, metatarsophalangeal (MTP)-interpha-langeal (IP) for the hallux, and MTP-IP for the lesser toes. Complications were also collected in our studies until the 12 months' follow-up.

Statistics

Statistical analyses were performed using STATA, version 10.0 (Stata Corporation, College Station, Texas, USA). We summarized continuous data with means and standard deviations (SDs). The two groups were com-pared with regards to continuous and categorical out-comes using the non-parametric T-test and Chi-square

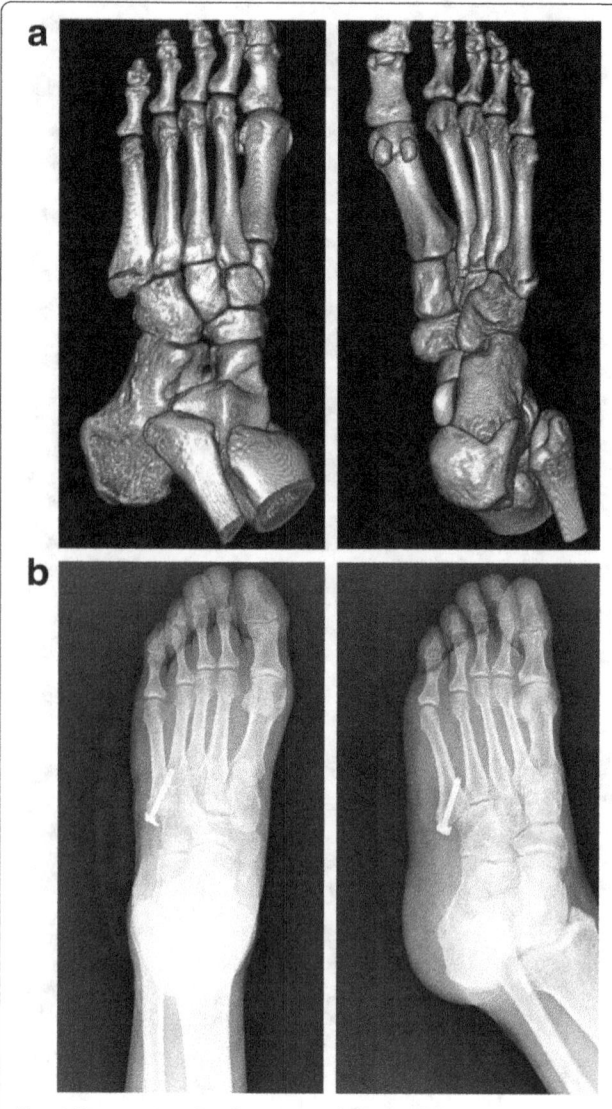

Fig. 4 Preoperative 3D reformations of CT scans (**a**) and postoperative (**b**) plain radiographs of a fifth metatarsal base fracture that was treated surgically using the Intramedullary Screw

Table 1 The baseline characters of patients

	PF $n = 18$	IMS $n = 25$	p-Value	Test
Age	39.89 ± 2.739	34.36 ± 1.977	0.4575	Unpaired T test
Male	27.78% (5)	60.00% (10)	0.5226	Chi-square test
Smoking	38.89% (7)	48.00% (12)	0.5528	Chi-square test

PF plate fixation, *IMS* Intramedullary screw

5.36 weeks, p < 0.001), full weight-bearing (6.52 and 8.48 weeks, p < 0.001), and bony union (7.49 and 9.64 weeks, $p = 0.0053$) was significantly less in patients with LCP distal ulna hook plate fixation cohort compared to IMS cohort. There was no significant difference in the time for return to daily life (12 and 12.52 weeks, $p = 0.4192$), pain scores before surgery (7.72 and 8, $p = 0.2432$), pain scores at 3 (4.61 and 4.64, $p = 0.9072$), 6 (3.56 and 3.68, $p = 0.4589$), 9 (2.39 and 2.68, $p = 0.0856$), and 12 weeks (0.44 and 0.52, $p = 0.6346$) after surgery, AOFAS before surgery (43.61 and 44.24, $p = 0.4554$), AOFAS at 3 (74.17 and 74.16, $p = 0.9931$), 6 months (76.67 and 76.6, $p = 0.7879$) after surgery between the two cohorts. While, the AOFAS scores at 9 (82.06 and 78.64, $p < 0.0001$), 12 months (93.56 and 87.8, p < 0.0001) after surgery were significantly higher in patients with LCP distal ulna hook plate fixation cohort (Table 2). One patient immigrates to Canada, we missed the follow up. There was no significant difference in the complications after surgery between the two cohorts.

Discussion

The main finding of this study is the efficacity of the fixation using a LCP distal ulna hook plate for a novel approach. There were only 4 studies studied the plate in the treatment of FMBFs [13, 15–17]. Three studies had evaluated the results of surgical treatment of zones I and II FMBFs using a mini-hook plate [13, 15, 16]. The fourth investigated the biomechanical comparison of IMS versus Low-Profile Plate fixation of a jones fracture [17]. There has been no previous comparison study investigating pain and functional outcome following treatment with LCP distal ulna hook plate and IMS, and our study is the first comparative retrospective cohort study to compare LCP distal ulna hook plate and IMS in displace evulsion FMBFs. Our finding showed that LCP distal ulna hook plate fixation as an alternative fixation method was better therapy for the displaced avulsion FMBFs than IMS fixation. LCP distal ulna hook plate fixation had a short surgery time and improved functional performance.

FMBFs can be challenging because of its subcutaneous location [18]. IMS as a precuneus technical was widely used in clinic and accepted as the standard of surgical treatment of these fractures [12]. Meanwhile, the screw

test respectively. We considered the conventional level of statistical significance as $p < 0.05$.

Results

18 patients treated with IMS and 25 patients treated with LCP distal ulna hook plate fixation were included in the study. All the raw data was in the Additional file 1. The two cohorts had similar baseline characteristics, including mean age (39.89 and 34.36 years, $p = 0.4575$), gender distribution (27.78% and 60.00% male, $p = 0.5226$), and smoking rates (38.89% and 48.00%, $p = 0.5528$) (Table 1). For both cohorts, the surgery time was significantly less in patients with LCP distal ulna hook plate fixation cohort (40.94 and 53.5 min, $p < 0.001$). Time for partial weight-bearing (3.67 and

Table 2 Surgical Results of patients with Fifth Metatarsal Base Fracture

	PF (n = 18)	IMS (n = 25)	P	Test
Time for surgery*	40.94 ± 1.18	53.52 ± 0.66	**<0.0001**	Unpaired T test
Time to partial weight-bearing*	3.67 ± 0.14	5.36 ± 0.13	**<0.0001**	Unpaired T test
Time to full weight-bearing*	6.52 ± 0.12	8.48 ± 0.19	**<0.0001**	Unpaired T test
Time for bony union*	7.49 ± 0.10	9.64 ± 0.61	0.0053	Unpaired T test
Time for return to daily life	12 ± 0.45	12.52 ± 0.42	0.4192	Unpaired T test
Pain before surgery	7.72 ± 0.21	8 ± 0.13	0.2432	Unpaired T test
Pain 3 weeks	4.61 ± 0.18	4.64 ± 0.16	0.9072	Unpaired T test
Pain 6 weeks	3.56 ± 0.15	3.68 ± 0.10	0.4589	Unpaired T test
Pain 9 weeks	2.39 ± 0.14	2.68 ± 0.10	0.0856	Unpaired T test
Pain 12 weeks	0.44 ± 0.12	0.52 ± 0.10	0.6346	Unpaired T test
AOFAS before surgery	43.61 ± 0.56	44.24 ± 0.57	0.4554	Unpaired T test
AOFAS 3 months	74.17 ± 0.63	74.16 ± 0.46	0.9931	Unpaired T test
AOFAS 6 months	76.67 ± 0.19	76.6 ± 0.15	0.7879	Unpaired T test
AOFAS 9 months*	82.06 ± 0.12	78.64 ± 0.11	**<0.0001**	Unpaired T test
AOFAS 12 months*	93.56 ± 0.25	87.8 ± 0.17	**<0.0001**	Unpaired T test
Complication delayed union	2	3	>0.9999	Fisher's exact test
Complication nonunion	0	0	–	–
Complication infection	0	0	–	–

PF plate fixation, IMS Intramedullary screw, AOFAS American Orthopedic Foot and Ankle Society
*and bold means P < 0.05

system was developed, allowing surgeons to choose among 4.5-, 5.5-, and 6.5-mm solid stainless steel screws. However, it was difficulty to fix the small avulsion fractures with screws and there were several complications associated with them, such as irritability of screws head, injury of peripheral nerve, bone nonunion because of small diameter, and secondary fractures because of large diameter [12]. Alternatively, LCP distal ulna hook plate may be a good choice. This plate has several advantages: (1) the fifth metatarsal tuberosity can be grasped tightly by the plate hook to maintain the stability of the peroneal tendons adhesion; (2) as a checkered plate, the re-displaced of fractures can be reduced. Joint surface collapse can be prevented by the support function of this plate; (3) this plate had good histocompatibility; (4) the fifth metatarsal's bending curvature fitted to the LCP distal ulna hook plate; and (5) low profile, obtuse edge and polishing surface can reduce the irritability of the soft tissue [17]. Vorlat, Achtergael and Haentjens reported that the most significant predictor of a poor functional outcome after these injuries was a prolonged period of non-weight-bearing [19]. The advantage functional outcome of LCP distal ulna hook plate was related to the early weight-bearing.

The retrospective cohort design of this study has several strengths. All cases were performed by a single senior surgeon (ZHF) using the same surgical approach, and all functional outcome evaluations were completed by a single senior physical therapist (SJZ) for precision. In addition, complications in both groups minimal. Limitations of this study include only twelve months of outcomes postoperatively, the total number of patients were small, and the radiographic evaluation was incomplete. Nowadays, we are focus on the effectively of the fifth metatarsal fractures anatomy plate.

Conclusions

This study suggests that the use of LCP distal ulna hook plate fixation improves patients' outcomes postoperatively.

Additional file

Additional file 1: The file contains the raw data of the age, gender, smoking, time for surgery, time for partial weight-bearing, time for full weight-bearing, time for bone union, return to daily life, pain before surgery, pain 3 weeks, pain 6 weeks, pain 6 weeks, pain 12 weeks, AOFAS before surgery, AOFAS 3 months, AOFAS 6 months, AOFAS 9 months, AOFAS 12 months, delayed union, nonunion, and infection. (XLSX 32 kb)

Abbreviations
AOFAS: American Orthopedic Foot and Ankle Society; FMBFs: Fifth Metatarsal Base Fractures; IMS: Intramedullary screw; LCP: Locking Compression Plate; PF: Plate Fixation

Acknowledgements
Not applicable.

Funding
The author(s) received no financial support for the research, authorship, and/or publication of this article.

Authors' contributions
ZHF and LX suggested the idea and were major contributors in writing the manuscript. XG and SJZ measured, analyzed and interpreted the patients' data. XG modified our manuscript. ZHF performed the surgery. All authors read and approved the final manuscript.

Competing interests
The authors declare that they have no competing interests.

References

1. Lawrence SJ, Botte MJ. Jones' fractures and related fractures of the proximal fifth metatarsal. Foot & ankle. 1993;14(6):358–65.
2. Petrisor BA, Ekrol I, Court-Brown C. The epidemiology of metatarsal fractures. Foot Ankle Int. 2006;27(3):172–4.
3. Egol K, Walsh M, Rosenblatt K, Capla E, Koval KJ. Avulsion fractures of the fifth metatarsal base: a prospective outcome study. Foot Ankle Int. 2007;28(5):581–3.
4. Mehlhorn AT, Zwingmann J, Hirschmuller A, Sudkamp NP, Schmal H. Radiographic classification for fractures of the fifth metatarsal base. Skelet Radiol. 2014;43(4):467–74.
5. Wiener BD, Linder JF, Giattini JF. Treatment of fractures of the fifth metatarsal: a prospective study. Foot Ankle Int. 1997;18(5):267–9.
6. Shahid MK, Punwar S, Boulind C, Bannister G. Aircast walking boot and below-knee walking cast for avulsion fractures of the base of the fifth metatarsal: a comparative cohort study. Foot Ankle Int. 2013;34(1):75–9.
7. Mahajan V, Chung HW, Suh JS. Fractures of the proximal fifth metatarsal: percutaneous bicortical fixation. Clinics in orthopedic surgery. 2011;3(2):140–6.
8. Mologne TS, Lundeen JM, Clapper MF, O'Brien TJ. Early screw fixation versus casting in the treatment of acute Jones fractures. Am J Sports Med. 2005;33(7):970–5.
9. Tan EW, Cata E, Schon LC. Use of a Percutaneous Pointed Reduction Clamp Before Screw Fixation to Prevent Gapping of a Fifth Metatarsal Base Fracture: A Technique Tip. J Foot Ankle Surg. 2016;55(1):151–6.
10. Wright RW, Fischer DA, Shively RA, Heidt RS Jr, Nuber GW. Refracture of proximal fifth metatarsal (Jones) fracture after intramedullary screw fixation in athletes. Am J Sports Med. 2000;28(5):732–6.
11. Roche AJ, Calder JD. Treatment and return to sport following a Jones fracture of the fifth metatarsal: a systematic review. Knee Surg Sports Traumatol Arthrosc. 2013;21(6):1307–15.
12. Ochenjele G, Ho B, Switaj PJ, Fuchs D, Goyal N, Kadakia AR. Radiographic study of the fifth metatarsal for optimal intramedullary screw fixation of Jones fracture. Foot Ankle Int. 2015;36(3):293–301.
13. Lee SK, Park JS, Choy WS. LCP distal ulna hook plate as alternative fixation for fifth metatarsal base fracture. Eur J Orthop Surg Traumatol. 2013;23(6):705–13.
14. Lorich DG, Fabricant PD, Sauro G, Lazaro LE, Thacher RR, Garner MR, Warner SJ. Superior Outcomes after Operative Fixation of Patella Fractures using a Novel Plating Technique: a Prospective Cohort Study. J Orthop Trauma. 2017;
15. Choi JH, Lee KT, Lee YK, Lee JY, Kim HR. Surgical results of zones I and II fifth metatarsal base fractures using hook plates. Orthopedics. 2013;36(1):e71–4.
16. Lee SK, Park JS, Choy WS. Locking compression plate distal ulna hook plate as alternative fixation for fifth metatarsal base fracture. J Foot Ankle Surg. 2014;53(5):522–8.
17. Huh J, Glisson RR, Matsumoto T, Easley ME. Biomechanical Comparison of Intramedullary Screw Versus Low-Profile Plate Fixation of a Jones Fracture. Foot Ankle Int. 2016;37(4):411–8.
18. O'Malley M, DeSandis B, Allen A, Levitsky M, O'Malley Q, Williams R. Operative Treatment of Fifth Metatarsal Jones Fractures (Zones II and III) in the NBA. Foot Ankle Int. 2016;37(5):488–500.
19. Vorlat P, Achtergael W, Haentjens P. Predictors of outcome of non-displaced fractures of the base of the fifth metatarsal. Int Orthop. 2007;31(1):5–10.

24

Prevalence and incidence of musculoskeletal extremity complaints in children and adolescents

Signe Fuglkjær[1]*[iD], Kristina Boe Dissing[1] and Lise Hestbæk[1,2]

Abstract

Background: It is difficult to gain an overview of musculoskeletal extremity complaints in childhood although this is essential to develop evidence-based prevention and treatment strategies. The objectives of this systematic review were therefore to describe the prevalence and incidence of musculoskeletal extremity complaints in children and adolescents in both general and clinical populations in relation to age, anatomical site and mode of onset.

Methods: MEDLINE and EMBASE were electronically searched; risk of bias was assessed; and data extraction was individually performed by two authors.

Results: In total, 19 general population studies and three clinical population studies were included with children aged 0-19 years. For most of the analyses, a division between younger children aged 0-12 years, and older children aged 10-19 years was used. Lower extremity complaints were more common than upper extremity complaints regardless of age and type of population, with the most frequent pain site changing from ankle/foot in the youngest to knee in the oldest. There were about twice as many non-traumatic as traumatic complaints in the lower extremities, whereas the opposite relationship was found for the upper extremities in the general population studies. There were relatively more lower extremity complaints in the general population studies than in the clinical population studies. The review showed no pattern of differences in reporting between studies of high and low risk of bias.

Conclusions: This review shows that musculoskeletal complaints are more frequent in the lower extremities than in the upper extremities in childhood, and there are indications of a large amount of non-traumatic low intensity complaints in the population that do not reach threshold for consultation. A meta-analysis, or even a simple overall description of prevalence and incidence of musculoskeletal extremity complaints in children and adolescents was not feasible, due to a large variety in the studies, primarily related to outcome measurements.

Keywords: Musculoskeletal injury, Musculoskeletal pain, Paediatrics, Prevalence, Incidence

* Correspondence: sfuglkjaer@health.sdu.dk
[1]Department of Sports Science and Clinical Biomechanics, Faculty of Health Sciences, University of Southern Denmark, Campusvej 55, DK-5230 Odense M, Denmark
Full list of author information is available at the end of the article

Background

Recently, the Global Burden of Disease studies reported musculoskeletal pain as one of the leading causes of years lived with disability [1] and this constitutes a substantial burden on society [2]. Therefore, it is important to design better prevention strategies and early effective treatment. To do that, more basic knowledge about the epidemiology of musculoskeletal complaints in children and adolescents must be obtained first.

The epidemiology of spinal pain in children is well-described [3–5], whereas less attention has been given to musculoskeletal extremity complaints (MEC) in children. Furthermore, musculoskeletal problems in childhood might not only lead to musculoskeletal complaints in adulthood, but could also be a barrier for physical activity and thus have a negative influence on general health [6]. It has been shown that physical activity is important for health in children and adolescents [6–9], and in addition the amount of physical activity in childhood is considered to be a predictor of the amount of physical activity in adults [9], which is important in prevention of many lifestyle disorders, e.g. diabetes and cardiovascular disease [8, 9].

Various terms have been used in relation to MEC, starting from the less severe ache to injury or more severe musculoskeletal disorders. Commonly, MEC are divided into traumatic and non-traumatic complaints, where a traumatic complaint has been defined as an injury resulting from a specific identifiable event, whereas a non-traumatic complaint is not related to an identifiable event [10]. In research of MEC, focus has traditionally been on either specific groups of athletes, or injuries reported at emergency departments, and patterns of paediatric injuries in relation to sport are therefore well described [11–13]. While this type of research provides valid information about specific injuries, mainly injuries of a traumatic onset, they do not represent the full picture of MEC in the general population. Specifically, none of these methods collect valid information about non-traumatic complaints in the general population, which has been shown to represent a large part, close to two thirds, of MEC [14, 15]. The prevalence and treatment strategies of some types of specific injuries, e.g. fractures [16] and ankle distortions [17–19] are well described, but such knowledge has not been accumulated for many other types of MEC, e.g. overuse injuries and non-specific minor complaints. To inform the development of evidence-based prevention and treatment strategies, the first step is to increase knowledge about types and frequency of MEC in childhood. At present it is difficult to gain an overview of the extent of various types of complaints in relation to mode of onset (traumatic vs. non-traumatic), different anatomical locations and histological involvement. Therefore, the objectives of this systematic review were to investigate the prevalence and incidence of musculoskeletal extremity complaints in children and adolescents in both general and clinical populations in relation to age, distribution between different complaint sites, and types of complaints (traumatic vs. non-traumatic). Furthermore, differences between general and clinical populations will be explored.

Methods

Case terminology

Different traditions and interest in different levels of complaint-severity are reasons for various terms used in research about musculoskeletal extremity complaints: injury, disorder, discomfort, complaint, pain, ache etc. In this review we analysed musculoskeletal extremity complaints in the general population, and therefore found a broad term of musculoskeletal extremity complaint (MEC) to be most comprehensive and this will be used throughout the rest of this article, regardless of the term used in the referenced articles. When possible, the MEC were divided according to causation, and were categorised as either traumatic or non-traumatic. A traumatic complaint was defined as an injury resulting from a specific identifiable event, whereas a non-traumatic episode was not related to an identifiable event [10]. For example, a traumatic complaint could be pain due to fall from a horse, and a non-traumatic complaint could be pain of unspecific origin developed over a longer period of time.

Identification of studies

The search was made in collaboration with a research librarian. Two electronic databases, MEDLINE and EMBASE, were searched for articles published before September 2015. The following search terms were used both as MeSH terms and free text in MEDLINE, and as Subject heading and abstract term in EMBASE: "prevalence", "incidence", "musculoskeletal disorder", "musculoskeletal injury", "musculoskeletal pain", "extremity", "limb", "children", "adolescents", "paediatric". As free text/abstract term "toddlers" and "teenager" were searched as well. Different forms of spelling and synonyms were used. The full search strategy is seen in Additional file 1. In addition, the reference lists of the relevant obtained articles were screened for additional relevant articles.

Inclusion criteria

The article had to report the prevalence or incidence of musculoskeletal disorders, complaints, injuries, pain or other description of complaints in the upper and/or lower extremities in general or clinical populations of children and adolescents. All levels of prevalence and incidence rates were included, and could be both parental reported or self-reported values. All study designs were included, but they had to be published in English, Swedish, Norwegian or Danish.

Exclusion criteria

Special settings or groups, e.g. children with other diseases such as diabetes or other chronic diseases, or children from a specific sport setting (e.g. football players) were excluded, because their pattern of injuries might not be comparable to rest of the population.

Selection of studies

The first and third author (SF and LH) reviewed the titles and abstracts and identified relevant articles to be read in full text. Inclusion of articles based on full text was decided by agreement between the first and third author (SF and LH).

Assessment of quality

We were not aware of quality assessment tools specifically designed for studies of prevalence and/or incidence, since most quality assessment tools are designed for studies of associations or comparative effectiveness in either observational studies [20–23] or randomised clinical trials [24]. Therefore the quality of the included articles was assessed by a modified version of the Quality In Prognosis Studies (QUIPS) tool (Additional file 2), which was originally developed to assess bias in studies of prognostic factors [25]. This tool identifies six domains to consider when evaluating risk of bias in studies of prognostic factors: 'Study Participation', 'Study Attrition', 'Prognostic Factor Measurement', 'Outcome Measurement', 'Study Confounding' and 'Statistically Analysis and Reporting' [25]. Three of these domains: 'Study Participation', 'Outcome Measurement' and 'Statistical Analysis and Reporting' were considered to be important, relevant and adequate for studies investigating prevalence, whereas the attrition domain was also included for studies investigating incidence, due to the main interest in relation to representativeness of the population of interest and the validity of the outcome measurement. In the 'Statistical Analysis and Reporting' domain, the items "strategy for model building is appropriate and is based on a conceptual framework or model" and "the selected statistical model is adequate for the design of the study" were not relevant and therefore ignored in the assessment. 'Study Attrition' is irrelevant for cross-sectional studies of prevalence and was therefore not included in the assessment of these studies, and 'Prognostic Factors Measurement' and 'Study Confounding' were not relevant either, since our results did not include analyses of prognosis or associations. The domains are described in detail by Hayden et al. [25].

Each of the three (four) domains was categorized as "yes", "partly" or "no" according to whether the level of quality was adequately fullfilled or not. In evaluation of risk of bias in studies of prevalence and incidence, the most important parameter to consider is whether the study sample is representative of the source population, thus leaving 'Study Participation' and 'Study Attrition' the most important domains in this review. This is supported by 'Study Participation' being the most frequently used parameter across different tools of evaluation of quality and susceptibility to bias in observational studies [26]. Therefore, 'Study Participation' and 'Study Attrition' (if included) needed to be considered as satisfactory ("yes") for the study to be classified in the low risk of bias category. Furthermore, the other two domains had to be at least partly fulfilled. If 'Study Participation' and 'Study Attrition' (if included) was not considered satisfactory ("no") the study was categorized as high risk of bias, regardless the judgements in the other domains. If 'Study Participation' and 'Study Attrition' (if included) was only partly fulfilled and both the other domains were not fulfilled, the study was classified as high risk as well. All other combinations were considered to be medium risk of bias.

Data extraction

The studies were divided into general population studies and clinical population studies. Data were extracted to a descriptive table, a modified version of the STROBE statement [27]. The following relevant items from the STROBE Statement were included in the table: study design, setting, age, study size including response rates, data sources/types of measurement, area of complaint and main results. In addition, type of prevalence or incidence, mode of data acquisition and the level of bias were added to the table.

Review process

Data extraction and assessment of quality were individually performed by two authors (SF and KBD) and results compared. In case of disagreement, the third author (LH) was consulted and consensus reached. The review was conducted according to the PRISMA guidelines, and the PRISMA checklist can be seen in Additional file 3.

Analyses

General population and clinical population studies

Obviously, clinical populations cannot be used to assess prevalence of disease. However, they can be used to identify the type of complaints, for which care is sought. Therefore both general population studies and clinical population studies were included in the review, but data were reported separately.

Follow-up studies considered as two cross-sectional studies

Some of the general population studies had a longitudinal design. Due to the focus on prevalence and incidence rates, these studies were considered as series of cross-sectional studies and each time point reported separately. If the study included any type of intervention, only baseline estimates were reported.

Data evaluated in relation to age

It is known that the prevalence of MEC change with age [28]. Therefore, to give the most relevant description, results were reported by age groups. Cut points between age groups were based on reporting in the included articles.

Prevalence and incidence of MEC reported by anatomical site

In *the general population studies* the use of self-reported questionnaires by children and parents did not make it possible to report specific diagnoses, and therefore the results in this review were simply reported by anatomic site. Wrist, hand and fingers were combined into one anatomic site called "wrist/hand/fingers", and likewise for the ankle and foot, called "ankle/ft".

To make the reported findings comparable to the general population studies, the diagnoses found in *the clinical population studies* were converted into similar anatomical sites.

Distribution of non-traumatic versus traumatic complaints

Where possible, the difference between rates of non-traumatic and traumatic complaints was reported.

Distribution of lower extremity complaints versus upper extremity complaints

Some of the studies reported combined prevalence or incidence rates of the complete upper or lower extremity regions. To identify a possible pattern in distribution of MEC, ratios between the prevalence or incidence rates of the upper and lower extremities were calculated.

Results

In total, 2660 titles were found in MEDLINE, EMBASE and by reference searches. After checking for duplicates and screening of titles and abstracts, 29 articles were found assessable for full-text review. Seven of these were subsequently excluded because results were not representative of the general population [16, 29–32], or because classification into anatomic region or site was not possible [33, 34], thus 22 studies were included in the final analyses (Fig. 1).

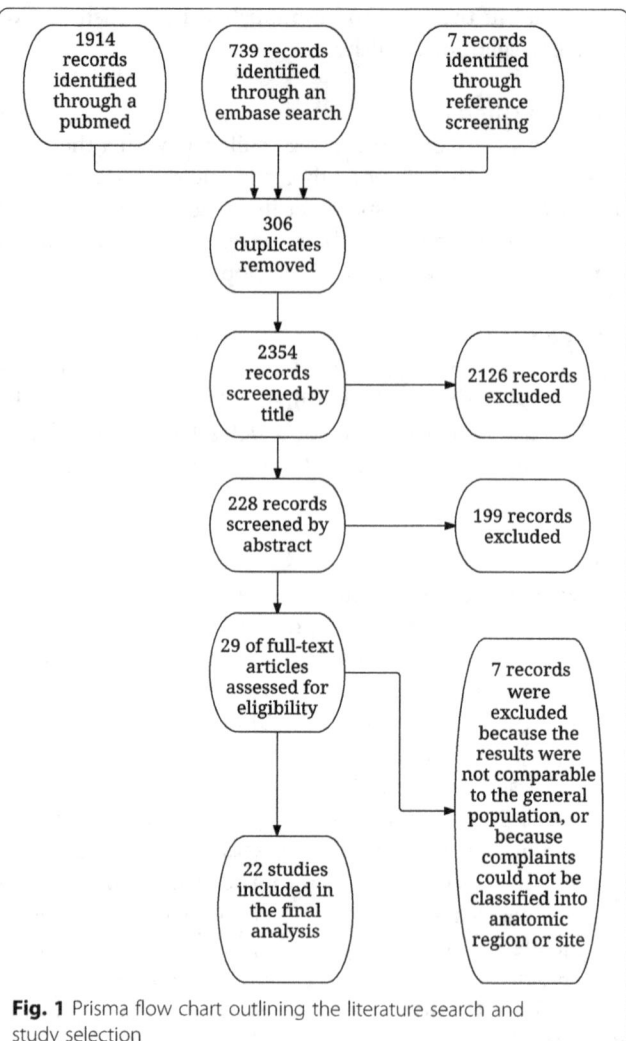

Fig. 1 Prisma flow chart outlining the literature search and study selection

Assessment of quality

The quality assessment categorized fourteen articles to have low risk of bias [14, 15, 35–46], two to have medium risk of bias [47, 48] and six as having high risk of bias [49–54] (Table 1). The clinical population studies were all in the low risk category. There was no disagreement in the independent quality assessments by the two authors (SF and KBD) regarding most of the articles, with the exception of two instances [47, 50] within the 'study participation' domain which were solved through discussion without need of mediation by the third author.

Description of included articles

The search resulted in 19 general population studies and three clinical population studies (Table 2). All the included studies covered children and adolescents of both sexes. Most of the studies were conducted in the northern part of Europe, but also other parts of the world were represented with three studies from North America [35, 43, 55], one from Australia [45] and one from India [49]. Of

Table 1 Results of the quality assessment of the 22 included articles

Author and year of publication	Study Participation	Study Attrition	Outcome Measurement	Statistical Analysis and Reporting	Risk of bias assessment
General population studies					
Abujam et al. 2014 [49]	No	N/A	Yes	Yes	High
Adams et al. 2013 [35]	Yes	N/A	Yes	Yes	Low
Auvinen et al. 2009 [50]	No	N/A	Partly	Yes	High
Bishop et al. 2012 [51]	No	N/A	Yes	Yes	High
Diepenmaat et al. 2006 [36]	Yes	N/A	Yes	Yes	Low
Ehrmann Feldman et al. 2002 [37]	Yes	Yes	Partly	Yes	Low
El-Metwally et al. 2006 [15]	Yes	N/A	Yes	Yes	Low
Hoftun et al. 2011 [38]	Yes	N/A	Yes	Yes	Low
Hulsegge et al. 2011 [47]	Partly	Yes	Partly	Yes	Medium
Jespersen et al. 2014 [14]	Yes	Yes	Yes	Yes	Low
Jespersen et al. 2015 [39]	Yes	N/A	Yes	Yes	Low
Krul et al. 2009 [40]	Yes	N/A	Yes	Yes	Low
Mikkelsson et al. 1997 [41]	Yes	N/A	Yes	Yes	Low
Molgaard et al. 2011 [48]	Partly	N/A	Yes	Yes	Medium
Rathleff et al. 2013 [42]	Yes	N/A	Yes	Yes	Low
Shrier et al. 2001 [43]	Yes	Yes	Partly	Yes	Low
Slowinska et al. 2015 [68]	No	N/A	Yes	Partly	High
Smedbraten et al. 1998 [52]	No	N/A	Yes	Yes	High
Verhagen et al. 2009 [54]	Yes	No	Yes	Yes	High
Clinical studies					
Bot et al. 2005 [44]	Yes	N/A[a]	Yes	Partly	Low
Henschke et al. 2014 [45]	Yes	N/A[a]	Yes	Yes	Low
Van der Waal et al. 2006 [46]	Yes	N/A[a]	Yes	Yes	Low

[a]Attrition bias may be present, but very small. If present, it will be on general practitioners level, and not on patient level

the 19 general population studies, seven were prospective, four with one follow up evaluation [37, 43, 50, 51], and three studies reporting incidence over time [14, 39, 54]. In most of the studies, data were collected via questionnaires, either self-reported or filled in by parents, but telephone interviews, mobile phone text messages and diagnoses from general practice were also used. The 22 studies used 14 different outcome measurements such as point prevalence, twelve month prevalence and incidence per 1000 exposure hours. Estimates are simply presented in the tables as they appear in the original articles because prevalence and incidence rates were reported in very different ways. For the same reason, meta-analysis was not possible, and even a reliable range of an estimate of frequency, i.e. incidence or prevalence, could not be presented either. However, the findings relating to *differences* in frequency between different age groups, between different anatomical sites and between different populations, are independent of the absolute prevalence or incidence rates and are therefore presented in detail. We attempted to report findings of younger children and older children separately, but

due to different cut points in age between the studies, it was not possible to do this. Throughout most of the analyses, a division between younger children aged 0–12, and older children aged 10–19 was used, but to accommodate all studies, some results were reported for the following age groups: 0–9, 9–12, 10–19, 6–17 and 2–19. A summary of findings is presented in Tables 3, 4, 5 and 6.

General population studies

In both the younger (aged 0–12) and the older children (aged 10–19), lower extremity complaints were more common than upper extremity complaints, and ankle/ft and knee were the most frequent sites of MEC. Among the younger children, two studies reported ankle/ft complaints to be about twice as frequent as knee complaints [39, 54], whereas the last study reported almost similar prevalence rates for the two sites [15] (Table 3). Among the older children, five of the six included studies reported 0.2 to 2.8 times more knee complaints than ankle/ft complaints [40, 42, 43, 50, 52] (Table 4). In the upper extremities, wrist/hand/fingers was the most

Table 2 Summary of study characteristics of the 22 included studies

Author and year of publication	Study Design	Setting	Age/ grade	Measurements (how did they ask?)	Study Size	Baseline response rate	Follow up response rate	Prevalence/ incidence	Type of complaints	Main result (text)	Bias
General population studies											
Abujam et al. 2014	Cross-sectional	India School based	6–17 yrs	Questionnaire filled in by children or parents if the child was less than 14 years	2059	?		Lifetime prevalence	Heel/ Ankle pain or swelling	N (%) 72 (3.5%)	High
Adams et al. 2013	Cross-sectional	US Cohort - Kaiser Permanente Southern California	2–19 yrs	ICD-9 codes	913,178			1 yrs. prevalence	Lower extremity Injuries or pain Upper extremity: Injuries or pain	5.8% 5.1%	Low
Auvinen et al. 2009	Prospective cohort	Finland 2-years Birth Cohort	16–18 yrs	Self-reported questionnaire	7344	7344/ 9215 (80%)	2012/ 2969 (68%)	6-month prevalence	Shoulder pain Elbow pain Wrist pain Knee pain Ankle pain	Prevalence % (N) F: female, M: male Age: 16 yrs. 18 yrs. F: 52 (506) 63 (616) M: 33 (253) 40 (307) F: 2 (22) 4 (35) M: 5 (37) 5 (37) F: 16 (156) 23 (219) M: 15 (114) 20 (150) F: 18 (178) 21 (201) M: 18 (141) 17 (129) F: 16 (150) 19 (179) M: 18 (142) 15 (116)	High
Bishop et al. 2012	Prospective cohort	England Cohort -Avon Longitudinal Study of Parents and Children	5–13 yrs	Questionnaire filled in by chief carer	9380	9380/ 13,988 (67%)	6502/ 13,988 (46%)	Often prevalence	Total replied, n(%) arms, n(%) leg(s), n(%) Total replied, n(%) arms, n(%) leg(s), n(%) Total replied, n(%) arms, n(%) leg(s), n(%)	Age 5* Age 6* 9380 (100.0) 8599 (100.0) 13 + 227 = 240 (2.6) 14 + 299 = 313 (3.6) 1142 + 227 = 1369 (14.6) 1204 + 299 = 1503 (17.5) Age 7* Age 8* 8325 (100.0) 7872 (100.0) 10 + 333 = 343 (4.1) 13 + 475 = 488 (6.2) 1226 + 333 = 1559 1188 + 475 = 1663 (21.1) Age 11* Age 13*6996 (100.0) 6502 (100.0) 22 + 635 = 657 (9.4) 33 + 730 = 763 (11.7) 1386 + 635 = 2021 1342 + 730 = 2072 (31.9)	High

Table 2 Summary of study characteristics of the 22 included studies (Continued)

Author and year of publication	Study Design	Setting	Age/grade	Measurements (how did they ask?)	Study Size	Baseline response rate	Follow up response rate	Prevalence/incidence	Type of complaints	Main result (text)	Bias
Diepenmaat et al. 2006	Cross-sectional	Holland School based questionnaire	12–16 yrs	Self-reported questionnaire	3485	3485/4898 (71%)		Monthly prevalence, pain lasting a day or longer	Arm pain	Male: 4.2% Female: 3.6%	Low
Ehrmann Feldman et al. 2002	Prospective cohort	Canada High school based	7.-9. grade	Self-reported questionnaire	810	810/948 (85%)	502/810 (62%)	6 months and 12 months Incidence	Upper limb Arm Shoulder	6 months[b] 12 months[b] 19.9% 13.3% 9% 7% 8% 5%	Low
El-Metwally et al. 2006	Cross-sectional	Finland 2-years Birth Cohort	9–11 yrs	Self-reported questionnaire	1756	1756/1823 (96%)		Weekly prevalence, within the last 3 months	Prevalence N(%) Lower limb pain Ankle-foot pain Knee pain Thigh pain Leg pain Hip pain	Traumatic Non-traumatic Both groups 105 (6.0) 216 (12.3) 321 (18.3) 32 (1.8) 154 (8.8) 186 (10.6) 37 (2.1) 181 (10.3) 218 (12.4) 15 (0.9) 166 (9.5) 181 (10.3) 30 (1.7) 89 (5.1) 119 (6.8) 13 (0.7) 47 (2.7) 60 (3.4)	Low
Hoftun et al. 2011	Cross-sectional	Norway Health Study	13–18 yrs	Self-reported questionnaire	7373	7373/7913 (93%)		Weekly prevalence, within the last 3 months	Upper extremity Lower extremity	13–15 yrs. (n % 95% CI): 16–18 yrs. (n % 95% CI): 163 4.0 (3.4–4.6) 129 3.9 (3.3–4.6) 522 12.8 (11.8–13.8) 282 8.6 (7.6–9.6)	Low
Hulsegge et al. 2011	Cross-sectional	Holland Cohort of pregnant women - Prevention and Incidence of Asthma and Mite Allergy	11 yrs	Questionnaire answered by parents and child	2638	2638/3963 = (67%)		1-year prevalence	Upper extremity Lower extremity	4.8% (Boys: 3.1%, girls: 6.3%) 10,9% (Boys: 10.4%, Girls: 11.2%)	Medium
J espersen et al. 2014	Prospective	Denmark School based cohort - Childhood Health, Activity and Motor Performance School Study	6–12 yrs	Repeated text messages and ICD-10 diagnosis given by clinicians	1259	90% for sports schools 71% for normal schools		Weekly mean incidence Weekly mean prevalence	Upper extremity Lower extremity Upper extremity Lower extremity	Injury: 0.2 (± 4.0) Overuse injury: 0.04 (± 2.0) Traumatic injury: 0.1 (± 3.5) Injury: 1.0 (± 9.7) Overuse injury: 0.7 (± 8.2)	Low

Table 2 Summary of study characteristics of the 22 included studies (*Continued*)

Author and year of publication	Study Design	Setting	Age/grade	Measurements (how did they ask?)	Study Size	Baseline response rate	Follow up response rate	Prevalence/incidence	Type of complaints	Main result (text)	Bias
										Traumatic injury: 0.3 (± 5.2) Injury: 0.5 (± 7.2) Overuse injury: 0.2 (± 4.9) Traumatic injury: 0.3 (± 5.8) Injury: 4.1 (± 19.9) Overuse injury: 3.2 (± 17.7) Traumatic injury: 1.1 (± 10.4)	
Jespersen et al. 2015	Prospective	Denmark School based cohort - Childhood Health, Activity and Motor Performance School Study	6–12 yrs	Repeated text messages and ICD-10 diagnosis given by clinicians	1259	90% for sportsschools 71% for normal schools		Incidence Rate	Shoulder/ Upper Arm Elbow/under Arm Hand/wrist Finger Hip/Groin Thigh Knee Lower leg Achilles Heel Ankle Foot	Overuse Traumatic0.03 (0.02–0.05) 0.03 (0.02–0.04) 0.01 (0.00–0.02) 0.02 (0.01–0.03)0.01 (0.00–0.01) 0.08 (0.06–0.10) 0.00 (0.00–0.01) 0.05 (0.03–0.07)0.05 (0.04–0.07) 0.01 (0.00–0.01) 0.04 (0.03–0.06) 0.03 (0.02–0.04)0.31 (0.27–0.35) 0.09 (0.07–0.11) 0.05 (0.03–0.06) 0.01 (0.00–0.02) 0.06 (0.04–0.08) 0.000.36 (0.31–0.4) 0.000.01 (0.00–0.01) 0.18 (0.15–0.21)0.09 (0.07–0.11) 0.07 (0.05–0.09)	Low
Krul et al. 2009	Cross-sectional	Holland -Second Dutch National Survey in generel practice	2–17 yrs	Interview aboutself-reported musculoskeletal symptoms. In children younger than 12 years interview was carried out with a parent.	2459	2459/2719 (90%)		2 weeks prevalence	Upper extremity All ages 2–11 y 12–17 y Lower extremity All ages 2–11 y 12–17 y Hip and knee All ages 2–11 y 12–17 y Ankle and foot All ages 2–11 y 12–17 y	% (n) 1.2 (26) 0.4 (5) 2.7 (21) 6.9 (147) 4.1 (57) 12.4 (90) 3.5 (75) 1.8 (25) 6.5 (50) 3.4 (72) 2.4 (32) 5.5 (40)	Low

Table 2 Summary of study characteristics of the 22 included studies *(Continued)*

Author and year of publication	Study Design	Setting	Age/ grade	Measurements (how did they ask?)	Study Size	Baseline response rate	Follow up response rate	Prevalence/ incidence	Type of complaints	Main result (text)	Bias
Mikkelsson[a] et al. 1997	Cross-sectional	Finland -School based cohort	3.-5. grade	Self-reported questionnaire	1756	1756/ 2141 (82%)	1628/ 1756 (92%)	Weekly prevalence Relative frequency (%) with 95% CI	Upper extremity Lower extremity	Boys: 7 (6–9)[b] Girls: 5.5 (4–7)[b] Boys: 19 (16–22)[b] Girls: 18 (15–20)[b]	Low
Molgaard et al. 2011	Single-blind case control (case-cohort)	Denmark High School based	16– 18 yrs	Self-reported questionnaire	299	227/ 299 (76%)		Monthly-prevalence	Non-traumatic knee pain	57/227 = (25%)	Medium
Rathleff et al. 2013	Cross-sectional	Denmark – Cohort – Adolescent Pain in Aalborg 2011,	12– 19 yrs	Self-reported questionnaire	4007	2953/ 4007 (73%)		Point prevalence	Knee Shoulder Foot Shin Hip/groin Forearm/hand Thigh Elbow	Any frequency: 32.3 (30.6–34.0) 13.3 (12.1–14.5) 11.5 (10.4–12.7) 6.2 (5.4–7.1) 5.9 (5.0–6.7) 4.4 (3.7–5.1) 2.7 (2.2–3.2) 2.6 (2.1–3.2)	Low
Shrier et al. 2001	Prospective cohort	Canada High School based	12– 18 yrs	Self-reported questionnaire	810	810/948 (85%)	502/810 (62%)	Incidence 6 months 12 months (once a week the last 6 months)	Lower extremity Foot/ankle Knee Leg Hip	6 months[b] 12 months[b] % % 21 16 14 8 13 11 11 6 7 4	Low
Smedbraten et al. 1998	Cross-sectional	Norway School based	10– 15 yrs	Self-reported questionnaire	569	569/661 (86%)		Prevalence Usually pain	Shoulder Elbow Hand Hip Knee Ankle Foot	Boys (n = 282) Girls (n = 287) % % 6 14 4 4 5 7 5 7 32 29 7 12 8 11	High
Slowinska et al. 2015	Cross-sectional	Poland School based	6– 7 yrs	Questionnaire filled in by parents	1509	1509/ 2748 (55%)		Prevalence often	Knee Hands	Often 11% 3%	High
Verhagen et al. 2009	Prospective cohort	Holland school based (iplay study)	10– 12 yrs	Injuries during physical activity monitored by teachers	996/ (996 + 95) (91%)			Incidence Rate	Shoulder Upper arm/ elbow Lower arm/wrist/ hand Upper leg/hip Knee	$0.03 \times 0.48 = 0.01$[c] $0.03 \times 0.48 = 0.01$[c] $0.22 \times 0.48 = 0.11$[c] $0.06 \times 0.48 = 0.03$[c] $0.11 \times 0.48 = 0.05$[c] $0.25 \times 0.48 = 0.12$[c] $0.15 \times 0.48 = 0.07$[c]	High

Table 2 Summary of study characteristics of the 22 included studies (Continued)

Author and year of publication	Study Design	Setting	Age/grade	Measurements (how did they ask?)	Study Size	Baseline response rate	Follow up response rate	Prevalence/incidence	Type of complaints	Main result (text)	Bias
									Lower leg/ankle Foot		
Clinical population studies											
Bot et al. 2005	Cross-sectional	Holland Second Dutch National Servey of generel practice	0– 19 yrs	ICPC codes	375,899(all ages)			Incidence per 1000 person years	L08 Shoulder complaint L09 Arm complaint L10 Elbow complaint L11 wrist complaint L12 Hand/finger complaint L92 Shoulder syndrome	Age group (years) Sex 0-9 (95% CI) 10-19 (95% CI) M: 0.6 (0.3–0.9) M: 4.0 (3.2–4.9) F: 0.7 (0.4–1.1) F: 4.8 (3.9–5.7) M: 2.0 (1.4–2.6) M:2.3 (1.7–3.0) F:2.3 (1.7–2.9) F: 2.8 (2.1–3.5) M: 1.3 (0.9–1.8) M: 2.3 (1.7–3.0) F: 1.7 (1.2–2.3) F: 1.9 (1.3–2.4) M: 1.8 (1.3–2.4) M: 6.3 (5.3–7.4) F: 2.1 (1.5–2.7) F: 7.9 (6.8–9.1) M: 5.0 (4.1–5.9) M: 8.7 (7.5–9.8) F: 3.9 (3.1–4.7) F: 9.1 (7.8–10.3) M: 0.1 (0.0–0.3) M: 1.4 (0.9–1.9) F: 0.0 ((0.0–0.1) F: 1.9 (1.3–2.4)	Low
Henschke et al. 2014	Cross-sectional	Australia national study in general practice – Bettering the Evaluation and Care of Health	5– 17 yrs	ICPC-2 codes	65,279 encounters			Management rate per 100 encounters (encs.)	Lower Limb Upper Limb Lower Limb Upper Limb Lower Limb Upper Limb	Age: 5–9 Boys Girls Number 118121 Rate/100 encs. 1.72 1.85 (95% CI) (1.39–2.06) (1.51–2.19) Number 89 90 Rate/100 encs. 1.30 1.38 (95% CI) (1.02–1.58) (1.09–1.66) Age: 10–14 Boys Girls Number 311254 Rate/100 encs 5.33 4.40	Low

Table 2 Summary of study characteristics of the 22 included studies (*Continued*)

Author and year of publication	Study Design	Setting	Age/ grade	Measurements (how did they ask?)	Study Size	Baseline response rate	Follow up response rate	Prevalence/ incidence	Type of complaints	Main result (text)	Bias
										(95% CI) (4.72–5.95) (3.85–4.96) Number 257188 Rate/100 encs 4.41 3.26 (95% CI) (3.85–4.97) (2.76–3.76) Age: 15–17 Boys Girls Number 169134 Rate/100 encs 4.55 2.26 (95% CI) (3.84–5.26) (1.87–2.65) Number 169 82 Rate/100 encs. 4.55 1.38 (95% CI) (3.83–5.27) (1.08–1.69)	
van der Waal et al. 2006	Cross-sectional	Holland Second Dutch National Servey of generel practice	0– 19 yrs	ICPC codes	375,899(all ages)			Incidence per 1000 person years	L13 Hip complaints L14 Leg/thigh complaints L15 Knee complaints L16 Ankle complaints L17 Foot/toe complaints L77 sprain of ankle/ft L78 sprain/strain of knees Acute meniscus/ ligament knee L97 Chronic int knee derangement	Age group (years) 0–9 (95% CI) 10–19 (95% CI) M: 4.0 (3.2–4.8) M: 2.1 (1.5–2.7) F: 4.9 (3.9–5.8) F: 2.2 (1.6–2.8) M: 4.1 (3.3–4.9) M: 5.1 (4.2–6.0) F: 4.2 (3.4–5.1) F: 4.3 (3.4–5.1) M: 3.6 (2.8–4.3) M: 17.0 (15.3–18.6) F: 2.7 (2.1–3.4) F: 16.7 (15.0–18.3) M: 2.4 (1.8–3.0) M: 5.3 (4.4–6.2) F: 1.9 (1.3–2.5) F: 5.0 (4.1–5.9) M: 9.2 (8.0–10.4) M: 16.2 (14.6–17.8) F: 8.5 (7.2–9.7) F: 14.3 (12.7–15.8) M: 3.6 (2.8–4.3) M: 15.4 (13.8–17.0) F: 3.8 (3.0–4.6) F: 16.4 (14.7–18.0) M: 0.9 (0.54–1.33) F: 6.0 (5.0–7.0)	Low

Table 2 Summary of study characteristics of the 22 included studies (*Continued*)

Author and year of publication	Study Design	Setting	Age/ grade	Measurements (how did they ask?)	Study Size	Baseline response rate	Follow up response rate	Prevalence/ incidence	Type of complaints	Main result (text)	Bias
										F: 0.4 (0.1–0.7) F: 3.7 (2.9–4.5) M: 0.1 (−0.03–0.2) F: 1.2 (0.8–1.7) F: 0 F: 0.8 (0.5–1.2) M: 0.4 (0.1–0.6) F: 4.3 (3.4–5.1) F: 0.6 (0.3–0.9) F: 7.0 (5.9–8.1)	

ICD-10: International Classification of Diseases – 10

ICPC: International Classification of Primary Care

[a] Only baseline were reported

[b] percentages taken from Fig. 1 in the original article

[c] percentage taken from Fig. 1 in the original article times the total incidence rate per 1000 exposure hours (0.48)

Table 3 General population studies. Prevalence and incidence rates of musculoskeletal extremity complaints in the younger age groups

	0–9 years of age					9–12 years of age			2–19 years of age
	Incidence		Prevalence, %			Incidence	Prevalence, %		Prevalence, %
Anatomic Region/ Site	Weekly, %	IR[a]	Often	Weekly	12 months	IR[a]	2 weeks	Weekly	12 months
Upper extremity in general	0.2 [14]		**2.6–6.2** [51]	0.5 [14]	4.8 [47]		0.4 [40]	5.5–7 [41]	5.1 [35]
Shoulder		0.06 [39]				0.01 [54]			
Elbow		0.03 [39]				0.01 [54]			
Wrist/hand/fingers		0.14 [39]	**3** [53]			0.11 [54][b]			
Lower extremity in general	1.0 [14]		**14.6–21.1** [51]	4.1 [14]	10.9 [47]		4.1 [40]	18.3 [15]18–19 [41]	5.8 [35]
Hip/groin		0.06 [39]				0.03 [54]		3.4 [15]	
Thigh		0.07 [39]						10.3 [15]	
Knee		0.40 [39]	**11** [53]			0.05 [54]	1.8 [40][c]	12.4 [15]	
Shin		0.12 [39]							
Ankle/ft		0.71 [39]				0.19 [54][d]	2.4 [40]	10.6 [15]	

[x]: reference number of included study
Bold: the study received high risk of bias in the quality assessment
[a] Incidence Rate per 1000 physical activity units
[b] Anatomical site relates to both lower arm, wrist, hand and fingers
[c] Anatomical site relates to both hip and knee
[d] Anatomical site relates to both shin and ankle/ft

common site of complaint in younger children [39, 54] (Table 3), whereas shoulder complaints were more common among older children [42, 50, 52] (Table 4). The least frequent anatomical site of complaint reported in both younger and older children was the elbow (Tables 3 and 4).

Clinical population studies
Also in the clinical population studies, lower extremity complaints were more frequent than complaints from the upper extremities [44–46]. Two of the three clinical population studies were based on data from the same cohort of children, but one reported on upper

Table 4 General population studies. Prevalence and incidence rates of musculoskeletal extremity complaints in the older age groups

	10–19 years of age								6–17 years of age
	Incidence, %		Prevalence, %						Prevalence, %
Anatomic Region/Site	6 months	12 months	Point	Often/ usually	Weekly	2 weeks	Monthly	6 months	Lifetime
Upper extremity in general	19.9 [37]	13.3 [37]		**9.4–11.7** [51]	3.9–4.0 [38]	2.7 [40]	3.6–4.2 [36]		
Shoulder	8 [37]	5 [37]	13.3 [42]	**6–14** [52]				**33–63** [50]	
Arm	9 [37]	7 [37]							
Elbow			2.6 [42]	**4** [52]				**2–5** [50]	
Wrist/hand/fingers			4.4 [42]	**5–7** [52]				**15–23** [50]	
Lower extremity in general	21 [43]	16 [43]		**28.9–31.9** [51]	8.6–12.8 [38]	12.4 [40]			
Hip/groin	7 [43]	4 [43]	5.9 [42]	**5–7** [52]					
Thigh			2.7 [42]						
Knee	13 [43]	11 [43]	32.3 [42]	**29–32** [52]		6.5 [40][a]	25 [48]	**17–21** [50]	
Shin			6.2 [42]						
Ankle/ft	14 [43]	8 [43]	11.5 [42]	**7–12** [52]		5.5 [40]		**15–19** [50]	3.5 [49]

[x]: reference number of included study
Bold: the study received high risk of bias in the quality assessment
[a] Anatomical site is relates to both hip and knee

Table 5 Clinical population studies. Prevalence and incidence rates of musculoskeletal extremity complaints in children by age group

Anatomic Region/Site	0–9 years of age		10–19 years of age	
	Incidence, %		Incidence, %	
	Per 1000 person years	Management rate per 100 encounters[a]	Per 1000 person years	Management rate per 100 encounters[a]
Upper extremity in general		1.30–1.38 [45]		1.38–4.55 [45]
Shoulder	0.0–0.7 [44]		1.4–4.8 [44]	
Arm	2.0–2.3 [44]		2.3–2.8 [44]	
Elbow	1.3–1.7 [44]		1.9–2.3 [44]	
Wrist/hand/finger	1.8–5.0 [44]		6.3–9.1 [44]	
Lower extremity in general		1.72–1.85 [45]		2.26–5.33 [45]
Hip/groin	4.0–4.9 [46]		2.1–2.2 [46]	
Thigh	4.1–4.2 [46]		4.3–5.1 [46]	
Knee	0.0–3.6 [46]		0.8–17.0 [46]	
Ankle/ft	1.9–9.2 [46]		5.0–16.2 [46]	

[x]: reference number of included study
[a] Management rate per 100 encounters: diagnoses recorded at general practitioners per 100 consecutive encounters

extremities [44] and the other on lower [46]. In the younger children the incidence rate of ankle/ft complaints was about three times higher than for the knee, whereas the incidence rates were almost equal for the two pain sites in the older children [46]. In the upper extremity, wrist/hand/fingers was the most common site in both age groups [44]. The least frequent site of

Table 6 Results from three population based studies including a distinction between traumatic or non-traumatic mode of onset

Anatomic Region/Site	Non-traumatic	Traumatic	Ratio Non-traumatic: Traumatic
Upper extremity in general	0.04 [14][a] 0.2 [14][b]	0.1 [14][a] 0.3 [14][b]	1:2.5 1:1.5
Shoulder	0.03 [39][c]	0.03 [39][c]	1:1
Elbow	0.01 [39][c]	0.02 [39][c]	1:2
Hand/wrist/fingers	0.01 [39][c]	0.13 [39][c]	1:13
Lower extremity in general	12.3 [15][b] 0.7 [14][a] 3.2 [14][b]	6.0 [15][b] 0.3 [14][a] 1.1 [14][b]	1:0.5 1:0.4 1:0.3
Hip	2.7 [15][b] 0.05 [39][c]	0.7 [15][b] 0.01 [39][c]	1:0.3 1:0.2
Thigh	9.5 [15][b] 0.04 [39][c]	0.9 [15][b] 0.03 [39][c]	1:0.1 1:0.8
Knee	10.3 [15][b] 0.31 [39][c]	2.1 [15][b] 0.09 [39][c]	1:0.2 1:0.3
Shin	0.11 [39][c]	0.01 [39][c]	1:0.01
Ankle/Foot	8.8 [15][b] 0.46 [39][c]	1.8 [15][b] 0.25 [39][c]	1:0.2 1:0.5

[x]: reference number of included study
[a] weekly incidence
[b] weekly prevalence
[c] Incidence Rate - per 1000 physical activity units

complaint was the shoulder in the younger group, and shoulder and hip/groin in the older age group (Table 5).

Traumatic versus non-traumatic complaints

In the younger children, three of the general population studies classified the complaints of the lower extremities into traumatic or non-traumatic mode of onset [14, 15, 39], but two of these were based on the same cohort of children [14, 39]. All three reported about two times more non-traumatic complaints compared to traumatic complaints (1:0.5 [15], 1:0.3 and 1:0.4 [14], respectively). One of the studies also reported mode of onset in upper extremities and found the opposite relationship, with non-traumatic complaints less frequently reported than traumatic complaints (1:1.5 and 1:2.5, for prevalence and incidence respectively) [14] (Table 6). There were no reports of mode of onset in other studies, neither in the older age group nor in the clinical population studies.

General population studies versus clinical population studies

Comparing lower and upper extremities in general, MEC were reported up to ten times more often from the lower than from the upper extremities (mean ratio 1:4.0; range 1:1.1 to 1:10.3) in the general population studies (Tables 3 and 4), whereas the difference was much smaller in the clinical population studies with ratios from 1:1.2 to 1:1.6 (mean 1:1.4) (Table 5). In the general population studies, the difference was more significant in the younger children (mean ratio 1:5.1; range 1:2.3 to 1:10.3) than in the older children (mean ratio 1:2.5; range 1:1.1 to 1:4.6).

Consequences of quality

No pattern of differences in reporting could be detected between studies of high and low risk of bias.

Discussion

In the general population studies, ankle/ft and knee were the most frequently reported anatomical complaint sites. We found relatively more ankle/ft complaints in the younger children and more knee complaints in the older age group, and this pattern has to our knowledge not been reported before. The dominance of ankle/ft and knee complaints was similar to what was found in a review of sports-related injuries in children and adolescents [11] indicating either that many of these complaints often are related to sport, or that sports participation actually reveals otherwise unnoticed injuries. A possible explanation for the changing complaint pattern with age could be the development of the musculoskeletal system due to pubertal growth including a general rapid physical growth [56]. One consequence of this could be that the calcaneal growth plate is stressed by the Achilles tendon (Sever's disease) in younger children whereas, when the child matures, the growth of the immature skeleton more commonly leads to apophysitis around the anterior knee located to the tibial tubercle or the inferior patellar pool, leading to more knee complaints in older child. Another shift with age was the relatively high occurrence of shoulder complaints in older children, whereas this was very rare in younger children. One explanation could be that teenagers in general spend more time in front of desktops or tablets, which might lead to posture related pain especially in the neck/shoulder region [57]. Whether these complaints actually relate to the shoulder joint or whether it is more related to the upper spine or the trapezius muscle is uncertain. It might be difficult for children and adolescents to distinguish between those two sources of pain, and it has been documented previously that neck and back pain increase with age during adolescence [4, 58]. If that is the case, the self-reported shoulder complaints are overestimated. To gain more reliable knowledge in this area, detailed questionnaires, including mannequin drawings, or interviews should be used in future studies.

In the clinical population studies, a similar pattern was seen for the lower extremities, but wrist/hand/fingers was the second most frequently reported site among young children, and the third most frequent in the older age group. However, this was based on only one study [44], albeit of high quality. In a review of fractures, Clark et al. also reported this area (the distal radius, fingers and carpal bones) to be the most common [16], indicating a certain susceptibility to both severe and more trivial injuries in the hand and wrist.

We found that lower extremity complaints were much more common than upper extremity complaints in the general population studies, whereas the clinical population studies showed a smaller difference in frequency between the two regions. Furthermore, the three studies reporting mode of onset, reported twice as many non-traumatic compared to traumatic complaints in the lower extremities. These two findings might indicate an overrepresentation of less severe complaints and/or more non-traumatic complaints in the lower extremities. In sports medicine, data collection traditionally has been based on diagnoses from emergency departments or among athletes requiring medical attention or time-loss definitions, and therefore reports of minor complaints have not been collected [59, 60]. In 1989, Backx et al. found that only 31% of all sports injuries led to health care usage [61], e.g. were serious enough to warrant consultation.

Recently Clarsen et al. developed a new tool to register overuse injuries in sport and compared it to the traditional time-loss registration of injuries. They found a completely different pattern of injuries in sport with especially more shoulder, knee and low back injuries [62], which support the thesis that some shoulder and knee complaints do not reach the threshold for health care consultation. In relation to reports of shoulder complaints, we also noted that prevalence rates were relatively high compared to incidence rates, which might indicate that these complaints are more long-lasting than other complaints which have smaller differences between prevalence and incidence rates. However, it could also be due to the misclassification mentioned earlier and actually relate to the neck or Trapezius area.

Most of the studies were conducted in the northern part of Europe and different patterns of complaints could possibly be present in other parts of the world. The type of injury might be related to the prevalent type of sport, and obviously there are large geographical differences in sport activities. Likewise, the threshold for reporting pain and the pattern of health care consumption are strongly culturally dependent, and therefore caution should be exercised when extrapolating results to other parts of the world.

The largest challenge of this review was the heterogeneity of outcomes; pooling of results to obtain reliable combined estimates of prevalence and incidence was impossible to conduct. The included 22 articles in this review used 14 different outcome measures, and this prevented meaningful combined estimates of prevalence or incidence.

The variation in outcome measurement and lack of knowledge in this area, also made it difficult to assess the risk of bias in the 'Outcome measurement' domain, which might have resulted in a too positive bias rating. Although the QUIPS tool has been validated [25] the modified version tool used in this review has not, which might be considered as a limitation of this review. Finally, it would have been appropriate to repeat the literature search in other databases. However, it is our experience that epidemiological articles can be found in the two databases that were used, MEDLINE and EMBASE, and therefore we do believe that the performed literature search can be justified, although we realize that potential relevant articles can have be missed.

Another issue in relation to heterogeneity is that there are challenges with use of questionnaires within this age group. In seven of the 19 general population studies, questionnaires or text messages were answered by parents [14, 39, 40, 47, 49, 51, 53]. Therefore, the concordance between parents' and children's reporting is important to understand. In general, agreement between children and parents is poor, especially in relation to minor complaints, whereas more severe complaints result in a better agreement [63–65]. Another potential problem is that the questionnaires have rarely been validated in the appropriate age groups, and finally the risk of recall bias might differ between children and adults. Harel et al. evaluated recall periods of 2 weeks to 12 months in children and adolescents in the US and found that reporting of severe injuries are not strongly affected by recall bias [66]. Another study by Moshiro et al., with a recall period of twelve months, found the same in an all-age cohort from Tanzania [67]. On the other hand, Harel et al. also concluded that reporting of minor complaints *are* affected by memory, especially if the recall period exceeds five months [66]. This indicates that to collect reliable estimates of minor symptoms the recall period needs to be relatively short. On this note, severity of complaint also needs to be considered, and this was often not the case in the included studies. In four of the 19 general population studies, participants were asked to categorize the complaints according to either severity or frequency, e.g. if the complaint was experienced never, once a month or once a week [15, 38, 41, 42], and in three other studies, consulting a physician was used as a measure of severity [47, 50, 54], but in the remaining studies no severity measures were reported.

Thus, in future studies data should be collected in a standardized way with due consideration to demarcation of the area, the parent/child reporting relationship, the severity and the frequency of pain. It became apparent during this review, that there is a strong need for better and more homogenous data collection methods. We therefore think it is time to make an effort to standardize future studies in relation to data collection with due to consideration to demarcation of the area, the severity and frequency of pain, and the parent/child reporting relationship. Furthermore, common age group definitions should be agreed upon. This could for example be

obtained through a Delphi process followed by a cross-cultural adaption of age-standardized questionnaires.

Fortunately, the profound heterogeneity did not affect the comparisons between anatomical sites, age groups etc. However, another difficulty encountered was that different terms of MEC complicated the literature search and therefore we are aware that there might be articles missing. Hopefully, the assistance of a research librarian and a wide search strategy has minimized the effect of this difficulty.

Conclusion

In general, ankle/ft and knee were the most frequent sites of musculoskeletal extremity complaints regardless of age and type of population. However, in the general population studies, there were relatively more non-traumatic complaints of the lower extremities than in the clinical population studies, indicating a large amount of non-traumatic low intensity complaints in the general population that do not reach threshold for consultation.

We intended to describe the prevalence and incidence of musculoskeletal extremity complaints in children and adolescents, but a meta-analysis, or even a simple overall description of prevalence and incidence, was not feasible, due to study heterogeneity, primarily related to outcome. Future research should use standardised and validated outcome measures and investigate the possible consequences of the low intensity complaints in large longitudinal cohorts to establish if there is a potential for prevention of long-term sequelae through early detection and intervention.

Abbreviation
KBD: Kristina Boe Dissing; LH: Lise Hestbæk; MEC: Musculoskeletal extremity complaint; QUIPS: Quality In Prognosis Studies; SF: Signe Fuglkjær

Acknowledgements
We would like to acknowledge research librarians Johan Wallin and Majbritt Johansen for their help with the literature search.

Funding
Not applicable.

Authors' contributions
LH and SF conceived the study idea. SF, LH and KBD participated in the interpretation of the results and for the first draft of the manuscript. All authors read, revised and approved the final version of the manuscript.

Competing interests
The authors declare that they have no competing interests.

Author details

[1]Department of Sports Science and Clinical Biomechanics, Faculty of Health Sciences, University of Southern Denmark, Campusvej 55, DK-5230 Odense M, Denmark. [2]Nordic Institute of Chiropractic and Clinical Biomechanics, Campusvej 55, DK-5230 Odense M, Denmark.

References

1. Disease GBD, Injury I, Prevalence C. Global, regional, and national incidence, prevalence, and years lived with disability for 310 diseases and injuries, 1990-2015: a systematic analysis for the global burden of disease study 2015. Lancet. 2016;388(10053):1545–602.

2. Martin BI, Deyo RA, Mirza SK, Turner JA, Comstock BA, Hollingworth W, Sullivan SD. Expenditures and health status among adults with back and neck problems. JAMA. 2008;299(6):656–64.

3. Jeffries LJ, Milanese SF, Grimmer-Somers KA. Epidemiology of adolescent spinal pain: a systematic overview of the research literature. Spine (Phila Pa 1976). 2007;32(23):2630–7.

4. Aartun E, Hartvigsen J, Wedderkopp N, Hestbaek L. Spinal pain in adolescents: prevalence, incidence, and course: a school-based two-year prospective cohort study in 1,300 Danes aged 11-13. BMC Musculoskelet Disord. 2014;15:187.

5. Dissing KB, Hestbaek L, Hartvigsen J, Williams C, Kamper S, Boyle E, Wedderkopp N. Spinal pain in Danish school children - how often and how long? The CHAMPS study-DK. BMC Musculoskelet Disord. 2017;18(1):67.

6. Janssen I, Leblanc AG. Systematic review of the health benefits of physical activity and fitness in school-aged children and youth. Int J Behav Nutr Phys Act. 2010;7:40.

7. Ekblom B, Astrand PO. Role of physical activity on health in children and adolescents. Acta Paediatr. 2000;89(7):762–4.

8. Andersen LB, Riddoch C, Kriemler S, Hills AP. Physical activity and cardiovascular risk factors in children. Br J Sports Med. 2011;45(11):871–6.

9. Expert Panel on Integrated Guidelines for Cardiovascular H, Risk Reduction in C, Adolescents, National Heart L, Blood I. Expert panel on integrated guidelines for cardiovascular health and risk reduction in children and adolescents: summary report, Pediatrics. 2011. 128 Suppl 5:S213–56.

10. Fuller CW, Ekstrand J, Junge A, Andersen TE, Bahr R, Dvorak J, Hagglund M, McCrory P, Meeuwisse WH. Consensus statement on injury definitions and data collection procedures in studies of football (soccer) injuries. Clin J Sport Med. 2006;16(2):97–106.

11. Caine D, Caine C, Maffulli N. Incidence and distribution of pediatric sport-related injuries. Clinical journal of sport medicine : official journal of the Canadian Academy of Sport Medicine. 2006;16(6):500–13.

12. Fernandez WG, Yard EE, Comstock RD. Epidemiology of lower extremity injuries among U.S. high school athletes. Acad Emerg Med Off J Soc Acad Emerg Med. 2007;14(7):641–5.

13. van Mechelen W, Hlobil H, Kemper HC. Incidence, severity, aetiology and prevention of sports injuries. A review of concepts. Sports medicine (Auckland, NZ). 1992;14(2):82–99.

14. Jespersen E, Holst R, Franz C, Rexen CT, Klakk H, Wedderkopp N. Overuse and traumatic extremity injuries in schoolchildren surveyed with weekly text messages over 2.5 years. Scand J Med Sci Sports. 2014;24(5):807–13.

15. El-Metwally A, Salminen JJ, Auvinen A, Kautiainen H, Mikkelsson M. Risk factors for traumatic and non-traumatic lower limb pain among preadolescents: a population-based study of Finnish schoolchildren. BMC Musculoskelet Disord. 2006;7:3.

16. Clark EM. The epidemiology of fractures in otherwise healthy children. Current osteoporosis reports. 2014;12(3):272–8.

17. Doherty C, Delahunt E, Caulfield B, Hertel J, Ryan J, Bleakley C. The incidence and prevalence of ankle sprain injury: a systematic review and meta-analysis of prospective epidemiological studies. Sports medicine (Auckland, NZ). 2014;44(1):123–40.

18. Seah R, Mani-Babu S. Managing ankle sprains in primary care: what is best practice? A systematic review of the last 10 years of evidence. Br Med Bull. 2011;97:105–35.

19. Kerkhoffs GM, Struijs PA, Marti RK, Assendelft WJ, Blankevoort L, van Dijk CN. Different functional treatment strategies for acute lateral ankle ligament injuries in adults. The Cochrane database of systematic reviews. 2002;3: CD002938.

20. Gallo V, Egger M, McCormack V, Farmer PB, Ioannidis JP, Kirsch-Volders M, Matullo G, Phillips DH, Schoket B, Stromberg U, et al. STrengthening the reporting of OBservational studies in epidemiology-molecular epidemiology (STROBE-ME): an extension of the STROBE statement. Eur J Epidemiol. 2011; 26(10):797–810.

21. Dreyer NA, Velentgas P, Westrich K, Dubois R. The GRACE checklist for rating the quality of observational studies of comparative effectiveness: a tale of hope and caution. J Manag Care Spec Pharm. 2014;20(3):301–8.

22. Meader N, King K, Llewellyn A, Norman G, Brown J, Rodgers M, Moe-Byrne T, Higgins JP, Sowden A, Stewart G. A checklist designed to aid consistency and reproducibility of GRADE assessments: development and pilot validation. Systematic reviews. 2014;3:82.

23. [http://methods.cochrane.org/bias/sites/methods.cochrane.org.bias/files/ uploads/Tool to Assess Risk of Bias in Cohort Studies.pdf 'data accessed'].

24. Higgins JP, Altman DG, Gotzsche PC, Juni P, Moher D, Oxman AD, Savovic J, Schulz KF, Weeks L, Sterne JA, et al. The Cochrane Collaboration's tool for assessing risk of bias in randomised trials. BMJ. 2011;343:d5928.

25. Hayden JA, van der Windt DA, Cartwright JL, Cote P, Bombardier C. Assessing bias in studies of prognostic factors. Ann Intern Med. 2013; 158(4):280–6.

26. Sanderson S, Tatt ID, Higgins JP. Tools for assessing quality and susceptibility to bias in observational studies in epidemiology: a systematic review and annotated bibliography. Int J Epidemiol. 2007; 36(3):666–76.

27. von Elm E, Altman DG, Egger M, Pocock SJ, Gotzsche PC, Vandenbroucke JP, Initiative S. The Strengthening the reporting of observational studies in epidemiology (STROBE) statement: guidelines for reporting observational studies. Lancet. 2007;370(9596):1453–7.

28. Picavet HS, Schouten JS. Musculoskeletal pain in the Netherlands: prevalences, consequences and risk groups, the DMC(3)-study. Pain. 2003; 102(1–2):167–78.

29. Kaspiris A, Zafiropoulou C. Growing pains in children: epidemiological analysis in a Mediterranean population. Joint, bone, spine : revue du rhumatisme. 2009;76(5):486–90.

30. Sorensen L, Larsen SE, Rock ND. The epidemiology of sports injuries in school-aged children. Scand J Med Sci Sports. 1996;6(5):281–6.

31. Abou El-Soud AM, Gaballa HA, Ali MA. Prevalence of osteochondritis among preparatory and primary school children in an Egyptian governorate. Rheumatol Int. 2012;32(8):2275–8.

32. El-Metwally A, Salminen JJ, Auvinen A, Kautiainen H, Mikkelsson M. Lower limb pain in a preadolescent population: prognosis and risk factors for chronicity–a prospective 1- and 4-year follow-up study. Pediatrics. 2005; 116(3):673–81.

33. Menz HB, Jordan KP, Roddy E, Croft PR. Characteristics of primary care consultations for musculoskeletal foot and ankle problems in the UK. Rheumatology. 2010;49(7):1391–8.

34. Siivola SM, Levoska S, Latvala K, Hoskio E, Vanharanta H, Keinanen-Kiukaanniemi S. Predictive factors for neck and shoulder pain: a longitudinal study in young adults. Spine. 2004;29(15):1662–9.

35. Adams AL, Kessler JI, Deramerian K, Smith N, Black MH, Porter AH, Jacobsen SJ, Koebnick C. Associations between childhood obesity and upper and lower extremity injuries. Inj Prev. 2013;19(3):191–7.

36. Diepenmaat AC, van der Wal MF, de Vet HC, Hirasing RA. Neck/shoulder, low back, and arm pain in relation to computer use, physical activity, stress, and depression among Dutch adolescents. Pediatrics. 2006;117(2):412–6.

37. Ehrmann Feldman D, Shrier I, Rossignol M, Abenhaim L. Risk factors for the development of neck and upper limb pain in adolescents. Spine (Phila Pa 1976). 2002;27(5):523–8.

38. Hoftun GB, Romundstad PR, Zwart JA, Rygg M. Chronic idiopathic pain in adolescence–high prevalence and disability: the young HUNT study 2008. Pain. 2011;152(10):2259–66.

39. Jespersen E, Rexen CT, Franz C, Moller NC, Froberg K, Wedderkopp N. Musculoskeletal extremity injuries in a cohort of schoolchildren aged 6-12: a 2.5-year prospective study. Scand J Med Sci Sports. 2015;25(2):251–8.

40. Krul M, van der Wouden JC, Schellevis FG, van Suijlekom-Smit LW, Koes BW. Musculoskeletal problems in overweight and obese children. Ann Fam Med. 2009;7(4):352–6.

41. Mikkelsson M, Salminen JJ, Kautiainen H. Non-specific musculoskeletal pain in preadolescents. Prevalence and 1-year persistence. Pain. 1997;73(1):29–35.

42. Rathleff MS, Roos EM, Olesen JL, Rasmussen S. High prevalence of daily and multi-site pain–a cross-sectional population-based study among 3000 Danish adolescents. BMC Pediatr. 2013;13:191.

43. Shrier I, Ehrmann-Feldman D, Rossignol M, Abenhaim L. Risk factors for development of lower limb pain in adolescents. J Rheumatol. 2001;28(3):604–9.

44. Bot SD, van der Waal JM, Terwee CB, van der Windt DA, Schellevis FG, Bouter LM, Dekker J. Incidence and prevalence of complaints of the neck and upper extremity in general practice. Ann Rheum Dis. 2005;64(1):118–23.

45. Henschke N, Harrison C, McKay D, Broderick C, Latimer J, Britt H, Maher CG. Musculoskeletal conditions in children and adolescents managed in Australian primary care. BMC Musculoskelet Disord. 2014;15:164.

46. van der Waal JM, Bot SD, Terwee CB, van der Windt DA, Schellevis FG, Bouter LM, Dekker J. The incidences of and consultation rate for lower extremity complaints in general practice. Ann Rheum Dis. 2006;65(6):809–15.

47. Hulsegge G, van Oostrom SH, Picavet HS, Twisk JW, Postma DS, Kerkhof M, Smit HA, Wijga AH. Musculoskeletal complaints among 11-year-old children and associated factors: the PIAMA birth cohort study. Am J Epidemiol. 2011; 174(8):877–84.

48. Molgaard C, Rathleff MS, Simonsen O. Patellofemoral pain syndrome and its association with hip, ankle, and foot function in 16- to 18-year-old high school students: a single-blind case-control study. J Am Podiatr Med Assoc. 2011;101(3):215–22.

49. Abujam B, Mishra R, Aggarwal A. Prevalence of musculoskeletal complaints and juvenile idiopathic arthritis in children from a developing country: a school-based study. Int J Rheum Dis. 2014;17(3):256–60.

50. Auvinen JP, Paananen MV, Tammelin TH, Taimela SP, Mutanen PO, Zitting PJ, Karppinen JI. Musculoskeletal pain combinations in adolescents. Spine (Phila Pa 1976). 2009;34(11):1192–7.

51. Bishop JL, Northstone K, Emmett PM, Golding J. Parental accounts of the prevalence, causes and treatments of limb pain in children aged 5 to 13 years: a longitudinal cohort study. Arch Dis Child. 2012;97(1):52–3.

52. Smedbraten BK, Natvig B, Rutle O, Bruusgaard D. Self-reported bodily pain in schoolchildren. Scand J Rheumatol. 1998;27(4):273–6.

53. Słowińska IKM, Jednacz E, Mańczak M, Rutkowska-Sak LRF. Pain associated with the musculoskeletal system in children from Warsaw schools. Reumatologia. 2015;52(3):4.

54. Verhagen E, Collard D, Paw MC, van Mechelen W. A prospective cohort study on physical activity and sports-related injuries in 10-12-year-old children. Br J Sports Med. 2009;43(13):1031–5.

55. Feldman DE, Shrier I, Rossignol M, Abenhaim L. Risk factors for the development of low back pain in adolescence. Am J Epidemiol. 2001; 154(1):30–6.

56. Patton GC, Viner R. Pubertal transitions in health. Lancet. 2007; 369(9567):1130–9.

57. Brink Y, Louw QA. A systematic review of the relationship between sitting and upper quadrant musculoskeletal pain in children and adolescents. Man Ther. 2013;18(4):281–8.

58. Kjaer P, Wedderkopp N, Korsholm L, Leboeuf-Yde C. Prevalence and tracking of back pain from childhood to adolescence. BMC Musculoskelet Disord. 2011;12:98.

59. Fuller CW, Ekstrand J, Junge A, Andersen TE, Bahr R, Dvorak J, Hagglund M, McCrory P, Meeuwisse WH. Consensus statement on injury definitions and data collection procedures in studies of football (soccer) injuries. Br J Sports Med. 2006;40(3):193–201.

60. Bahr R. No injuries, but plenty of pain? On the methodology for recording overuse symptoms in sports. Br J Sports Med. 2009;43(13):966–72.

61. Backx FJ, Erich WB, Kemper AB, Verbeek AL. Sports injuries in school-aged children. An epidemiologic study. Am J Sports Med. 1989;17(2):234–40.

62. Clarsen B, Myklebust G, Bahr R. Development and validation of a new method for the registration of overuse injuries in sports injury epidemiology: the Oslo sports trauma research Centre (OSTRC) overuse injury questionnaire. Br J Sports Med. 2013;47(8):495–502.

63. Sundblad GM, Saartok T, Engstrom LM. Child-parent agreement on reports of disease, injury and pain. BMC Public Health. 2006;6:276.

64. Singer AJ, Gulla J, Thode HC Jr. Parents and practitioners are poor judges of young children's pain severity. Acad Emerg Med Off J Soc Acad Emerg Med. 2002;9(6):609–12.

65. Kroner-Herwig B, Morris L, Heinrich M, Gassmann J, Vath N. Agreement of parents and children on characteristics of pediatric headache, other pains, somatic symptoms, and depressive symptoms in an epidemiologic study. Clin J Pain. 2009;25(1):58–64.

66. Harel Y, Overpeck MD, Jones DH, Scheidt PC, Bijur PE, Trumble AC, Anderson J. The effects of recall on estimating annual nonfatal injury rates for children and adolescents. Am J Public Health. 1994;84(4):599–605.

67. Moshiro C, Heuch I, Astrom AN, Setel P, Kvale G. Effect of recall on estimation of non-fatal injury rates: a community based study in Tanzania. Inj Prev. 2005;11(1):48–52.

68. Slowinska I, Kwiatkowska M, Jednacz E, Manczak M, Rutkowska-Sak L, Raciborski F. Pain associated with the musculoskeletal system in children from Warsaw schools. Reumatologia. 2015;53(3):139–42.

25

A qualitative study of patient education needs for hip and knee replacement

Deborah Kennedy[1,2,3*], Amy Wainwright[1,3], Lucy Pereira[1], Susan Robarts[1], Patricia Dickson[1,4], Jennifer Christian[5] and Fiona Webster[6]

Abstract

Background: Quality health information is key to patient engagement, self-management and an enhanced healthcare experience. There is strong evidence to support involving patients and their families in the development and evaluation of health-related educational material. These factors were the impetus for our high volume joint replacement centre to undertake a qualitative study to elicit patient experiences to inform the development of effective strategies and education along the care continuum for hip and knee replacement.

Methods: Purposively selected patients from postoperative follow-up clinics were recruited to participate in a focus group or telephone interview. We developed a semi-structured interview guide that addressed four specific aspects of the patient's experience with educational material: pre-surgery, hospital stay, recovery period and future recommendations. The focus groups and interviews continued to the point of saturation and were audio-recorded and transcribed verbatim. Interview transcripts were coded and then inductively organized into larger categories using thematic analysis.

Results: Six focus groups and seven telephone interviews were conducted, totalling 32 participants. One of the key themes that emerged was a need for more education concerning pain management post-operatively; specifically, patients wanted more information on expected levels of pain, pain medication usage, management of side effects and guidelines for weaning off the medication. There was surprising variability in patients' descriptions of their pre-surgery, surgery and recovery experiences. These corresponded to an equally diverse range of preferences for educational content, delivery and timing. Many patients reported using the web while others preferred traditional formats for information delivery. There was some interest in receiving education using mobile technology.

Conclusions: Our findings validate the importance of multi-modal patient education tailored to individual preferences and experiences, which may differ according to such characteristics as gender and age. The gap in pain management information is a critical finding for healthcare providers working with patients undergoing joint replacement. Developing pain management education in different formats that addresses frequently asked questions will enhance patient engagement and, their overall experience and recovery.

Keywords: Patient engagement, Hip and knee replacement, Education, Pain management, Person-centred care

---

* Correspondence: Deborah.kennedy@sunnybrook.ca
[1]Sunnybrook Holland Orthopaedic and Arthritic Centre, 43 Wellesley Street East, Toronto, ON M4Y 1H1, Canada
[2]School of Rehabilitation Science, McMaster University, 1400 Main St. W, Hamilton, ON L8S 1C7, Canada
Full list of author information is available at the end of the article

Background

In our increasingly complex healthcare environment, patients require high quality information to successfully manage their health. Although access to information on the web and other sources has increased, it has not necessarily translated to increased understanding. Often patient health information has been created from the lens of the providers without patient consultation.

In 2015, the World Health Organization released a global strategy on people-centred and integrated health services calling for a fundamental shift in the way health services are managed and delivered [1]. The current focus for healthcare organizations is a person-centred care approach, where the patient's values, knowledge, preferences and needs are central to their care. There is strong evidence to support the importance of involving patients and their families in the development and evaluation of educational material for health purposes [2, 3].

Currently, there is limited literature exploring the education needs of patients and their families in many patient populations including that of hip and knee replacement. This information would be extremely useful in the design of effective strategies that support and educate patients both prior to, in hospital and after discharge. Given the growing prevalence of this surgery, along with shortening lengths of stay, patients need this type of information for shared decision-making.

These factors were the impetus for our team to undertake a qualitative study at our high volume joint replacement centre and seek the voice of our patients about their educational needs and preferences. Our study question was, "What are the informational needs and delivery preferences for education of families and patients undergoing hip or knee replacement?"

Methods

Design and setting

The study was conducted in a large Canadian orthopaedic centre specialized in joint replacement surgery. Using descriptive qualitative methods [4], purposefully selected patients were recruited from outpatient clinics at their 6 week to one-year follow-up visits post joint replacement.

Sampling

Using purposeful sampling, a small percentage of patients were invited to participate in the study to explore their experiences and preferences for education following hip or knee replacement surgery [5]. Maximum variation sampling was used to ensure we had participants who differed by age, gender, affected joint, and marital status. This helped to ensure that the patients we interviewed were similar to those regularly seen at our facility. We did not collect information about socio-

economic status. We conducted focus groups as well as telephone interviews to accommodate those who did not reside within the urban setting of the hospital. One spouse attended a focus group at the participant's request as she did not feel sufficiently comfortable with English but wanted to share her story. One focus group was composed entirely of men. Six focus groups and seven telephone interviews were conducted totalling 32 participants, at which point our team decided we had generated sufficient data to reach saturation while maintaining a manageable final dataset within this project's timeframe. The mean age of the 32 participants was 67.9 (standard deviation ±7.82; min 46, max 78) years. There was equal distribution of men and women ($n = 16$ each) and similarly, hip and knee replacements. Regarding time point of participation, 44% of the patients were up to 3 months postoperatively, another 44% between 3 months to 9 months and 12% greater than 9 months up to 1 year.

Ethics

Local Research Ethics Board approval was obtained for this study. Patients were approached for consent during their follow-up visits. The clinic secretary asked the patient if they would be willing to receive a consent form, and have someone from research speak to them about participating in a focus group or interview.

Focus groups

We developed a focus group guide to address four specific aspects of the patient's experience with educational material [6]. The guide (see Additional file 1) began with open, broader questions about the patient's educational needs and experiences leading up to surgery and then questions were asked about each stage of the hospital and recovery process. Finally, a series of questions were asked in relation to the patient's preferences for future educational materials, including videos and internet resources. All questions were meant to be exploratory and relied on probes to allow differences between patients in perceptions and experiences to emerge during the course of the interview. The focus group guide was pilot tested with one patient identified by our research team. The objective of pilot testing was to confirm the length of each interview and to ensure that the questions were clear and comprehensible. FW, who is a trained qualitative interviewer, performed the pilot interview with one patient and facilitated several of the focus groups and telephone interviews; other focus groups were conducted by an experienced Research Associate, JC. Members of the healthcare team did not solicit or conduct interviews. All interviews and focus groups were audio-taped and professionally transcribed verbatim.

Data analysis

Data collection and analysis were conducted concurrently. Three members of the research team (DK, FW and JC) read transcriptions of the pilot interview independently to identify codes. The researchers then met to compare their independent analyses and develop a coding framework for use in the subsequent analysis. JC then coded the remaining interviews, keeping memo notes of any potential changes to the coding framework that she identified. After all interviews had been coded, the larger research team held several meetings in which they interpreted the data to identify similarities and differences across the interviews. We combined our codes into themes and identified predominant ones. The relationships between the themes were also summarized in these team meetings.

Our team performed several steps to ensure rigour [6]. To ensure *reliability*, more than one investigator performed each key step. Our analysis was *reflexive* as our team was multidisciplinary, consisting of clinicians, educators and researchers, which allowed us to consider our personal biases during data analysis throughout the memoing and data summarizing steps [6].

Results

Although some people preferred to be interviewed one-on-one rather than in a focus group, we did not find any significant differences in their accounts. For the purposes of this study, using both data collection approaches allowed us to achieve both depth and breadth, increasing the number of participants we could speak with over a relatively short period of time [7]. While qualitative interviews and focus groups are not inter-changeable we did not find significant differences in the data we obtained across using the two approaches. We organized our findings into four main themes: 1) education gaps relating to pain management 2) participant's validation of existing organizational education materials; 3) informal sources of information; and 4) interest in new delivery modes for education, such as mobile health applications.

Theme 1: Educational gaps around pain management

An important finding that emerged from our interviews and focus groups was an identified need to have more education around pain management post-operatively. In particular, participants expressed an interest in education related to expected levels of post-operative pain, the purpose of the prescribed medications, information on how to take the medications, their side effects and how to "wean off" pain medications. In the following account, the patient describes how she needed more information to manage her pain,

"Well, if there was possibility to deal with the pain part more effectively ... that might have been of help. I think [the surgeon] did say if I had any questions ... I could phone them, I just don't think I did because I thought there wasn't really much they could do about, you know, the pain stuff ..." (Participant #1, Interview #4, Female)

Another participant describes his perception of other people's negative experiences of medication side effects. In the following excerpt, he is suggesting that patients are both afraid to ask about medication and are without recourse regarding pain medication once they leave the hospital. He says,

"I mean, I got off those white little pills as fast as I possibly could. I took Tylenol Extra Strength for whatever, and now maybe once a week or so I'll take a couple Tylenol Extra Strength. But two things, one is a lot of the people that go to rehab, they get sick from them, they get sick from those white little pills, whatever they are, OxyContin or oxy-something, they get sick, but the doctor told them to take them and they continue to take them ... but there's no recourse back, and they're afraid to ask, they're definitely afraid to ask about the pills ... So again it's education about medication."
(Participant #1, Focus Group #1, Male)

Participants suggested that nobody provided them with information about how to "wean" themselves off their pain medication once they were back at home.

"...The first time around I expected someone to say to me, "Once you get your pain medication here's a method of getting off of it. Here's a way of weaning yourself off of that," but nobody did this. ..., it was maybe at six weeks I was still taking Oxy. The first time [the pharmacist] go, "You gotta stop doing this," I go, "What do you mean?" No one had told me [that]. ... even this time when I had my hip nobody would give me a method of weaning myself off of it, I had to go back to the pain specialist." (Participant #3, Focus Group #1, Male)

While participants did acknowledge they received information that they would need to reduce their pain medication, they frequently felt that these instructions lacked crucial information about how they would accomplish this in terms of practical steps. As one participant shared,

"I think I started to wean off on my own without realizing it. It was every four hours, I think, if I remember. And then I realized afterwards I had

forgotten one time, and I thought, "Oh, okay, I've been an hour without it," so I took it then because I felt pain. So the next day I really tested it out … Now, I was fortunate … But it was a nurse here, before I left, when I got the prescription, who said to me, "You'll want to wean yourself off," but not how." (Participant #6, Focus Group #1, Female)

Theme 2: Participants' validation of existing materials

Despite identifying a gap in pain management education, patients did validate the usefulness of the existing patient education tools (www.sunnybrook.ca/holland) offered in different mediums both pre and post-operatively. These included a comprehensive guide (organized into preoperative, hospital stay and post discharge sections), a preoperative education class, as well as, a short animated educational YouTube video developed by our organization in partnership with Dr. Mike Evans. Of note, not all participants attended the workshop or recalled seeing the video.

2a) guide for patients having hip or knee replacement

The following participant highlights that the Guide is useful across various stages of the pre to post surgery process and was something she referred to throughout her recovery.

"I like having the book because you don't remember everything you read the first time, and you don't remember everything a month later, so I could go back to the book, especially about preparing and getting ready. So it was nice to have the printed material that I could look at."
(Participant #1, Interview #2, Female)

2b) the preoperative education class

Participants commented on the benefits of attending the Preoperative Education class. They commented on how appropriate preparation *"built their confidence"* (Participant #1, Focus Group #1, Male). This confidence building was important given how many people were initially fearful of having surgery. In the following account, the participant stresses the importance of hearing from another patient and described how valuable it was to have the expertise of the rehabilitation staff.

"I was terrified like I think most people are, and there was a person who'd gone through the surgery who was able to answer any questions that most people had. The physiotherapist and the OT were, you know, incredibly gracious and able to sit down and really, you know, relax most of the patients there." (Participant #1, Pilot Interview, Female)

2c) Dr. Mike Evans' 'preparing you for your hip or knee replacement surgery' (www.sunnybrook.ca/holland/hipknee)

Participants who had viewed the Dr. Mike Evans' video expressed that they had found it helpful, especially as it emphasized and was consistent with the information they had received in the Guide.

"…I think it repeated a lot of what was in the pamphlet, but you could see it. You know, it's concrete, tangible, you see it, very step-by-step, and so it helped me…" (Participant #2, Focus Group #4, Female)

Theme 3: Favoured sources of patient information

Patients identified several sources of information that they drew on most frequently. Not surprisingly, and consistent with other studies, these included family and friends; information they found on the internet (referred to by several participants as "Dr. Google") as well as surgeons.

3a) family and friends

Patients frequently identified friends and families as an important source of information. Hearing stories from other people that their surgeries had been successful seemed to go a long way toward reassuring participants, as the following account exemplifies,

"I think my bigger source was other people that had the same operation…what you do is you gather information, which is all part of the decision-making process, but you gather information from multiple sources and you start to get confident in the things that are consistently heard from everybody, so that's where I got my information."
(Participant #1, Focus Group #2, Female)

At the same time, they voiced their concern that experiential accounts were not necessarily medically valid. Related to this, many voiced a desire to access a bank of patient "testimonials" that the hospital could curate, hence increasing its reliability from a patient perspective. Several noted that they wanted to hear both "good and indifferent" experiences from others:

"What I think is going to be helpful for me is testimonials, good and indifferent … so testimonials from past patients who have had whatever type of surgery, whether it's hip or knee …"
(Participant #3, Focus group #2, Male)

3b) "Dr. Google"

The majority of participants had searched Google for information on the surgery or recovery process. Many did not question the validity or accuracy of this information.

For some participants, mostly men, they wanted to actually watch the surgery *"to see what goes on in the operating room"*.

Women were more likely to indicate that they specifically did not want to view the surgery online, as the following quote exemplifies:

"I just kind of Googled "total knee replacement surgery" or, "required devices required after total knee replacements." "... I didn't look up what the procedure looked like because I thought I might chicken out then." "No, I don't want to see that!""
(Participant#1, Interview #4, Female)

Not all people thought that accessing information on the internet was useful and in some instances it reinforced the fear they already felt about the upcoming surgery.

3c) surgeons as a source of education
Some participants identified the surgeon as their main source of information. While patients felt that surgeons were an important source of knowledgeable information, they often described mixed experiences of how much time they felt surgeons could or did provide.

Theme 4: Interest in new delivery modes for education, such as social media
Several participants were interested in accessing information from newer technologies including mobile health applications and social media. A small number of people said that they would in the future use an app. As one participant noted,

"[It would be] easy access to information to compare notes with other patients who've gone through it ... either from apps or ...Twitter ..."
(Participant #4, Focus group #2, Male)

Other participants, however, were uncertain as to how social media would be useful for them. Some noted that they were comfortable with the computer but did not own smartphones or other technology that would enable them to use newer forms of social media/mobile apps. The following quotes were typical of what we heard during the focus groups.

"I use a computer extensively and I look up a lot of stuff on the Internet, so a website that I can go to is fine, I just don't do the social media, I don't want to get involved, and I don't have a smartphone, don't want one. So for me, you know, that's just my level and my choice. But it might benefit somebody else. We're not dealing too often with younger people who are more into those things." (Participant #3, Focus Group

#3, Female)*"I'm not sure. I'm still learning all these apps. Right now it's information overload."* (Participant #6, Focus Group #1, Female)

Discussion
Our experiences and findings with this study have validated the importance of engaging our patients to fully understand their educational needs and delivery preferences. The largest gap that patients identified related to pain medication education, especially for the time-period after they had left the hospital and were at home recovering. This finding was very interesting to the team as historically, we had been very intentional to include information about pain management in our comprehensive guide and preoperative education classes. However, upon reviewing our materials, we realized that although we covered some core concepts, we did not provide enough details around specific medications or weaning steps.

Chan et al. [8] found that more than half of patients after knee replacement reported the first 2 weeks at home as being the most painful time-period after surgery. Poorly managed pain decreases patient satisfaction, the ability to progress functionally [8, 9] and has been found to increase the likelihood of persistent pain following joint replacement [10]. Chan et al's study of over one hundred patients following knee replacement, after hospital discharge found there was suboptimal use of pain medication and non-pharmacological strategies, misconceptions of pain medication usage, disturbing side effects and inadequate information provided to manage pain at home [8]. Similarly, our patients voiced a need for more information on pain medication usage, side effects and how to wean off at the appropriate time. Given the shortening lengths of stay, these topics are becoming even more important as patients are managing acute pain while at home.

The importance of multiple modalities (pamphlets, classes, videos, Apps) available to patients in plain, clear language has been demonstrated in other populations [11]. Our findings also supported the importance of providing multi-modal education to patients that can be tailored to their individual learning preferences and experiences. Prior research investigating the information needs of patients undergoing arthroplasty found that although a core set of questions could be defined; the information needs across patients was quite variable [12, 13]. While this idea is not novel, we still have to broaden our understanding of the social and cultural differences between patients and how to address these in education.

Participants valued the organization's educational materials, including the comprehensive guide, the YouTube video and the pre-operative education classes. The guide enabled patients to review materials at different stages of recovery. All participants described using this guide repeatedly along the continuum of care. The preoperative education session was highly regarded and reduced fears by enabling patients to ask questions, clarify issues and interact with others undergoing similar surgeries. Several studies have shown the importance of preoperative education in reducing anxiety and improving satisfaction, however study findings are variable as demonstrated in a recent meta-analysis [14–16].

Other sources of information patients accessed included; families and friends, the internet and their surgeons. They strongly favoured learning from the experiences of other patients; often these were friends. For this reason, many suggested that having access to a curated set of patient vignettes or "stories" available on a hospital website would be useful. This would allow them to learn from peer experiences while having the added benefit of providing legitimacy to these accounts, an issue many struggled with in relation to the medical validity of the lay accounts they heard from others or by browsing the web. There was interest in using technology to deliver education such as mobile health apps. Although, not all patients have access to smartphones or tablets, the use of mobile technology is increasing annually. The latest Government of Canada statistics indicated that in 2014, 66% of Canadians owned a smartphone and 49% owned a tablet [17].

The study findings have been the impetus for a number of quality improvement projects. We have strengthened the role of patient and family advisors to improve the care experience. To address the gap in our pain management education, patient advisors and team members co-designed new materials in multimodal formats. We introduced a new brochure and video addressing the top 10 questions about pain medication after joint replacement, the information of which is also available online (www.sunnybrook.ca/hipkneepain). Concurrently, we provided widespread staff education about the new resources.

These experiences have reinforced the importance of including the patient voice, as the healthcare team's focus was not always reflective of patients' preferences. We have also launched a mobile app (with a web-based version to follow shortly) that includes a daily health check with recommendations based on responses and a library of resources on key patient identified topics to empower patients to better manage their recovery. The new pain management information is located in the education library of the mobile app.

Our study had several limitations. Due to resource implications, we recruited only English speaking patients (except in one instance in which an English-speaking spouse participated); future studies might focus on non-English speaking patients. We did not specifically target younger patients for whom the use of mobile technology and social media might be more relevant. Finally, we did

not collect data about individual participant's demographic details such as home support, occupation, marital status and level of education and therefore did not stratify our analysis across these differences. We did however obtain rich, in-depth information about the experiences of our patients, with the goal of providing insight into their experiences, rather than on obtaining statistical generalizability. For this reason, the core concepts from our research should be transferable to other centres wanting to develop more patient-centred education materials.

Conclusion

Patients undergoing hip and knee replacement have a wide range of preferences for educational content, modes of delivery and timing to successfully engage and manage their recovery. The findings of our study underscore the importance of multi-modal patient education that can be tailored to individual preferences and experiences. It is important to offer traditional formats for information delivery as well as alternatives using web and mobile technology.

Patients emphasized the need for more comprehensive education concerning pain management following discharge from hospital. Management of acute postoperative pain remains a significant challenge, particularly for those undergoing knee replacements. Given the trend of shortening lengths of stay, patients are coping with acute pain at home; therefore, they require more information on pain medication usage, side effects and guidelines for weaning off the medications. Since completing this study, our site has introduced a new pain management brochure and video, which are also available online and through our new mobile App.

Acknowledgements
Funding for this study was provided by the Canadian Orthopaedic Foundation whose mission is to achieve excellence in bone and joint health, mobility, and function for all Canadians through the advancement of research, education, and care.
We are grateful to the interprofessional team members for all of their contributions to developing patient-centred educational materials. Of course, without our patients this study would not have been possible, and we thank them for all their support and willingness to participate.

Funding
Funding for this study was provided by the Canadian Orthopaedic Foundation. The Canadian Orthopaedic Foundation was not involved in the design, conduct, data interpretation or publication.

Authors' contributions
DK conceived the idea, designed the study, supervised data collection, assisted with data analysis, and prepared and wrote the manuscript with AW. AW was also involved in qualitative data analysis. LP, SR, PD were involved in study conception and design as well as manuscript review. JC conducted the focus groups and interviews and assisted in the qualitative data analysis

and manuscript preparation. FW was involved in study conception, design, conducted and/or supervised focus groups and interviews, led the qualitative data analysis and contributed to writing the manuscript. All authors read and approved the final manuscript.

Competing interests

The authors declare that they have no competing interests.

Author details

[1]Sunnybrook Holland Orthopaedic and Arthritic Centre, 43 Wellesley Street East, Toronto, ON M4Y 1H1, Canada. [2]School of Rehabilitation Science, McMaster University, 1400 Main St. W, Hamilton, ON L8S 1C7, Canada. [3]Department of Physical Therapy, University of Toronto, 500 University Avenue, Toronto, ON M5G 1V7, Canada. [4]Department of Occupational Science and Occupational Therapy, University of Toronto, 500 University Avenue, Toronto, ON M5G 1V7, Canada. [5]Centre for Addiction and Mental Health, 33 Russell Street, Toronto, ON M5S 2S1, Canada. [6]Institute of Health Policy Management and Evaluation, Dalla Lana School of Public Health, University of Toronto, 155 College Street, Toronto, ON M5T 3M7, Canada.

References

1. World Health Organization global strategy on integrated people-centred health services 2016–2026 [http://www.who.int/servicedeliverysafety/areas/people-centred-care/global-strategy/en/]. Accessed 29 June 2016.
2. Making the Case for Information: The evidence for investing in high quality health information for patients and the public [http://www.pifonline.org.uk/the-case-for-information-investment-in-patient-information-improves-outcomes-and-reduces-costs/]. Accessed 23 Sept 2015.
3. Macdonnell M, Darzi A. A key to slower health spending growth worldwide will be unlocking innovation to reduce the labor-intensity of care. Health Aff (Millwood). 2013;32(4):653–60.
4. Sandelowski M. Whatever happened to qualitative description? Res Nurs Health. 2000;23(4):334–40.
5. Coyne IT. Sampling in qualitative research. Purposeful and theoretical sampling; merging or clear boundaries? J Adv Nurs. 1997;26(3):623–30.
6. Guba EG. Criteria for assessing the trustworthiness of naturalistic inquiries. Educ Commun Technol. 1981;29:75–91.
7. Morgan DL. Focus groups. Ann Rev Sociol. 1996;22:129–52.
8. Chan EY, Blyth FM, Cheow SL, Fransen M. Postoperative pain following hospital discharge after knee replacement surgery: a patient survey. Pain Manag. 2013;3(3):177–88.
9. Chan EY, Blyth FM, Nairn L, Fransen M. Acute postoperative pain following hospital discharge after total knee arthroplasty. Osteoarthr Cartil. 2013;21(9):1257–63.
10. Clarke H, Woodhouse LJ, Kennedy D, Stratford P, Katz J. Strategies aimed at preventing chronic post-surgical pain: comprehensive Perioperative pain management after Total joint replacement surgery. Physiother Can. 2011;63(3):289–304.
11. Gaglio B, Glasgow RE, Bull SS. Do patient preferences for health information vary by health literacy or numeracy? A qualitative assessment. J Health Commun. 2012;17(Suppl 3):109–21.
12. Macario A, Schilling P, Rubio R, Bhalla A, Goodman S. What questions do patients undergoing lower extremity joint replacement surgery have? BMC Health Serv Res. 2003;3(1):11.
13. Soever LJ, Mackay C, Saryeddine T, Davis AM, Flannery JF, Jaglal SB, Levy C, Mahomed N. Educational needs of patients undergoing total joint arthroplasty. Physiother Can. 2010;62(3):206–14.
14. McDonald S, Page MJ, Beringer K, Wasiak J, Sprowson A. Preoperative education for hip or knee replacement. Cochrane Database Syst Rev. 2014;5:CD003526.
15. McGregor AH, Rylands H, Owen A, Dore CJ, Hughes SP. Does preoperative hip rehabilitation advice improve recovery and patient satisfaction? J Arthroplast. 2004;19(4):464–8.
16. Spalding NJ. Reducing anxiety by pre-operative education: make the future familiar. Occup Ther Int. 2003;10(4):278–93.
17. Go C. Smartphone and tablet ownership on the rise. Ottawa, Canada: Government of Canada; 2015.

Permissions

All chapters in this book were first published in BMC MD, by BioMed Central; hereby published with permission under the Creative Commons Attribution License or equivalent. Every chapter published in this book has been scrutinized by our experts. Their significance has been extensively debated. The topics covered herein carry significant findings which will fuel the growth of the discipline. They may even be implemented as practical applications or may be referred to as a beginning point for another development.

The contributors of this book come from diverse backgrounds, making this book a truly international effort. This book will bring forth new frontiers with its revolutionizing research information and detailed analysis of the nascent developments around the world.

We would like to thank all the contributing authors for lending their expertise to make the book truly unique. They have played a crucial role in the development of this book. Without their invaluable contributions this book wouldn't have been possible. They have made vital efforts to compile up to date information on the varied aspects of this subject to make this book a valuable addition to the collection of many professionals and students.

This book was conceptualized with the vision of imparting up-to-date information and advanced data in this field. To ensure the same, a matchless editorial board was set up. Every individual on the board went through rigorous rounds of assessment to prove their worth. After which they invested a large part of their time researching and compiling the most relevant data for our readers.

The editorial board has been involved in producing this book since its inception. They have spent rigorous hours researching and exploring the diverse topics which have resulted in the successful publishing of this book. They have passed on their knowledge of decades through this book. To expedite this challenging task, the publisher supported the team at every step. A small team of assistant editors was also appointed to further simplify the editing procedure and attain best results for the readers.

Apart from the editorial board, the designing team has also invested a significant amount of their time in understanding the subject and creating the most relevant covers. They scrutinized every image to scout for the most suitable representation of the subject and create an appropriate cover for the book.

The publishing team has been an ardent support to the editorial, designing and production team. Their endless efforts to recruit the best for this project, has resulted in the accomplishment of this book. They are a veteran in the field of academics and their pool of knowledge is as vast as their experience in printing. Their expertise and guidance has proved useful at every step. Their uncompromising quality standards have made this book an exceptional effort. Their encouragement from time to time has been an inspiration for everyone.

The publisher and the editorial board hope that this book will prove to be a valuable piece of knowledge for researchers, students, practitioners and scholars across the globe.

List of Contributors

Joon Ho Wang
Department of Orthopaedic Surgery, Samsung Medical Center, Sungkyunkwan University School of Medicine, Seoul 06351, South Korea
Department of Health Sciences and Technology, SAIHST, Sungkyunkwan University, Seoul, South Korea
Department of Medical Device Management and Research, SAIHST, Sungkyunkwan University, Seoul, South Korea

Eun Su Lee
Department of Orthopaedic Surgery, Dongbu Jaeil Hospital, Seoul, Republic of Korea

Byung Hoon Lee
Department of Orthopaedic Surgery, Kang-Dong Sacred Heart Hospital, Hallym University Medical Center, Gil-dong, Seoul 134-701, South Korea

Tetsuro Ohba, Shigeto Ebata and Hirotaka Haro
Department of Orthopaedics, University of Yamanashi, 1110 Shimokato, Chuo, Yamanashi 409-3898, Japan

So Kubota, Yutaka Inaba, Naomi Kobayashi, Hyonmin Choe, Taro Tezuka and Tomoyuki Saito
Department of Orthopaedic Surgery, Yokohama City University, 3-9Fukuura, Kanazawa-ku, Yokohama, Kanagawa 236-0004, Japan

Jessica DiVenere, Felix Dyrna, John Apostolakos, David Lam, Mark P. Cote and Augustus D. Mazzocca
Department of Orthopaedic Surgery, University of Connecticut Health Center, Farmington, CT, USA

Andreas Voss
Department of Orthopaedic Surgery, University of Connecticut Health Center, Farmington, CT, USA
Department of Orthopaedic Sports Medicine, Technical University of Munich, Munich, Germany

Knut Beitzel
Department of Orthopaedic Sports Medicine, Technical University of Munich, Munich, Germany

Department of Orthopedic Sports Medicine, Technische Universität München, Isamningerstr 22, 81675 Munich, Germany

Simone Cerciello
Department of Orthopaedic Surgery, Casa di Cura Villa Betania, Rome, Italy
Department of Orthopaedic Surgery, Marrelli Hospital, Crotone, Italy

Olga Solovyova
Department of Orthopaedic Surgery, NYU Hospital for Joint Disesases, New York, NY, USA

Paweł Skowronek and Paweł Olszewski
Clinic of Orthopedic and Traumatology, Regional Hospital and Kochanowski Medical University, Kielce, Poland

Wojciech Święszkowski
Faculty of Materials Science and Engineering, Warsaw University of Technology, Warsaw, Poland

Marcin Sibiński and Marek Synder
Clinic of Orthopedics and Pediatric Orthopedics, Medical University of Lodz, Lodz, Poland

Michał Polguj
Department of Angiology, Medical University of Łódź, ul Narutowicza 60, 90-136 Łódź, Polands

María Teresa Solis-Soto
Universidad San Francisco Xavier de Chuquisaca, Estudiantes, 96 Sucre, Bolivia
Institute for Occupational, Social and Environmental Medicine, Occupational and Environmental Epidemiology & Net Teaching Unit, University Hospital Munich (LMU), Munich. Ziemssenstr. 1, 80336 Munich, Germany

Anabel Schön, Manuel Parra and Katja Radon
Institute for Occupational, Social and Environmental Medicine, Occupational and Environmental Epidemiology & Net Teaching Unit, University Hospital Munich (LMU), Munich. Ziemssenstr. 1, 80336 Munich, Germany

Angel Solis-Soto
Centro de Diagnóstico Neurológico, Urriolagoitia, 354 Sucre, Bolivia

Shama R. Iyer, Mohit N. Gilotra and Richard M. Lovering
Department of Orthopaedics, University of Maryland School of Medicine, AHB, Rm 540, 100 Penn St., Baltimore, MD 21201, USA

Ana P. Valencia
Department of Orthopaedics, University of Maryland School of Medicine, AHB, Rm 540, 100 Penn St., Baltimore, MD 21201, USA
Department of Kinesiology, University of Maryland School of Public Health, College Park, USA

Espen E. Spangenburg
Department of Physiology, East Carolina Diabetes and Obesity Institute, Brody School of Medicine, East Carolina University, Greenville, USA

Jochen Markel, Tim Schwarting, Dominik Malcherczyk, Christian-Dominik Peterlein, Steffen Ruchholtz and Bilal Farouk El-Zayat
Center of Orthopaedics and Traumatology, University Hospital Marburg, Baldingerstrasse, 35033 Marburg, Germany

Marcel Leonardo Rodriguez and LePing Li
Department of Mechanical and Manufacturing Engineering, University of Calgary, 2500 University Drive, N.W, Calgary, AB T2N 1N4, Canada

Martin Kiechle and Matthias Militz
BG Unfallklinik Murnau, Prof. Küntscher Str. 8, Murnau 82418, Germany

Sven Hungerer and Christian von Rüden
BG Unfallklinik Murnau, Prof. Küntscher Str. 8, Murnau 82418, Germany
Institute of Biomechanics, Paracelsus Medical University Salzburg and BG Unfallklinik Murnau, Prof. Küntscher Str. 8, Murnau 82418, Germany

Mario Morgenstern
BG Unfallklinik Murnau, Prof. Küntscher Str. 8, Murnau 82418, Germany
Institute of Biomechanics, Paracelsus Medical University Salzburg and BG Unfallklinik Murnau, Prof. Küntscher Str. 8, Murnau 82418, Germany
Department of Orthopaedic Surgery and Traumatology, University Hospital Basel, Spitalstr 21, 4031 Basel, Switzerland

Markus Guehring, Ulrich Stoeckle and Patrick Ziegler
Department for Traumatology and Reconstructive Surgery, BG Trauma Center Tübingen, University of Tübingen, Schnarrenbergstr 95, 72076 Tuebingen, Germany

Simon Lambert
Shoulder and Elbow Service, Royal National Orthopaedic Hospital, Stanmore HA7 4LP, UK

Sascha J. Baettig, Karl Wieser and Christian Gerber
Orthopaedic Department, Balgrist University Hospital, University of Zurich, Forchstrasse 340, 8008 Zurich, Switzerland

Mélanie Cogné
Service de Médecine Physique et de Réadaptation, hôpital Raymond Poincaré, 92380 Garches, France
Service de Médecine Physique et de Réadaptation, CHU de Bordeaux, 33076 Bordeaux, France
EA4136 Handicap, Activité, Cognition, Santé, Bordeaux University, Bordeaux, France

Hervé Petit, Alexandre Creuzé and Dominique
Service de Médecine Physique et de Réadaptation, CHU de Bordeaux, 33076 Bordeaux, France

Mathieu de Seze
Service de Médecine Physique et de Réadaptation, CHU de Bordeaux, 33076 Bordeaux, France
EA4136 Handicap, Activité, Cognition, Santé, Bordeaux University, Bordeaux, France

Liguoro
Neurosurgical Unit, University Hospital, Bordeaux, France

Guo-Chun Zha, Shuo Feng, Xiang-Yang Chen and Kai-Jin Guo
Department of Orthopedic Surgery, the Affiliated Hospital of Xuzhou Medical University, No. 99 Huaihai West Road, Xuzhou, Jiangsu 221002, People's Republic of China

Xue-Mei Yang
Hyperbaric Oxygen Treatment Center, the Affiliated Hospital of Xuzhou Medical University, No. 99 Huaihai West Road, Xuzhou, Jiangsu 221002, People's Republic of China

Jun-Ying Sun
Orthopaedic Department, the First Affiliated Hospital of Soochow University, 188 Shizi Street, Suzhou, Jiangsu 215006, People's Republic of China

Xingchen Li, Yang Xu, Yuan Zhu and Xiangyang Xu
Orthopaedic Department, Ruijin Hospital, Ruijin Er Road No.197, Shanghai 200025, China

Naoki Hayami, Akio Iida, Takamasa Shimizu, Kenji Kawamura and Yasuhito Tanaka
Department of Orthopedic Surgery, Nara Medical University, 840 Shijo-cho, Kashihara City, Nara Prefecture, Japan

Shohei Omokawa
Department of Hand Surgery, Nara Medical University, 840 Shijo-cho, Kashihara City, Nara Prefecture, Japan

Jirachart Kraisarin
Department of Orthopedic Surgery, Faculty of Medicine, Chiang Mai University, Chiang Mai 50200, Thailand

Hisao Moritomo
Department of Physiotherapy, Osaka Yukioka College of Health Science, 41,1,1, Soujiji, Ibaraki City, Osaka, Japan

Pasuk Mahakkanukrauh
Department of Anatomy, Faculty of Medicine, Chiang Mai University, Chiang Mai 50200, Thailand Excellence in Osteology Research and Training Center (ORTC), Chiang Mai University, Chiang Mai 50200, Thailand

Ryo Ueno, Tomoya Ishida, Masanori Yamanaka, Shohei Taniguchi, Mina Samukawa, Hiroshi Saito and Harukazu Tohyama
Faculty of Health Sciences, Hokkaido University, North 12, West 5, Kitaku, Sapporo 060-0812, Japan

Ryohei Ikuta
Hachioji Sports Orthopaedic Clinic, Hachioji-Nakacho-Bldg3, 5-1, Nakacho, Hachioji, Tokyo 192-0085, Japan

Chang Ho Shin, Wan Kee Hong, Doo Jae Lee, Won Joon Yoo and In Ho Choi
Department of Orthopaedic Surgery, Seoul National University College of Medicine, Seoul, Republic of Korea

Tae-Joon Cho
Department of Orthopaedic Surgery, Seoul National University College of Medicine, Seoul, Republic of Korea
Division of Pediatric Orthopaedics, Seoul National University Children's Hospital, 101 Daehak-ro Jongno-gu, Seoul 03080, Republic of Korea

Qing Wang and Dejun Zhong
Department of Spine Surgery, the Affiliated Hospital of South-west Medical University, No.25 Taiping St, Luzhou, Sichuan 646000, China

Guangzhou Li
Department of Spine Surgery, the Affiliated Hospital of South-west Medical University, No.25 Taiping St, Luzhou, Sichuan 646000, China
Department of orthopedics, Sichuan University West China Hospital, Sichuan Province, Chengdu, China

Hao Liu
Department of orthopedics, Sichuan University West China Hospital, Sichuan Province, Chengdu, China

Fiona L. Hamilton
E-Health Unit, Research Department of Primary Care and Population Health, Upper Third Floor UCL Medical School (Royal Free Campus), Rowland Hill Street, NW3 2PF, London, UK

Emma Dunphy
E-Health Unit, Research Department of Primary Care and Population Health, Upper Third Floor UCL Medical School (Royal Free Campus), Rowland Hill Street, NW3 2PF, London, UK
Homerton University Hospital NHS Trust, Homerton Row E96SR, London, UK

Irena Spasić
School of Computer Science & Informatics, Cardiff University, Queens Building, 5 The Parade, Cardiff CF24 3AA, UK

Kate Button
School of Healthcare Sciences, Cardiff University, Eastgate House, Newport Road, Cardiff CF24 0AB, UK
Cardiff & Vale University Health Board, Health Park, Cardiff CF14 4XW, UK

Jan Hartvigsen and Lise Hestbæk
Department of Sports Science and Clinical Biomechanics, Faculty of Health Sciences, University of Southern Denmark, Campusvej 55, 5230 Odense M, Denmark
Nordic Institute of Chiropractic and Clinical Biomechanics, Campusvej 55, 5230 Odense M, Denmark

Eleanor Boyle
Department of Sports Science and Clinical Biomechanics, Faculty of Health Sciences, University of Southern Denmark, Campusvej 55, 5230 Odense M, Denmark
Dalla Lana School of Public Health, University of Toronto, 155 College St, Toronto, ON M5T 3M7, Canada

Eva Jespersen
Department of Sports Science and Clinical Biomechanics, Faculty of Health Sciences, University of Southern Denmark, Campusvej 55, 5230 Odense M, Denmark
Department of Rehabilitation, Odense University Hospital, Odense, Denmark and National Centre of Rehabilitation and Palliation, University of Southern Denmark, Odense, Denmark

Tina Junge
Department of Sports Science and Clinical Biomechanics, Faculty of Health Sciences, University of Southern Denmark, Campusvej 55, 5230 Odense M, Denmark
Health Sciences Research Centre, University College Lillebaelt, Niels Bohrs Allé 1, 5230 Odense M, Denmark

Niels Wedderkopp
Institute of Regional Health Services Research, University of Southern Denmark, Winsloewparken 193, 5000 Odense C, Denmark
Sports Medicine Clinic, Orthopaedic Department, Hospital Lillebaelt, Østre Hougvej 55, 5500 Middelfart, Denmark

Lisbeth Runge Larsen
Research and Innovation Center for Human Movement and Learning, Inter-Faculty Educational Resources, University College Lillebælt, Niels Bohrs Alle 1, 5230 Odense M, Denmark

Hsiu-Ho Wang
Department of Nursing, Yuanpei University of Medical Technology, 306 Yuanpei Street, Hsinchu 30015, Taiwan

Li-Huan Chen
Department of Nursing, Yuanpei University of Medical Technology, 306 Yuanpei Street, Hsinchu 30015, Taiwan
Graduate Institute of Clinical Medical Sciences, Chang Gung University, 259 Wenhua 1st Road, Guishan District, Taoyuan 33302, Taiwan

Jersey Liang
Department of Health Management and Policy, School of Public Health, University of Michigan, 1415 Washington Heights M3007 SPH II, Ann Arbor, MI 48109, USA
Institute of Gerontology, University of Michigan, 1415 Washington Heights, M3007 SPH II, Ann Arbor, MI 48109, USA

Min-Chi Chen
Department of Public Health & Biostatistics Consulting Center, Chang Gung University, 259 Wenhua 1st Road, Guishan District, Taoyuan 33302, Taiwan

Chi-Chuan Wu
Department of Orthopedic Surgery, Chang Gung Memorial Hospital, Linkou, 5 Fu-Hsing Street, Guishan District, Taoyuan 33305, Taiwan

Huey-Shinn Cheng
Department of Internal Medicine, Chang Gung Memorial Hospital, Linkou, 5 Fu-Hsing Street, Guishan District, Taoyuan 33305, Taiwan

Yea-Ing Lotus Shyu
Department of Orthopedic Surgery, Chang Gung Memorial Hospital, Linkou, 5 Fu-Hsing Street, Guishan District, Taoyuan 33305, Taiwan
School of Nursing, College of Medicine, and Healthy Aging Research Center, Chang Gung University, 259 Wenhua 1st Road, Guishan District, Taoyuan 33302, Taiwan
Department of Nursing, Kaohsiung Chang Gung Memorial Hospital, 123 Dapi Road, Niaosng District, Kaohsiung 83301, Taiwan

Department of Gerontological Care and Management, Chang Gung University of Science and Technology, 261 Wenhua 1st Road, Guishan District, Taoyuan 33303, Taiwan

Lin Xie, Xin Guo, Shu-Jun Zhang and Zhen-Hua Fang
Department of Orthopedic Surgery, Wuhan Orthopedic Hospital, Wuhan Puai Hospital, Huazhong University of Science and Technology, Hanzheng Street 473#, Wuhan City, Hubei Province 430033, China

Signe Fuglkjær and Kristina Boe Dissing
Department of Sports Science and Clinical Biomechanics, Faculty of Health Sciences, University of Southern Denmark, Campusvej 55, DK-5230 Odense M, Denmark

Lucy Pereira and Susan Robarts
Sunnybrook Holland Orthopaedic and Arthritic Centre, 43 Wellesley Street East, Toronto, ON M4Y 1H1, Canada

Deborah Kennedy
Sunnybrook Holland Orthopaedic and Arthritic Centre, 43 Wellesley Street East, Toronto, ON M4Y 1H1, Canada
School of Rehabilitation Science, McMaster University, 1400 Main St. W, Hamilton, ON L8S 1C7, Canada

Department of Physical Therapy, University of Toronto, 500 University Avenue, Toronto, ON M5G 1V7, Canada

Amy Wainwright
Sunnybrook Holland Orthopaedic and Arthritic Centre, 43 Wellesley Street East, Toronto, ON M4Y 1H1, Canada
Department of Physical Therapy, University of Toronto, 500 University Avenue, Toronto, ON M5G 1V7, Canada

Patricia Dickson
Sunnybrook Holland Orthopaedic and Arthritic Centre, 43 Wellesley Street East, Toronto, ON M4Y 1H1, Canada
Department of Occupational Science and Occupational Therapy, University of Toronto, 500 University Avenue, Toronto, ON M5G 1V7, Canada

Jennifer Christian
Centre for Addiction and Mental Health, 33 Russell Street, Toronto, ON M5S 2S1, Canada

Fiona Webster
Institute of Health Policy Management and Evaluation, Dalla Lana School of Public Health, University of Toronto, 155 College Street, Toronto, ON M5T 3M7, Canada

Index